ANNALS OF THE NEW YORK ACADEMY OF SCIENCES

Volume 819

EDITORIAL STAFF

Executive Editor
BILL BOLAND

Managing Editor
JUSTINE CULLINAN

Associate Editor
STEVEN E. BOHALL

The New York Academy of Sciences
2 East 63rd Street
New York, New York 10021

THE NEW YORK ACADEMY OF SCIENCES
(Founded in 1817)

BOARD OF GOVERNORS, October 1996 — October 1997

MARTIN L. LEIBOWITZ, *Chairman of the Board*
RICHARD A. RIFKIND, *Vice Chairman of the Board*
RODNEY W. NICHOLS, *President and CEO* [ex officio]

Honorary Life Governors

WILLIAM T. GOLDEN   JOSHUA LEDERBERG

JOHN T. MORGAN, *Treasurer*

Governors

ELEANOR BAUM   D. ALLAN BROMLEY   LAWRENCE B. BUTTENWIESER
PRAVEEN CHAUDHARI   EDWARD COHEN   RONALD L. GRAHAM
BILL GREEN   JACQUELINE LEO   WILLIAM J. McDONOUGH
SANDRA PANEM   CHARLES RAMOND
WILLIAM C. STEERE, JR.   TORSTEN WIESEL

HENRY M. GREENBERG, *Past Chairman of the Board*

HELENE L. KAPLAN, *Counsel* [ex officio]   CRAIG PURINTON, *Secretary* [ex officio]

NUTRITIONAL IMPLICATIONS OF MACRONUTRIENT SUBSTITUTES

ANNALS OF THE NEW YORK ACADEMY OF SCIENCES
Volume 819

NUTRITIONAL IMPLICATIONS OF MACRONUTRIENT SUBSTITUTES

Edited by G. Harvey Anderson, Barbara J. Rolls, and Daniel G. Steffen

The New York Academy of Sciences
New York, New York
1997

Copyright @ 1997 by the New York Academy of Sciences. All rights reserved. Under the provisions of the United States Copyright Act of 1976, individual readers of the Annals *are permitted to make fair use of the material in them for teaching and research. Permission is granted to quote from the* Annals *provided that the customary acknowledgment is made of the source. Material in the* Annals *may be republished only by permission of the Academy. Address inquiries to the Executive Editor at the New York Academy of Sciences.*

Copying fees: *For each copy of an article made beyond the free copying permitted under Section 107 or 108 of the 1976 Copyright Act, a fee should be paid through the Copyright Clearance Center, Inc., 222 Rosewood Drive, Danvers, MA 01923. The fee for copying an article is $3.00 for nonacademic use; for use in the classroom it is $0.07 per page.*

∞ *The paper used in this publication meets the minimum requirements of American National Standard for Information Sciences – Permanence of Paper for Printed Library Materials. ANSI Z39.48-1984.*

Library of Congress Cataloging-in-Publication Data

Nutritional implications of macronutrient substitutes / edited by G. Harvey Anderson, Barbara J. Rolls, and Daniel G. Steffen.
    p.   cm. — (Annals of the New York Academy of Sciences ; v. 819)
    Includes bibliographical references and index.
    ISBN 1-57331-084-0 (alk. paper). — ISBN 1-57331-085-9 (pbk. : alk. paper)
    1. Nutrition—Congresses.   2. Fat substitutes—Congresses.
3. Food preferences—Congresses.   I. Anderson, G. Harvey, 1941-   .
II. Rolls, Barbara J.   III. Steffen, Daniel G.   IV. Series.
Q11.N5 vol. 819
[QP141.A1]
500 s—dc21
[613.2'84]   97-19405
                                                                                                               CIP

PCP
Printed in the United States of America
ISBN 1-57331-084-0 (cloth)
ISBN 1-57331-085-9 (paper)
ISSN 0077-8923

ANNALS OF THE NEW YORK ACADEMY OF SCIENCES

Volume 819
May 23, 1997

NUTRITIONAL IMPLICATIONS OF MACRONUTRIENT SUBSTITUTES [a]

Editors
G. HARVEY ANDERSON, BARBARA J. ROLLS,
and DANIEL G. STEFFEN

Conference Organizers

TECHNICAL COMMITTEE ON MACRONUTRIENT SUBSTITUTION OF THE
INTERNATIONAL LIFE SCIENCES INSTITUTE NORTH AMERICA

CONTENTS

Preface. By DANIEL G. STEFFEN	ix
Summary of the Conference. By the Technical Committee on Macronutrient Substitution	xi

Part I. Macronutrient Substitutes: Definition and Rationale

Nutritional and Health Aspects of Macronutrient Substitution. By G. HARVEY ANDERSON	1
Macronutrient Substitutes: Description and Uses. By GILBERT A. LEVEILLE and JOHN W. FINLEY	11
Regulatory Aspects of the Introduction of New Macronutrient Substitutes. By ALAN M. RULIS, LINDA S. PELLICORE, and HELEN R. THORSHEIM	22

Part II. Regulation of Energy Balance

Energy Balance: Role of Genetics and Activity. By F. XAVIER PI-SUNYER	29
Effect of Fat Intake on Energy Balance. By P. ANTONIO TATARANNI and ERIC RAVUSSIN	37

[a] This volume is the result of a conference, entitled **Nutritional Implications of Macronutrient Substitutes,** held in Arlington, Virginia on October 27–29, 1996, by the New York Academy of Sciences. The conference was also sponsored by the International Life Sciences Institute North America Technical Committee on Macronutrient Substitution.

Carbohydrates and Energy Balance. *By* R. JAMES STUBBS, A. M.
PRENTICE, and W. P. T. JAMES 44

Part III. Macronutrient Modification and Food Selection

Impact of Macronutrient Substitutes on the Composition of the Diet
and the U.S. Food Supply. *By* REBECCA MORGAN, MADELEINE
SIGMAN-GRANT, DENISE S. TAYLOR, KRISTIN MORIARTY,
VALERIE FISHELL, and PENNY M. KRIS-ETHERTON............ 70

Impact of Macronutrient-substituted Foods on Food Choice and
Dietary Intake. *By* DAVID J. MELA......................... 96

Impact of the Use of Reduced-fat Foods on Nutrient Adequacy. *By*
JAMES T. HEIMBACH, BROOKE E. VAN DER RIET, and
S. KATHLEEN EGAN 108

Part IV. Macronutrient Substitutes: Consumer Knowledge, Attitudes, and Practices

Consumer Attitudes and Practices. *By* LYN O'BRIEN NABORS....... 115

Social Determinants of Food Intake. *By* LOUIS E. GRIVETTI 121

Macronutrient Substitutes and Weight-reduction Practices of Obese,
Dieting, and Eating-disordered Women. *By* ADAM
DREWNOWSKI 132

Part V. Macronutrient Substitutes: Clinical and Experimental Evaluation

Dietary Fiber: Nutritional Lessons for Macronutrient Substitutes. *By*
KAY M. BEHALL 142

Appropriate Animal Models for Clinical Studies. *By* RUTH B. S.
HARRIS 155

Nutritional Aspects of Macronutrient-substitute Intake. *By* JOHN C.
PETERS 169

Fat and Sugar Substitutes and the Control of Food Intake. *By*
BARBARA J. ROLLS 180

Food Intake Regulation in Children: Fat and Sugar Substitutes and
Intake. *By* LEANN L. BIRCH and JENNIFER O. FISHER 194

Beyond Calories: Other Benefits of Macronutrient Substitutes—
Effects on Chronic Disease. *By* JUDY S. HANNAH............. 221

Observations on the Conference Proceedings and Future Research
Directions: Luncheon Remarks. *By* CUTBERTO GARZA......... 229

Part VI. Poster Papers

Replacement of Dietary Fat with Fat-free Margarine Alters Vitamin
E Storage in Rats. *By* G. V. MITCHELL, E. GRUNDEL, and
M. Y. JENKINS 236

Assessment of the Caloric Value of a Fat Substitute Using a New Tracer Method. *By* B. MITTENDORFER, Y. ZHENG, D. CHINKES, and R. R. WOLFE 239

Oil-soluble Vitamin Content of New Reduced-fat and Fat-free Margarines: Potential Implications for Vitamin E Intake. *By* JEANNE I. RADER.. 242

The Evolution of Carbohydrate Intake in the Slovak Republic during the Economic Transformation. *By* ROBERT ŠIMONČIČ . 247

Weight Gain of Rats Consuming Full-fat versus Reduced-fat Foods. *By* ZOE S. WARWICK, KATHLEEN J. BOWEN, and MICKA ROY . 251

***

Index of Contributors 255

Financial assistance was received from:
The International Life Sciences Institute North America Technical Committee on Macronutrient Substitution

The New York Academy of Sciences believes it has a responsibility to provide an open forum for discussion of scientific questions. The positions taken by the participants in the reported conferences are their own and not necessarily those of the Academy. The Academy has no intent to influence legislation by providing such forums.

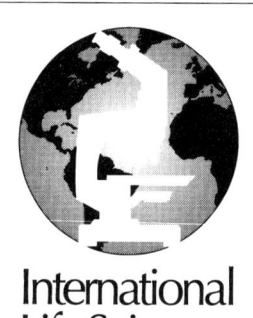

Preface

This volume of the *Annals* summarizes a conference entitled *Nutritional Implications of Macronutrient Substitutes* held on October 27-29, 1996, in Arlington, Virginia under the auspices of the International Life Sciences Institute North America and the New York Academy of Sciences. The conference organizers sought to enhance the understanding of the impact of macronutrient substitutes on energy and nutrient intake, food selection, and dietary patterns. For the purpose of this conference, it was assumed that macronutrient-substitute ingredients would be safe for their intended use in foods; speakers could then concentrate on health and nutrition issues. This approach was not intended to lessen the importance of safety approval of these new food ingredients, but rather recognized the extensive debate of macroingredient safety issues already underway in other forums.

The substitution of macroingredients in the diet is an old concept. Fiber-rich foods and ingredients have long been used to reduce dietary energy, and intense sweeteners have replaced sugars in many food products. Newer ingredients have advanced efforts to replace fat while still maintaining its characteristic functions in the modified food. These fat substitutes represent novel ingredients with unique properties, such as limited digestibility. Thus, many speakers addressed the nutritional importance of fat substitutes, particularly the fat-based fat substitutes, which will soon enter the food supply.

The order of the papers in this book follows the conference structure, with the addition of a summary and the poster papers. In the introductory papers, the role of macronutrient substitutes in promoting public health and nutrition goals is discussed, followed by a summary of the variety of substances available for use by the food industry (Anderson, Leveille). Regulatory hurdles faced by new macroingredients are next described, as well as the role of nutritional data in the approval process (Rulis). Consideration of the association between macronutrient substitutes and energy balance provides the framework for papers on genetics and obesity, fat and carbohydrate intake, and the heterogeneity of responses to dietary changes (Pi-Sunyer, Tataranni, Stubbs). Presentations evaluating food selection with fat-modified foods suggest that several strategies may lead to reduction in energy and fat intake (Kris-Etherton, Mela, Heimbach). A series of papers on consumer attitudes and reactions toward dietary trends suggest that acceptance of modified foods may require education to decrease the possibility of rejection of new foods (Nabors, Grivetti). However, taste is still important, and macronutrient substitutes offer a unique approach to offset a seemingly inexorable trend for the energy (and fat) density of the diet to increase with wealth (Drewnowski). The last group of papers considers clinical and experimental approaches to evaluate macronutrient substitutes; in particular, food intake of adults and children in response to a fat-based fat substitute is explored (Behall, Harris, Peters, Rolls, Birch). Potential applications of macronutrient substitutes to achieve benefits beyond calorie reduction completes the session (Hannah). The concluding luncheon address (Garza) offers a contemporary summary of the proceedings and a perspective for future research.

The timely topics covered here will be of interest to nutrition researchers, health professionals, and food technologists from government, academia, industry, and consumer areas. The reader will recognize a recurrent theme in these papers: Macronutrient substitutes are but one tool for individuals to use in an overall strategy to tailor diets to meet public health goals. The volume captures this important message that bears remembering as the field of macronutrient substitutes continues to unfold.

DANIEL G. STEFFEN

Summary of the Conference

TECHNICAL COMMITTEE ON MACRONUTRIENT SUBSTITUTION

The conference entitled Nutritional Implications of Macronutrient Substitutes was sponsored by the Technical Committee on Macronutrient Substitution of the North American branch of the International Life Sciences Institute (ILSI N.A.) and the New York Academy of Sciences.

The purpose of this conference was to present the current state of scientific knowledge on the nutritional impact of macronutrient substitutes, including intense sweeteners and fat replacers, and to identify future directions for research based on gaps in scientific knowledge. Although some aspects of the safety of macronutrient substitutes were discussed, the focus of the conference was on nutrition. Topics included the science-based aspects of energy balance, the potential impact of macronutrient substitutes on the diet, and consumer practices.

MACRONUTRIENT SUBSTITUTES: DEFINITION AND RATIONALE

G. Harvey Anderson (University of Toronto) reviewed the association between consumption of a high-fat diet and the increased incidence of a variety of diseases, including heart disease, diabetes, and certain types of cancer. Further, he summarized nutritional goals and a proposed role for achieving them through the use of macronutrient substitutes. Noteworthy potential benefits of macronutrient substitutes include reduced energy density of foods, decreased fat intake, maintenance of dietary pattern, maintenance of healthy weight, and increased nutrient density. The potential for adverse effects may also exist, including the potential to develop abnormal eating behaviors.

One response to public health recommendations for decreased fat intake has been an increase in the number of low- and no-fat foods available. Gilbert A. Leveille (Nabisco Inc.) discussed the definition and some proposed uses of macronutrient substitutes. Macronutrient substitutes include replacers of carbohydrates, such as sugar replacers (polyols and reduced-starch hydrolysates) and bulk fillers. Three categories of fat replacers include fat mimetics, low-calorie fats, and fat substitutes. By definition, these agents have similar goals (reduction of caloric density), but the goals may be reached through different means. The substitute may contain fewer calories because it is not metabolized as well as the component it replaces, or it may be free of calories because it is not absorbed.

Safety and regulatory aspects of macronutrient substitutes were discussed by Alan M. Rulis (FDA). Any macronutrient substitute, before being approved for use in food in this country, must be shown to present a "reasonable certainty of no harm" to the consumer. A typical petition includes a chemical profile for the food additive, including identification, composition, proposed uses, intended effect, a method for quantification, and sometimes, toxicologic information. For food additives, the range of exposure should include doses intended to mimic very low exposure (indirect additives) and higher exposure (direct additives). A clear distinction between a petition for a macronutrient substitute and a petition for a food additive is the need for nutritional evaluation. Every macronutrient should be tested under conditions that will provide meaningful information as to what the nutritional impact will be on consumers.

REGULATION AND ENERGY BALANCE

Genetics as well as environmental conditions play important roles in the development of obesity. The role of genetics was discussed by F. Xavier Pi-Sunyer (Columbia University). At least 20 different genes have demonstrated an association with a high body mass index (BMI), but many more are likely to be involved. Genetic associations have been demonstrated for *ob*-protein and hypothalamic *ob*-protein receptors, leptin, and some neurotransmitters. Although individual genes specifically predict obesity, a better predictor may be resting metabolic rate (RMR). Energy expenditure is predicted to be based on RMR (60-70%), physical activity (15-30%), and thermogenesis (5-10%).

A multitude of epidemiologic studies have shown a positive correlation between consumption of dietary fat and obesity. Pietro Antonio Tataranni (NIH) discussed the role of fat intake on energy balance. The importance of genetics was also discussed. In particular, some reports have demonstrated that lean persons have a propensity to remain lean even when their intake of fat increases. Lean persons may actually increase fat oxidation upon consumption of greater amounts of fat.

As with the consumption of increased amounts of dietary fat, increased consumption of carbohydrates does not necessarily lead to an increase in daily energy expenditure. Consumption of carbohydrates may further promote fat storage by decreasing fat oxidation and possibly even increasing *de novo* synthesis of fat. R. James Stubbs (Rowett Research Institute) discussed the role of carbohydrate intake on energy balance. Energy intake may remain constant regardless of the composition of the actual intake (*e.g.,* high versus low fat), suggesting that, in some people, decreasing the proportion of fat in the diet can lead to compensation for the decreased calories by the increased consumption of other foods.

MACRONUTRIENT MODIFICATION AND FOOD SELECTION

Penny Kris-Etherton (Pennsylvania State University) discussed the potential impact of macronutrient substitutes on the U.S. diet based on computer modeling. Minor dietary modifications using fat-modified products had the potential to impact the consumption of dietary fat but appeared to be most effective when more than one product was used. The computer modeling also showed that if a very low-fat diet were designed (< 15% of energy), then intakes of zinc and vitamin E would be significantly decreased. She also reported on an analysis of dietary intake data that looked at people who used either skim milk, lean meats, or fat-modified products.

SUMMARY OF THE CONFERENCE xiii

These individuals had a lower fat intake, and most had a lower energy intake than the rest of the population.

David J. Mela (Institute of Food Research) discussed the effect of macronutrient substitutes on food choice. Consumption of intense sweeteners appears to cause increased consumption of calories from other sources in males but not in females. Ad libitum human feeding studies have demonstrated that consumption of low-fat foods, while effective in the short term at reducing fat and caloric intake, eventually may be overridden by caloric compensation from another source in some people. In summary, casual use of low- /no-fat foods may have a significant effect on fat intake, but efficacy from the use of sugar replacers is less clear.

The potential impact of macronutrient substitutes on nutritional adequacy in children was discussed by James T. Heimbach (Technical Assessment Systems Inc.). Self-reported consumption of more than two low-fat foods per day was common, but the upper end limit was five per day. The total percentage of dietary fat was estimated at 35% for those not using low-fat products, but the use of low-fat foods effectively reduced the intake of dietary fats (32% for those using 1 or 2 substitutes). The strategy was more effective when used in combination (26% in persons using 3-5 per day). Reduced-fat consumption tended to be compensated for by an increased consumption of carbohydrates. The portion size was the same or smaller for fat-modified products versus their full-fat counterparts. There was no associated change in protein intake or in micronutrient profile on a population basis. One issue that needs further clarification is that of substitution versus supplementation.

MACRONUTRIENT SUBSTITUTES: CONSUMER KNOWLEDGE, ATTITUDES, AND PRACTICES

Lyn O'Brien Nabors (Calorie Control Council) discussed industry response to consumer concerns about dietary fat. The number and variety of products available has increased by a factor of greater than three since 1989. Surveys indicate that 88% of adults consume reduced-fat food and that 78% use low-calorie or reduced-fat foods at least once in a two-week period; of the 12% that do not, the primary self-reported reason is taste. For weight control, the self-reported incidence of dietary modification is ahead of exercise.

Social determinants of food intake were summarized by Louis E. Grivetti (University of California, Davis). The primary components can be reduced to four determinants: availability, familiarity, selectivity, and anticipation/expectation. Food rejection is a learned behavior based on danger, disgust, and distaste (the 3 Ds) often triggered by odd food combinations or timing of ingestion. Sociocultural analysis may be useful in gauging consumer response to macronutrient substitutes as "technofixes"; they are likely to be rejected by those who fear technology (neophobia) but accepted by those who embrace new technical advances (neophilia). Testing of these new substances requires caution because of the "professional effect," whereby the presence of an expert alters the response of the consumer.

Behavioral differences in food consumption were discussed by Adam Drewnowski (University of Michigan). Consumption of sugar and fat are associated with socioeconomic status. Increased fat consumption is nearly always at the expense of carbohydrates rather than protein. Further influences on fat consumption include the Gross

National Product (GNP); as the GNP increases so does the intake of calories from fat. Although increased GNP is not specifically noted with change in the quantity of protein consumed, it is associated with a shift in protein source from plants to animals. Additionally, increased GNP is nearly always associated with an increased incidence of deaths from cardiovascular disease and cancer. He also noted that once a society achieves a high degree of dietary variety, it is nearly impossible to revert back to a simpler diet. Therefore, modifying the food supply is a logical approach to improving the quality of the diet. Macronutrient substitutes represent a grand attempt to reduce the energy density of a highly varied diet associated with an advanced socioeconomic society.

MACRONUTRIENT SUBSTITUTES: CLINICAL AND EXPERIMENTAL EVALUATION

The use of dietary fiber as a macronutrient substitute was discussed by Kay M. Behall (USDA). Fiber-containing foods have long been used to dilute the energy and fat content of the diet. Much research points to benefits of fiber consumption, specifically related to soluble fiber, such as improved serum lipid profile and glycemic response. Certain fiber and starch sources are metabolized in the large bowel to short-chain fatty acids, which are an energy source for colonocytes and may affect cholesterol metabolism. Abdominal discomfort associated with high-fiber diets generally disappears after the first week. Significant negative mineral balance has not been reported in high-fiber feeding studies or among vegetarians.

The selection of appropriate animal models and the advantages and disadvantages of animal toxicology testing was discussed by Ruth B. S. Harris (Louisiana State University). Advantages include lower cost, increased compliance, and potential to test for more invasive end points. However, disadvantages include different responses to sensory stimulation and differences in gastrointestinal systems.

Overall energy status is a balance between the amount of energy consumed and energy used. John C. Peters (the Procter & Gamble Company) discussed the nutritional aspects of macronutrient substitutes. Energy expenditure is often constant regardless of the diet, but variables do exist. For example, overconsumption of carbohydrates is associated with increased oxidation of carbohydrates, whereas overconsumption of fat is more frequently associated with increased storage of fat. One of the dietary goals of macronutrient substitutes is to decrease calorie density with the goal of decreasing energy intake, thereby promoting a better fat balance. The assumption that reduction of dietary fat will automatically cause weight loss is incorrect, but that does not mean that macronutrient substitutes are unsuccessful. These agents are only tools as part of an overall strategy to promote a better fat balance.

Barbara J. Rolls (Pennsylvania State University) discussed the role of sugar and fat replacers in the control of food intake. There is a distinction between satiety and satiation. Satiety refers to inhibition of further intake after consumption of a certain amount of food. Intense sweeteners tend not to increase food intake. However, covert fat substitution in some cases may cause compensation for total calories but not specifically for fat. Products with labels declaring low or no fat are often consumed in greater quantities whether or not the descriptor is accurate. This suggests that the packaging can influence consumption patterns. Comparison of ad libitum potato chip consumption (fat-substituted versus full-fat brand) demonstrated that satiety was dependent more on mass than calories. Both groups consumed approximately the same quantity in grams daily over a 10-day period. However, those consuming the fat-substituted chips cut their fat and calorie intake considerably (30 cal/day vs. 150 cal/day).

Leann L. Birch (Pennsylvania State University) discussed the potential impact of fat and sugar substitution in children. As with adults, the dietary recommendation for children older than two is to consume less than 30% of calories from fat. However, self-selection of fat in children can range from 25-42 percent. A caloric-compensation model demonstrated that children consistently compensate for sugar replacement, but always with less than 100% of the calories. The results for fat replacement are inconsistent, but when compensation did occur, it was over a two-day period rather than at the next meal.

Judy S. Hannah (Medlantic Research Institute) discussed the potential for benefits of macronutrient substitutes other than calorie reduction. Consumption of a diet high in fat is associated with numerous diseases, including atherosclerosis, noninsulin-dependent diabetes mellitus, and certain types of cancer. Some studies have demonstrated a reduced incidence of these diseases with the reduction of fat intake. However, the potential for fat substitutes to actually decrease the incidence of any disease has not been fully demonstrated, nor has it been claimed.

Nutritional and Health Aspects of Macronutrient Substitution

G. HARVEY ANDERSON [a]

Department of Nutritional Sciences
FitzGerald Building
University of Toronto
Toronto, Ontario, Canada, M5S 3E2

Obesity, cardiovascular disease, and cancer are major public health problems in North America. All have been attributed to inactivity combined with diets of the wrong composition selected from a generous supply of foods. Since the 1970s, dietary guidelines have urged reductions in fat intake as one strategy toward achieving healthier diets.

To help consumers achieve dietary change, the food industry, over the past ten years, has developed many foods low in calories and low in fat. In 1995, approximately 80% of the new food items introduced to the marketplace bearing health claims were in the reduced/low-fat or reduced/low-calorie categories.[1] Many processing techniques and new formulations substitute the macronutrients fat and carbohydrate with compounds that deliver their taste and other functional properties, but that have fewer calories.

This paper will discuss the potential role for macronutrient substitutes in achieving dietary change that is consistent with dietary guidelines.

RATIONALE FOR DIETARY CHANGE

The motivating force behind macronutrient substitutes is the worldwide consensus that an excess of energy intake and diets high in fat calories create health risks.[2] Virtually every developed country has government-initiated dietary guidelines that encourage its population to maintain healthy body weights and to reduce fat intake, as a proportion of energy, from an average of 38% to 30% or below.[3-5] Dietary guidelines emphasize following an eating pattern that includes a variety of foods: cereals, breads, other grain products, vegetables, fruits, low-fat dairy products, lean meats, fish, and foods prepared with little or no fat. Dietary guidelines for people in the U.S. are shown in TABLE 1.[6]

These recommendations for dietary change arise from changing patterns of morbidity and mortality in the past 50 years. Infectious diseases have given way to chronic degenerative diseases as the cause of morbidity and mortality. Successful control of infectious diseases has lengthened life expectancy, so that people die of chronic degenerative diseases, mainly cardiovascular disease and cancer. Both disease

---

[a] Tel: (416) 978-1832; fax: (416) 978-5882; e-mail: harvey.anderson@utoronto.ca.

TABLE 1. Dietary Guidelines for People in the U.S.[6]

Eat a variety of foods.
Balance the food you eat with physical activity; maintain or improve your weight.
Choose a diet with plenty of grain products, vegetables, and fruits.
Choose a diet low in fat, saturated fat, and cholesterol.
Choose a diet moderate in sugars.
Choose a diet moderate in sodium.
If you drink alcoholic beverages, do so in moderation.

categories appear to be influenced by diet, especially excesses of energy and fat intake. Although proof of cause-and-effect relationships between diet and chronic disease are difficult to obtain, there is general acceptance that positive dietary change will lead to a reduction in the incidence of chronic disease. Thus, programs aimed at achieving dietary goals have been set up by health agencies and governments at the federal, state, territorial, and municipal levels, in cooperation with food and food-service industries, nutrition and health professionals, and professional and nongovernmental organizations.

Of recent concern is the sharp increase in the prevalence of obesity. Between 1980 and 1990 obesity increased by 25% in adults and 21% in 12- to 19-year-olds. In 1990, 33% of adults had a body mass index over 27,[7] and 21% of 12- to 19-year-olds were overweight.[8]

ACHIEVING DIETARY CHANGE

To achieve healthier diets, nutrition educators want people to make appropriate food choices from the traditional food supply. Dietary guidelines suggest changes for the average diet and indicate quantitative goals. However, most people need this dietary guidance translated into foods and servings of foods. These are shown in the current food guides of the United States[9] and Canada.[10] The guides indicate that necessary dietary change can be achieved by appropriate selection from the traditional food supply.[11] They emphasize foods high in complex carbohydrates, including fruits, vegetables, and grains. They discourage foods high in fat, including most snack foods; whole milk and cheeses; fatty meats; and fats and oils, including salad dressings, butter, and margarine. An individual following this pattern of food selection and consumption will have a nutrient-adequate diet, and will be eating according to the dietary guidelines.

Although the dietary guidelines and nutrition education messages, including the food guides, have been in use since the 1970s, it is clear that nutrition education alone does not accomplish the difficult task of modifying people's food choices significantly. Dietary change is a difficult task for the individual because of the immutable fact that the choice of food and quantity consumed are determined by a complex array of physiological and cognitive variables.

Physiological determinants of food intake are strong.[12] Total food intake is governed rather precisely, for most individuals, by mechanisms that give a high priority to matching energy intake with expenditure and, possibly, by the body mass setpoint. These mechanisms create strong determinants of whether or not food is eaten. Energy deficit is expressed in the form of hunger, an unpleasant, physiologically determined sensation. For most individuals, this physiologically regulated system is the primary determinant of the quantity of food they eat.[13]

Contrary to lay perceptions of the system, energy intake regulation is remarkably precise for most individuals, ensuring that energy requirements are met during periods of several days or weeks. The system is not easily fooled, and the quantity of food consumed is ultimately adjusted according to its energy content. For example, in an analysis of the dietary records of 29 adults for one year, day-to-day food intake was found to be extremely variable even though body weight changed little.[14] Each individual, however, had a characteristic pattern, likely due to environmental factors, life-style, and personality traits. Such variation does not rule out regulation, but challenges our understanding of the mechanisms operating.

In contrast to our understanding of the forces guiding intake of food energy, we do not yet know any physiological determinants of the intake of nutrients. The selection of nutrient-adequate diets is dependent upon a wide range of relatively uncontrolled and poorly understood factors.[15,16] There are many cognitive influences on food preferences and selection. These include health beliefs, tolerance, price, convenience, and prestige. Physiological and cognitive factors interact and, with the possible exceptions of taste and price, their effects on food choices and dietary patterns are poorly understood and somewhat unpredictable. Their importance to the individual is modified by cultural origins, economic and society status, and by heredity, sex, age, and activity. Nutrition educators and advertisers focus on altering food selection and dietary patterns by strategies touching on one or more of these determinants of food selection.

For some consumers, knowledge of the diet–health relationship is a strong motivator of food choice,[15] and consumer surveys show that our education messages to reduce fat are being heard. A recent survey of Canadian consumers asked them what would be the top three items of nutrition information that they would want on the food label.[17] Sixty-two percent listed fat content. Only 42% thought calorie content should be in these top three items. Nutrition monitoring in the United States also provides evidence that nutrition education messages are being heard. North Americans have made changes in food selection in the past decade that suggest attempts to move toward healthier diets.[18] Dietary changes over 12 years from 1977–1978 to 1989–1990 include approximately 40% decreases in the average amount consumed per day of whole milk, pork, and beef. Low-fat and skim milk consumption increased by 120%, grain product and carbonated soft-drink consumption increased by over 20%, and dark green vegetable consumption increased by nearly 40 percent.

Unfortunately, nutrition messages and these changes in food selection do not appear to have impacted greatly on the amount of fat consumed. Depending on the database one uses, it can be concluded that fat intake in the average diet has, or has not, decreased between the early 1970s and the late 1980s, the time period when a great deal of effort was made to educate individuals about reductions in fat intake. There has been a small decline from peak dietary fat energy concentrations of approximately 42%, reported by participants in dietary surveys in the 1960s and early 1970s, to approximately 36% in 1984.[19] However, as shown in TABLE 2, the

TABLE 2. Percent of Food Energy from Dietary Fat, 1965–1988[18]

	NFCS[a] 1965–66	NHANES I[b] 1971–74	NHANES II 1976–80	NFCS 1977–78	CSFII[c] 1985–86	NFCS 1987–88
Percent of food energy from fat	42.1	36.5	36.1	40.1	36.0	36.3

[a] NFCS, Nationwide Food Consumption Survey.
[b] NHANES, National Health and Nutrition Examination Survey.
[c] CSF, Continuing Survey of Food Intakes.

NHANES studies of the 1970s showed fat intakes to be 36% of energy. This is very similar to that reported in the CSFII and NFCS surveys in the 1980s. Furthermore, per capita availability of food fats and oils increased by 15 pounds from 1970 to 1985 and has been quite stable at 60-65 pounds per capita to 1990, indicating that the demand for use of edible fats remains high.[18] More recent information from the NHANES III survey of 1988–1991 suggests that fat intake has dropped to 34% of energy.[20] This decrease, if it continues, may be reflecting the availability of fat-reduced products in the marketplace, not the success of nutrition education. Low-fat and fat-reduced foods began to appear in significant numbers in the late 1980s.

BENEFITS AND RISKS ASSOCIATED WITH DIETARY CHANGE

Implicit in dietary recommendations is the notion that reducing consumption of fat calories and the replacement of them with complex carbohydrates is without risk. This is a reasonable assumption, inasmuch as the majority of evidence shows that risk of chronic disease is lower in populations consuming diets lower in dietary fat than that of the average North American. However, there is no proof that individuals will make the appropriate food choices to achieve the goal of 30% or less of dietary calories from fat, without health risk. For example, consumers have heard the message that animal fat is bad, and the consumption of red meat, butter, whole milk, and eggs has decreased. Paradoxically, however, the consumption of heavy cream, cheese, frozen desserts, full-fat yogurts, and vegetable oil has increased. Many people may be selecting nutrient-inadequate diets by shifting from nutrient-rich foods, such as meat, milk, and eggs, to less nutritious foods that contain as much, or more, fat. The cause of this inappropriate shift in food choice is unknown but may be confusion caused by inconsistent nutrition messages.

There are other risks to the nutritional health of individuals who partially adopt the dietary guidelines. For example, a shift away from animal products toward complex carbohydrate foods reduces intakes of calcium, highly available iron and other trace minerals, including zinc and copper, and vitamins A and D. Unless vitamin- and mineral-supplemented breakfast cereals are part of an individual's eating pattern, it is unlikely that the requirements for these nutrients will be met.[21]

The major problem faced by nutrition educators in achieving the dietary goals is that the change in dietary pattern required of most individuals is large. Reversal of a dietary pattern that has developed over decades does not occur easily. Thus it is logical that macronutrient substitutes should have a supporting role in achieving the goal of a healthier diet.

NUTRITIONAL ASPECTS OF MACRONUTRIENT-MODIFIED FOODS

Operating on the knowledge that traditional and familiar food preferences are very difficult to alter, food scientists and the food industry have applied science and technology to assist in achieving dietary goals. They have moved quickly to modify the composition of familiar foods, specifically by reducing energy density, fat, and carbohydrate content. For example, in 1989, there were 626 new products in the reduced-fat/low-fat category, and in 1995, 1914 were introduced, along with 1161 foods reduced in fat and energy.[1] Approximately 6600 foods are now available in these categories.

Fewer calories and less fat in foods and beverages can be achieved by the two primary approaches to reducing energy density, or by replacement of one of the macronutrients with a substance that is less physiologically available. The energy density of a food, for example, ice cream or margarine, can be reduced by dilution techniques, in which water or air is added. Macronutrient substitution can be achieved by replacing a major energy-producing component, such as fat, with a nonmetabolizable substance or with a lower energy-producing component, such as a carbohydrate or protein. The food industry has pursued the reduction of the energy content of carbohydrate foods by developing high intensity sweeteners and by adding bulking agents and dietary fiber. Fat substitutes may be carbohydrate-, protein- or fat-based. They behave like fat in the food system with all its functional and organoleptic properties but provide significantly fewer calories than fat.[22,23]

Macronutrient-substituted foods are readily available. High-intensity sweeteners are widely used, especially in beverages, to provide taste and variety without the calories contained in nutritive sweeteners. Adding dietary fiber to breakfast cereals and breads maintains the taste, texture, and nutrient properties, but reduces caloric density by replacing some of the digestible carbohydrate. In salad dressings and other emulsion-based foods, using carbohydrates instead of fat is another form of macronutrient substitution that reduces the energy density of the familiar food. Similarly, protein emulsions instead of fat have been used in ice cream. Fat-based fat replacers may be either completely indigestible, for example, olestra, or partially digestible, for example, Salatrim. These are now available to the consumer in savory snack foods and chocolate-based items, respectively.

Consumer acceptance of energy-reduced and macronutrient-modified foods suggests that they are willing to use such foods to achieve a healthier diet, if they can do so without a change in dietary habits and lifestyles. Thus, the availability of macronutrient-modified foods contributes to healthier diets consistent with dietary goals. The societal benefits to encouraging these developments is a reduction in chronic disease.

PUTATIVE BENEFITS OF MACRONUTRIENT SUBSTITUTES

Macronutrient substitutes cannot replace the need for individuals to make dietary changes and wise food selections, but they can assist individuals to achieve healthier diets. However, several nutritional benefits of the judicious use of macronutrient substitutes can be proposed.

From a nutritional viewpoint, there is one clear theoretical benefit to macronutrient substitutes. By reducing the energy density of a food while maintaining its taste and nutrient properties, the nutrient-to-energy ratio of the food is enhanced. Of course, not all foods will have enhanced nutrient-to-energy ratios through these substitutions. Soft drinks, which do not contain vitamins or minerals, are examples of this. However, when examined in the context of a daily diet, these macronutrient-substituted foods have the potential to increase the nutrient density of the diet, which is a highly desirable feature. Obesity still occurs even though energy intakes have declined, primarily because inactivity has become a way of life.

A second benefit to fat replacement is the reduced intake of fat calories. Individuals following their usual dietary pattern will benefit if foods that are fat-reduced are substituted for the high-fat counterparts.[24,25] Based on one year of daily food records of 29 individuals and the within-subject variation in energy and macronutrient intake, Beaton et al.[24] predicted the expected impact of macronutrient substitutes on the diet of individuals without a strong motivation to control macronutrient or energy intake. A fundamental premise of the paper was that the individuals would replace a substantial part of the energy lost in the original substitution, and would maintain their usual food pattern. Based on a 2250 kcalorie diet, it was predicted that the use of noncaloric fat replacers to replace 20 g/day of fat would lead to a net decrease (although less than the original substitution) in fat intake of 11 g and net increases in carbohydrate and protein intakes (TABLE 3). Conversely, carbohydrate replacements in core foods (or the true replacement of 50 g of nutritive sweetener with a high-intensity sweetener, rather than as an add-on as currently occurs) would result in net increases in fat of about 10 g and in protein of 6 g, and a partial decrease of 32 g in carbohydrate intakes. It was noted, however, that simple availability of high-intensity sweeteners in drinks would not be expected to have this effect, because the soft drinks containing them appear to be used as add-ons to the diet, not as substitutes.

Gatenby et al.[25] support the prediction of Beaton et al.[24] In this experimental study, subjects were asked to use, for six weeks, reduced-fat foods *ad libitum* in

TABLE 3. Predicted Effect of Noncaloric Carbohydrate and Fat Replacements on Dietary Composition[a]

Noncaloric Replacements	Replaced (g)	Net Change			
		Macronutrients			Energy
		Protein	CHO	Fat	
Carbohydrate	50	+5.8	−31.7	+10.0	0
Fat	20	+5.0	+16.5	−11.0	0

[a] Based on a 2250 kcal/day diet.[24]

place of the traditional, high-fat items. A control group continued their usual diet. The experimental group reduced the percentage of energy from fat from 38 to 30% and increased the percentage of energy from protein and carbohydrate. Weight loss initially occurred in the experimental group, but the authors state that "long-term sustained reduction in energy intake may be limited if this dietary strategy is used in isolation." There is some indication that the availability of reduced fat/low-fat foods has sped up the trend to lower fat diets, possibly to be confirmed by recent surveys.

Third, implicit in the above is that with macronutrient substitution consumers do not need to make large changes in their habitual dietary pattern. Healthier diets will emerge by selecting familiar foods containing macronutrient substitutes guided by health claims. Educating even the most unaware consumer to make this choice will be easier than convincing him/her to select unfamiliar foods.

Fourth, a less clear but putative benefit to fat replacement may be its contribution to the maintenance of body weight within a desirable range. Low-fat diets offer theoretical benefits to reducing energy intake. They are less energy dense than high-fat diets, and current knowledge of regulatory mechanisms suggests that carbohydrate intake is more precisely regulated than fat intake.[26] A recent review of the literature, however, provides little support for this hypothesis.[27] It concludes that the relative contributions of energy density, fat and carbohydrate content, and variety and palatability of food to energy regulation have not been defined, that low-fat and sugar-free foods will coexist with their high-fat and sugar-containing counterparts, and that energy compensation will continue to be easily possible. Thus the consequence of fat replacements for the majority of consumers will likely be as predicted by Beaton *et al.*[24] and observed by Gatenby *et al.*[25] That is, they contribute to reduced fat intake, but not reduced energy intake. For the individual, reducing energy intake will require a conscious effort.

DISADVANTAGES OF MACRONUTRIENT SUBSTITUTION

The disadvantages of macronutrient substitution in the diet are difficult to identify based on quantitative data. On the other hand, the subject has led to considerable speculation. For example, in recent years the hypothesis has been put forward that beverages or foods containing high-intensity sweeteners create enhanced appetite and result in increased food intake.[28] The proposed physiologic mechanism explaining this behavior involves the cephalic phase response to food. The sight, taste, and smell of food involves central nervous system responses that in turn prepare the body's gastrointestinal and hormonal systems for the presence of food. It has been argued that beverages containing high-intensity sweeteners stimulate this response but do not provide the energy substrate required to satisfy this cephalic phase response. The hypothesis was that this anticipated, but undelivered, energy leaves the individual with an enhanced feeling of hunger, which is only satisfied by eating more food than would have been consumed without this stimulus. Further studies failed to support the notion that such beverages have a counterproductive effect on food intake.[29-31]

It is possible that macronutrient substitution will lead to altered behavior with respect to eating, but there is no evidence to date of adverse effects. It seems more likely that each individual will continue to make food choices based on health beliefs, cultural background, and the properties of the food, including taste and texture, convenience, and price. Sensory-specific satiety is a strong determinant, suppressing repetitive intake of any one particular food or beverage, no matter how appealing it may be. Nutrition education, emphasizing that a variety of foods is required to obtain a balanced diet, and that diet has a role in chronic disease, will continue to be an important activity in helping consumers to make appropriate food choices. Nutrition educators could be most helpful in preparing messages that enhance consumer knowledge of all opportunities for individuals to select foods contributing to a healthier diet, including macronutrient-substituted foods.

The extent to which macronutrient-substituted foods assist the population in achieving healthier diets consistent with dietary guidelines can be determined only by monitoring their use. Regulatory agencies currently demand that the safety of new food ingredients be established before their entry to the marketplace. However, with macronutrient substitutes there is a need to provide continued assurance of safety through postmarket surveillance, but perhaps more important, to confirm intakes.[32] Achieving their full benefit, however, will also depend on an informed consumer.

CONCLUSION

Based on current knowledge of the factors regulating human food intake and selection, macronutrient substitutes will make a useful contribution to the achievement of dietary goals. Incorporation of nonnutritive substitutes as replacement for nutritive macronutrients in foods that are energy dense will automatically increase their nutrient density, if all other factors remain the same. If this substitution is achieved, it is likely that the nutrient composition of the individual's total diet will be improved. Furthermore, the specific replacement of fat calories in foods will help the consumer reduce fat intake.

There is no reason to believe, a priori, that the substitution of a metabolically inert substance for an energy-producing component of a food will have any inherent potential to cause dietary problems. Humans adapt easily to a wide range of energy densities in diets, and more quantity (in terms of weight) is eaten of low-energy foods compared with high-energy foods, in order to meet energy requirements. Their impact on modulating the increase, or reducing the prevalence, of obesity remains to be determined.

REFERENCES

1. FRIEDMAN, M. 1996. New products come alive in '95. Prepared Foods **165**(5): 29–32.
2. TRUSWELL, A. 1987. Evaluations of dietary recommendations, goals and guidelines. Am. J. Clin. Nutr. **45**: 1060–1072.
3. NATIONAL RESEARCH COUNCIL (U.S.) COMMITTEE ON DIET AND HEALTH. 1989. Diet and Health: Implications for Reducing Chronic Disease Risk. National Academy Press. Washington, D.C.
4. KOOP, C. E. 1988. The Surgeon General's Report on Nutrition and Health. U.S. Gov. Printing Office. Washington, D.C.

5. HEALTH AND WELFARE CANADA. 1990. Nutrition Recommendations: The Report of the Scientific Review Committee. Canadian Government Publishing Center, Supplies and Services Canada. Ottawa, Canada.
6. U.S. DEPARTMENT OF AGRICULTURE AND U.S. DEPARTMENT OF HEALTH AND HUMAN SERVICES. 1995. Nutrition and Your Health: Dietary Guidelines for Americans. U.S. Government Printing Office. Washington, D.C.
7. KUCZMARSKI, R. J., K. M. FLEGAL, S. M. CAMPBELL & C. L. JOHNSON. 1994. Increasing prevalence of overweight among U.S. adults: the National Health and Nutrition Examination Surveys, 1960 to 1991. J. Am. Med. Assoc. **272**(20): 205–211.
8. CENTERS FOR DISEASE CONTROL AND PREVENTION. 1994. Prevalence of overweight among adolescents—United States, 1988–1991. Morb. Mortal. Wkly. Rep. **43**(44): 818–821.
9. UNITED STATES DEPARTMENT OF AGRICULTURE. HUMAN NUTRITION INFORMATION SERVICES. The Food Guide Pyramid. Home and Garden Bulletin No. 252.
10. HEALTH AND WELFARE CANADA. 1992. Canada's Food Guide to Healthy Eating for People Four Years and Older. Ministry of Supply and Services. Ottawa, Canada.
11. WELSH, C. S., C. DAVIS & A. SHAW. 1992. Development of the Food Guide Pyramid. Nutr. Today **27**(6): 12.
12. ANDERSON, G. H. 1988. Metabolic regulation of food intake. *In* Modern Nutrition in Health and Disease. M. E. Shils & V. R. Young, Eds.: 557–569. Lea & Febiger. Philadelphia, PA.
13. ANDERSON, G. H. 1996. Hunger, Appetite, and Food Intake. *In* Present Knowledge in Nutrition. E. E. Ziegler & L. J. Filer, Eds.: 13–18. ILSI Press. Washington, D.C.
14. TARASUK, V. & G. H. BEATON. 1991. The nature and individuality of within-subject variation in energy intake. Am. J. Clin. Nutr. **54**: 464–470.
15. KRONDL, M. 1990. Conceptual Models. *In* Diet and Behavior: Multidisciplinary Approaches. G. H. Anderson, N. A. Krassegor, G. D. Miller & A. P. Simopoulos, Eds.: 5–15. Springer-Verlag. New York, NY.
16. JOHNS, T. & H. V. KUHNLEIN. 1990. Cultural determinants of food selection and behavior. *In* Diet and Behavior: Multidisciplinary Approaches. G. H. Anderson, N. A. Krassegor, G. D. Miller & A. P. Simopoulos, Eds.: 17–31, Springer-Verlag. New York, NY.
17. FOOD AND CONSUMER PRODUCTS MANUFACTURERS OF CANADA. 1996. Consumerline Canada. Don Mills, Ontario.
18. INTERAGENCY BOARD FOR NUTRITION MONITORING AND RELATED RESEARCH. 1993. Nutrition Monitoring in the United States. Chartbook I: Selected Findings from the National Nutrition Monitoring and Related Research Program. Public Health Service. Hyattsville, MD.
19. STEPHEN, A. M. & N. J. WALD. 1990. Trends in individual consumption of dietary fat in the United States, 1920–1984. Am. J. Clin. Nutr. **52**: 457–469.
20. CENTERS FOR DISEASE CONTROL AND PREVENTION. 1994. Daily dietary fat and total food-energy intakes-NHANES III, Phase 1, 1988–91 Morb. Mortal. Wkly. Rep. **43**: 116–117, 123–125.
21. GENERAL MILLS NUTRITION DEPARTMENT. 1978–1990. General Mills Dietary Intake Study. General Mills: Minneapolis, MN.
22. DREWNOWSKI, A. 1990. The new fat replacements. A strategy for reducing fat consumption. Postgrad. Med. **87**(6): 1402–1407.
23. LYNCH, P. M. 1990. Sugar and fat substitutes: The challenge for today and tomorrow. The Diabetes Educator **16**: 101–105.
24. BEATON, G. H., V. TARASUK & G. H. ANDERSON. 1992. Estimation of possible impact on non-caloric fat and carbohydrate substitutes on macronutrient intake in the human. Appetite **19**: 87–103.
25. GATENBY, S. J., J. I. AARON, G. M. MORTON & D. J. MELA. 1995. Nutritional implications of reduced-fat food use by free-living consumers. Appetite **25**: 241–252.
26. LISSNER, L., D. A. LEVITSKY, B. J. STRUPP, H. J. KALKWARF & D. A. ROE. 1987. Dietary fat and the regulation of energy intake in human subjects. Am. J. Clin. Nutr. **46**: 886–892.

27. BELLISLE, F. & C. PEREZ. 1994. Low-energy substitutes for sugars and fats in the human diet: Impact on nutritional regulation. Neurosci. Biobehav. Rev. **18**(2): 197–205.
28. BLUNDELL, J. E. & A. J. HILL. 1986. Paradoxical effects of an intense sweetener (aspartame) on appetite. Lancet **1:** 1092–1093.
29. FOLTIN, R. W., M. W. FISCHMAN, C. S. EMURIAN & J. J. RACHLINSKI. 1988. Compensation for caloric dilution in humans given unrestricted access to food in a residential laboratory. Appetite **10**(1): 13–24.
30. BLACK, R. M., P. TANAKA, L. A. LEITER & G. H. ANDERSON. 1991. Soft drinks with aspartame: Effect on subjective hunger, food selection, and food intake of young adult males. Physiol. Behav. **49:** 303–310.
31. ROLLS, B. J., S. KIM & I. C. FEDEROFF. 1990. Effects of drinks sweetened with sucrose or aspartame on hunger, thirst, and food intake in men. Physiol. Behav. **48:** 19–26.
32. BORZELLECA, J. F. 1995. Post-marketing surveillance of macronutrient substitutes. Food Technol. **49**(9): 107–113.

Macronutrient Substitutes

Description and Uses

GILBERT A. LEVEILLE [a] AND JOHN W. FINLEY [b]

Nabisco Inc.
200 Deforest Avenue
East Hanover, New Jersey 07936

INTRODUCTION

American consumers have been bombarded with recommendations to reduce their fat intake and, if overweight, their caloric intake.[1,2] For individuals trying to lower weight through caloric reduction, it appears that eliminating fat calories is more effective than elimination of calories from other sources.[1,2] For example, exchange (on a weight basis) of fat for carbohydrate would appear to offer a caloric advantage of 2.25 (*i.e.*, 9 kcal/g for fat vs 4 kcal/g for carbohydrate). In fact, it appears that the advantage is really a factor of 3 inasmuch as about 25% of the energy of carbohydrates is expended in the conversion of carbohydrates to fat.[3,4] The health community is convinced of the health advantages of reducing fat intake, and the consumer has heard their message. However, implementing the recommendations is difficult without a modification of the food supply. Manufacturers have responded to this demand by introducing a wide array of new, low- or no-fat foods. The design and production of such products is dependent upon the availability of technologies and/or ingredients that permit reducing or replacing the fat- and calorie-supplying components of food. This paper will review the major available macronutrients and their uses. This topic has been reviewed earlier by Finley and Leveille.[5]

Macronutrients are the major components of food: water, protein, carbohydrate, and fat. Macronutrient substitutes are ingredients that can replace these components to achieve a specific purpose, such as caloric or fat reduction. The sweetening function of sucrose can be provided by an intense sweetener, leaving the need for a bulking agent to replace the mass usually provided by sucrose. Alternatively, sucrose can be replaced by another sugar having the desired attributes (*e.g.*, fewer calories, less fermentable). Replacement of starch also requires the addition of a bulking agent but one having different functional properties than a sucrose replacer.

Because fat is calorically dense, its replacement offers the greatest potential for caloric reduction. Two types of macronutrient substitutes have been developed for fat: mimetics, which are usually protein or carbohydrates that when hydrated provide some of the mouthfeel characteristics of fat, and fat substitutes that replace fat gram-for-gram but provide significantly fewer calories by virtue of being unabsorbed or only partially absorbed.

---

[a] Current address: 23 Cambridge Avenue, Denville, NJ 07834. Tel: (201) 366-7823; e-mail: gleveill@ix.netcom.com.

[b] Current address: 511 Eagles Nest Court, Wildwook, MO 63011.

TABLE 1. Caloric Value and Taste of Selected Polyols[5]

Compound	Energy Value (kcal/g)	Taste of Dry Sugar	Sweetness Relative to Sucrose
Sorbitol	1.8–3.3	Cool	0.70
Erythritol	0–0.4	Cool	0.65
Mannitol	1.6	Cool	0.50
Maltitol	2.8–3.5	None	0.75
Xylitol	~2.4	Very cool	0.90
Hydrogenated glucose syrups	2.8–3.2	None	0.75
Lactitol	2 or less	Slightly cool	0.40
Isomalt	2	None	0.60
Fructooligosaccahrides	2.0	~Sucrose	0.30
Polydextrose	1	None	None

CARBOHYDRATE REPLACEMENTS

In liquid products, such as soft drinks or sweeteners for coffee, sugar can be readily replaced by intense sweeteners, inasmuch as water is the bulk phase. In solid foods, such as confections, cookies, or cakes, sugar accounts for a considerable portion of the bulk phase. Thus, substitution with an intense sweetener would not replace the bulk missing from the food when sucrose is removed. Bulking agents are therefore required to make up this mass in product formulations.

POLYOLS

The simplest bulking agents are a group of sugar replacers referred to as polyols. Polyols are hydrogenated analogues of simple sugars that are generally less sweet than sucrose. TABLE 1 presents information for some properties of commonly used polyols. Currently the primary uses of polyols are in chewing gum, hard candies, and coatings for candies. There is still some controversy concerning the caloric values for individual polyols.[6-9] For example, in the United States the FDA now allows 2.6 kcal/g for sorbitol, 2.4 kcal/g for xylitol, and 2 kcal/g for isomalt. The European Community Nutritional Labeling Directive of 1990 assigned a caloric value of 2.4 kcal/g for all polyols. Japan, on the other hand, has set individual caloric values for the various polyols: isomalt = 1.9, lactitol = 1.6; mannitol, sorbitol, and xylitol = 2.8; and maltitol = 1.8. The sugar alcohols have physical properties similar to sugars, particularly liquid sugar systems, and function similarly in food systems. For most food applications sugar alcohols replace all or some of the sugar on an equal weight basis.

Sugar alcohols are poorly absorbed from the upper gastrointestinal tract but are readily fermented by the colon microflora. Fermentation in the colon generates less usable energy from the sugar alcohols than would be provided by the parent sugar. The range of absorption of monomeric sugar alcohols ranges from 50% for sorbitol to essentially zero for erythritol (TABLE 2). The dimeric sugar alcohols exhibit ranges of digestibility and absorption based on their monomeric constituents.

Sugar alcohols have been recognized as having a much lower cariogenic potential than sucrose or glucose[10] and, consequently, are appropriately used in chewing gum and hard candies.

REDUCED STARCH HYDROLYSATES

Reduced starch hydrolysates are mixtures of mono-, di- and oligomeric polyols prepared by partial hydrolysis of starch followed by hydrogenation. Commercially available products contain varying levels of sorbitol, maltitol, and oligosaccharides hydrogenated at the reducing end. Upon ingestion the reduced starch hydrolysates are hydrolyzed to glucose, sorbitol, and maltitol with insignificant portions of the hydrolysis products reaching the colon.[11] The Life Sciences Research Office[12] expert panel concluded that the net energy was probably below 3.2 kcal/g.

OLIGOFRUCTOSE

Fructo-oligosaccharides occur naturally in a variety of plants, such as onion, asparagus, wheat, rye, triticale, and the Jerusalem artichoke.[13] Similar oligosaccharides can be prepared industrially from sucrose or inulin. Functionally, fructo-oligosaccharides provide a sweet taste, with intensity about 30% that of sucrose but without the "cooling" effect experienced with crystalline sucrose. The water retention properties are slightly greater than for sucrose, similar to sorbitol. The oligosaccharides are stable to low pH and heat stable up to approximately 140° C.[14]

Fructo-oligosaccharides are not digested by the brush border enzymes of the small intestine.[15] The colonic microflora easily and quantitatively hydrolyze and use inulin and fructooligisaccharides, lowering the pH and increasing the fecal mass proportional to the intake of fructo-oligosaccharides or inulin.[16-19] Fructooligosaccharides appear to have a caloric value of between 1.0 and 1.5 kcal/g.[20]

POLYDEXTROSE

Polydextrose is a commercially available, water soluble, reduced calorie bulking agent of Cultor Science, Inc. Polydextrose is a randomly bound polymer of glucose containing minor amounts of sorbitol and citric acid. The product is only partially metabolized by humans, and, unlike sugar alcohols and fructooligosaccahrides, it is not fermented by the microflora in the gastrointestinal tract. Approximately 25% of polydextrose is metabolized, providing approximately 1 kcal/g.[21] Allingham[22] reported that polydextrose is well tolerated at normal ingestion levels. The average threshold for laxative effect was 90 g/day compared to 70 g/day for sorbitol.

COMPLEX CARBOHYDRATE BULKING AGENTS

Complex carbohydrates are frequently classified as dietary fiber and can also be considered low-calorie bulking agents. Materials falling into this category include

TABLE 2. Digestion and Absorption of Sugar Alcohols[5]

Sugar Alcohol	Type	Digested	Absorbed	Metabolized	Fermented
Mannitol	monomeric	no	~25%	negligible	+
Sorbitol	monomeric	no	~50%	up to 85% of absorbed	+
Xylitol	monomeric	no	25%	100% of absorbed	+
Erythritol	monomeric	no	none	negligible	+
Isomalt	dimeric	20% to 75%	up to 20%	+	+
Lactitol	dimeric	negligible	negligible	negligible	+
Maltitol	dimeric	partially	up to 40%	+	+
Hydrogenated starch hydrolysates	oligomeric	partially	incomplete	+	+

cellulose, hemicelluloses, pectins, gums, mucilages, and lignins. Unlike the lower molecular weight bulking agents, these materials are very complex mixtures of carbohydrate polymers. As a result of their complexity, they are frequently somewhat ill-defined, chemically. Because they come from a variety of food sources many are already common to our diets. The "natural" occurrence of these materials makes them attractive alternatives as bulking agents. It is more the new and different application of these materials rather than new exposure as food that raises interest.

POLYMERIC BULKING AGENTS

Polymeric low-calorie bulking agents, such as cellulose, pectins, hemicelluloses, and gums from a variety of sources, vary widely in composition and quality, which makes precise definition of any attribute difficult at best.

PECTINS

Pectins are complex galacturonoglycans composed primarily of polymers of D-galacturonic acid. Pectins occur primarily in the cell wall of plants. The most abundant natural sources of pectin are apples, citrus fruits, sunflower seeds, and sugar beets. Pectins are slowly degraded in the intestinal tract primarily by microflora in the large intestine and colon.[21] It has also been reported that pectin reduces total serum cholesterol without effecting the high-density lipoprotein cholesterol.[23]

β-GLUCANS

β-Glucans are glucose polymers containing both β-(1-3) and β-(1-4) linkages in various proportions, depending on the source.[24] Barley and oats are both excellent sources of β-glucans. Physiological effects associated with β-glucans are improved bowel activity and a lowering of serum cholesterol. These materials are not generally added to food directly but represent a portion of cereal bran fractions.

GALACTOMANNANS

Galactomannans are composed of β-(1-4)-D-mannopyranosyl chains with α-(1-6)-D galactopyranosyl units attached at carbon 6 of the mannose at various intervals, depending on the source.[25] Primary sources are guar gum and locust bean gum. Locust bean and guar gum are frequently used in low-calorie foods to emulate the texture of fat. Galactomannan in combination with carrageenan simulates the spreadability of some fat products.

CELLULOSE

Cellulose encompasses a variety of complex carbohydrates with the primary structure being β-(1-4)-glucan. It also includes a number of chemically modified celluloses, such as carboxymethyl cellulose, microcrystalline cellulose, and methyl cellulose. The derivitized celluloses can be used in foods as functional bulking agents, binders, stabilizers in frozen food systems, and thickeners. Cellulose acts as a noncaloric insoluble bulking agent in a variety of food applications.

RESISTANT STARCH

Heat processing of certain starchy foods causes a fraction of the starch to become resistant to digestive enzymes.[26] Starch has been classified on the basis of the probable rate of digestion in the small intestine, namely as rapidly digested starch, slowly digested starch, and resistant starch.[27]

Until relatively recently starch was thought to be completely digested in the small intestine. A number of studies[28-33] clearly show that significant amounts of dietary starch escape digestion in the small intestine and pass intact into the colon, where the starch is fermented by anaerobic bacteria and absorbed as volatile fatty acids. Although not conclusive, resistant starch in the large intestine may share many of the characteristics and health benefits attributed to dietary fiber, such as amelioration of diabetes, cardiovascular disease, and colon cancer.[34]

FAT REPLACEMENTS

There is an overall goal in the United States to reduce the amount of fat and the calories from fat provided by various foods. Fat replacers are intended to help achieve the goals of reducing the caloric contribution of fat in the diet as well as the absolute amount of fat. Fats and oils provide many important attributes in foods, including flavor, palatability, mouthfeel, creaminess, and lubricity. Frying oils are also important as heat transfer agents in the frying process, and, in fried foods, the fats provide part of the crispness in the products. Currently, available fat replacers serve these functions to varying degrees.

Generally fat replacers are ingredients that are designed to replace all or part of the fat normally in a product with minimum impact on the organoleptic quality of the food product. Examples include: increasing milk solids in reduced fat or skim milk and frozen desserts; using more lean meat in low-fat and processed meat products and baking, not frying, snack foods. Many low-fat baked products and other low-fat foods are currently available where the fat has been replaced by sugars and starches. Fat replacers can be classified in three categories: fat mimetics, fat substitutes, and low-calorie fats.

FAT MIMETICS

Fat mimetics are materials that replace the bulk, body, and mouthfeel of fats. Typical constituent categories of fat mimetics are starch, cellulose, pectin, protein, hydrophillic colloids, dextrins, or polydextrose. These materials are frequently microparticulated to emulate the particle size of fats and are usually highly hydrated. Many

TABLE 3. Selected Fat Mimetic Types and Suppliers[5]

Mimetic	Producer	Protein	Carbohydrate
Amalean	American Maize		corn starch
Dairy-Lo	Pfizer	whey	
Fibercel	Alpha-Beta Technology		yeast
Kelcogel	Kelco		gellan gum
Leanmaker	Quaker Oats		oat bran
Lita	Opta Food Ingredients	zein	
Litese	Pfizer		polydextrose
Maltrin	Grain Processing		maltodextrin
Methocel	Dow Chemical		cellulose
N-Lite	National Starch		starch + guar gum
N-Oil	National Starch		starch
Nutralean	Webb Technologies		oat bran
Oatrim	Quaker		oat dextrin
Optagrade	Opta Food Ingredients		starch
Paselli SA2	Avebe America Inc.		potato starch
Rhodilean SD	Rhone-Poulenc		xanthan gum oatrim
Simplesse	Nutrasweet	egg + milk proteins	
Slendid	Hercules, Inc.		pectin
Sta-Slim	A.E. Staley		potato starch
Stellar	A.E. Staley		corn starch
Trailblazer	Kraft Foods	egg + milk proteins	
Trim Choice	Conagra		oatrim
Ultra-Freeze	A.E. Staley	egg + milk proteins	
Wonderslim	Natural Food Technologies		plums

of the fat mimetic materials are fully digestible (*i.e.,* starch, dextrins, and protein) providing 4 kcal/g (dry weight). Because they are hydrated, the caloric reductions in products are even greater. Thus, the fat mimetics provide some textural replacement for fat and substantially reduce the caloric contribution. The fat mimetics are generally limited to products with a fairly high degree of hydration, such as desserts and spreads, and are not functional in frying applications. The basis for the fat mimetic category is macronutrients that exist in nature and often are modified to provide the desired technical effects. Some of the commercially available fat mimetics are listed in TABLE 3. The table includes the primary carbohydrate or protein source of the mimetic. It should be noted that mimetics based on cellulose, seaweed, and gums are noncaloric, whereas starch and protein-based mimetics provide 4 kcal/g (dry weight).

LOW-CALORIE FATS

Low-calorie fats are true triglycerides that are structured to provide fewer than 9 kcal/g. The low-calorie fats are commercially exemplified by medium-chain triglycerides (MCTs) (Stepan Corp.), Caprenin® (Procter and Gamble), and salatrim (Nabisco/Cultor). MCTs have been proposed for use in many food applications. Caprenin® is specifically designed for use as a cocoa butter substitute in confections. Salatrim is useful as a cocoa butter substitute as well as a shortening in baked products, a confectionary fat, or a butter fat replacer.

Stepan Corporation has filed a GRAS petition for MCTs. MCTs are triglycerides composed of fatty acids of 8-12 carbons that provide 7 to 8 kcal/gram MCTs are rapidly absorbed through the portal blood stream and are rapidly used as energy. MCTs provide little caloric advantage over conventional fats (7-8 kcal/g vs. 9 kcal/g), but they do provide meaningful metabolic advantages.[35,36]

Structurally Caprenin® is a triglyceride in which two fatty acids esterified to the glycerol backbone are medium-chain fatty acids (caprylic and capric), and the third is behenic acid. Caprylic and capric acids are primarily obtained by fractionation of palm kernel or coconut oil. Behenic acid is obtained from the complete hydrogenation of rapeseed oil. Behenic acid is very poorly absorbed by the body. The result is that Caprenin® provides 5 kcal/g, compared to 9 kcal/g for normal fats and oils.[37]

Salatrim represents a family of low-calorie fats developed by Nabisco and currently marketed by Cultor Food Science, Inc. as BENEFAT™. These fats have a variety of functional properties and thus have the potential for wide application in foods.[38,39] Salatrim is a randomized triglyceride containing short- and long-chain fatty acids. The short-chain fatty acids are acetic and/or propionic and/or butyric, whereas the long-chain fatty acid is predominately stearic acid. The long-chain fatty acids are obtained by complete hydrogenation of vegetable oils, such as canola or soy. The hydrogenation process converts the oleic, linoleic, and linoleic acids in the oils to stearic acid. Because these oils contain small amounts of fatty acids that are shorter than the C18s and small amounts of longer-chain fatty acids, Salatrim contains small amounts of palmitic, arachidic, and behenic acids. The stearic acid and longer-chain fatty acids are poorly absorbed. In rat-growth studies, Finley et al.[40] demonstrated the caloric availability for a range of Salatrim family members the average value was 5 kcal/g. Hayes et al.[41] reached similar conclusions in a radiolabeled study in rats. The metabolism of salatrim was shown to be completely predictable. The short-chain fatty acids were rapidly released and converted to carbon dioxide. Hayes et al.[41] also demonstrated that the stearic acid that was absorbed was largely converted to oleic acid. The caloric availability estimates were confirmed in human clinical studies by Finley et al.[42] to be approximately 5 Kcal/g based on stearic acid balance.

FAT SUBSTITUTES

The fat substitutes are materials that are physically similar to fats and oils but generally are not absorbed or metabolized. These materials can theoretically replace fat on a one-for-one basis in foods and are generally heat stable. Sucrose polyester or olestra, developed at Procter and Gamble over the last 20 years, has recently been approved for food use by the FDA. It is the only approved fat substitute commercially available in the United States. Olestra is a mixture of hexa-, hepta-, and octafatty acid esters of sucrose. The fatty acid distribution can range from 8 to 22 carbon fatty acids, either saturated or unsaturated. The wide range of available fatty acids allows the development of a variety of sucrose polyesters that can range from a liquid, to a plastic fat, to a hard fat. Taste, viscosity, heat stability, functionality, and appearance are claimed to be indistinguishable from normal triglyceride-based vegetable fats. Sucrose polyesters with at least six fatty acids esterified to the molecule are virtually indigestible. Olestra is not digested in the small intestine by mammalian enzymes, and it is also unreactive in the colon. The digestion and absorption of olestra are reviewed in detail by Swanson et al.[43]

Cultor Food Science, Inc. is investigating a noncaloric fat called sorbestrin. Sorbestrin is the hexafatty acid ester of sorbitol, and its functionality is determined by the fatty acid composition. Sorbestrin was assumed to be like olestra, that is, indigestible and therefore providing no available energy. However, Mittendorfer et al.[44] have presented evidence indicating a caloric value of 2.6 kcal/gm for sorbestrin.

Arco Chemical Corporation has developed a family of noncaloric fats that are esterified propoxylated glycerol esters (EPGs). The EPGs are made from naturally occurring fats with various numbers (1 to 4) of propylene oxide units inserted between the glycerol and the fatty acids. The EPGs can be made from any common fat or oil, including soy, cottonseed, corn, canola, tallow or lard. Depending upon the fatty acids used in manufacture, the physical properties range from oils through plastic fats to solid fats. Like olestra the EPGs are not significantly digested or fermented in the gastrointestinal tract. The potential benefits and negatives are similar to olestra.

CONCLUSIONS

There are a number of macronutrient substitutes currently available and many more on the horizon that offer immense potential for the production of reduced fat/calorie foods. With a population where over 30% are obese, there is a need for foods that provide satisfaction but a lower caloric density. If such foods are to provide public health benefit, the foods must taste good and have familiar textures. Macronutrient substitutes will help food processors to achieve these objectives.

REFERENCES

1. NATIONAL RESEARCH COUNCIL, COMMITTEE ON DIET AND HEALTH. 1989. Diet and Health: Implications for Reducing Chronic Disease Risk. National Academy Press. Washington, DC.
2. NATIONAL CHOLESTEROL EDUCATION PROGRAM. 1981. Report of the expert panel on population strategies for blood cholesterol reduction. Circulation **83:** 2154-2232.
3. DONATO, K. A. & D. M. HEGSTED. 1985. Efficiency of utilization of various energy sources for growth. Proc. Nat. Acad. Sci. USA **82:** 4866-4870.
4. GERSHOFF, S. N. 1995. Nutrition evaluation of dietary fat substitutes. Nutr. Rev. **53:** 305-313.
5. FINLEY, J. W. & G. A. LEVEILLE. 1996. Macronutrient substitutes. In Present Knowledge in Nutrition. E. E. Ziegler, & L. J. Filer, Jr. Eds.: 581-595. ILSI Press. Washington, DC.
6. BAR, A. 1990. Factorial calculation model for the estimation of the physiological caloric value of polyols. In Caloric Evaluation of Carbohydrates. N. Hosoya Ed.: 209-257. The Japan Association of Dietetic and Enriched Foods. Tokyo.
7. BERNIER J. & G. PASCAL. 1990. Valeur energetique des polyols (sucres alcools). Med. Nutr. **26:** 221-238.

8. Anonymous. 1987. The energy value of sugar alcohols. Recommendations of the Committee on Polyalcohols. Neth. Voeding. **48:** 357-365.
9. BORNET, F. R. J. 1993. Low calorie bulk sweeteners: Nutrition and metabolism. *In* Low Calorie Foods and Food Ingredients. R. Khan, Ed.: 36-52. Blackie Academic & Professional. New York.
10. BIRKHED, D., S. KALFAS, G. SVENSATER & S. EDWARDSSON. 1985. Microbiological aspects of some caloric sugar substitutes. Int. Dent. J. **35:** 9-17.
11. NGUYEN, N. U., G. DUMOULIN, M. T. HENRIET, S. BERTHELAY & J. REGNARD. 1993. Carbohydrate metabolism and urinary excretion of calcium and oxalate after ingestion of polyol sweetners. J. Clin. Endocrinol. Metab. **77:** 388-392.
12. Life Sciences Research Office. 1994. The evaluation of the energy of certain sugar alcohols used as food ingredients. Prepared for Calorie Control Council by the Life Sciences Research Office. Federation of American Societies for Experimental Biology. Bethesda, MD. June.
13. CLEVENGER, M. A., D. TURNBULL, H. INOUE, M. ENOMOTO, J. A. ALLEN, L. M. HENDERSON & E. JONES. 1988. Toxicological evaluation of neosugar: Genotoxicity and chronic toxicity. J. Am. Coll. Toxicol. **5:** 643-662.
14. DREVON, T. & F. BORNET, 1992. Les Fructo-oligosaccharides: ACTILIGHT®. *In* Les Sucre, Les Edulcorants et Les Glucides de Dharges dans Les IAA. J. L. Multon, Ed: 313-338. TEC & DOC Lavoisier.
15. OKU, T., R. TOKUNAGA & N. HOYSOYA. 1984. Non-digestibility of a new sweetener "Neosugar" in the rat. J. Nutr. **114:** 1574-1581.
16. TSUJI, Y., K. YAMADA, N. HOYSOYA & S. MORIUCHI. 1986. Digestion and absorption of sugars and sugar substitutes in rat small intestine. J. Nutr. Sci Vitaminol. **32:** 92-100.
17. TOKUNAGA, R. & T. OKU. 1989. Utilization and excretion of a new sweetener, fructooligosaccharide (Neosugar) in rats. J. Nutr. **119:** 553-559.
18. HIDAKA, H. 1983. Fructosyloligosaccharides. A new material for dietary food. Attention to the improvement, balance, and the effect of lowering cholesterol in the blood. Kagaku to Seibustu **21:** 291.
19. HIDAKA, H., T. EIDA T. TAKIZAWA, T. TOKUNAGA & Y. TASHIRO. 1986. Effects of fructooligosacharides on intestinal flora and human health. Bifido-bacteria. Microflora **5:** 37.
20. ROBERFOID, M. 1993. Dietary fiber, inulin, and oligofructose: A review comparing their physiological effects. Crit. Rev. Food Sci. Nutr. **33:** 103-148.
21. ANNISON, G., C. BERTOCCHI & R. KHAN. 1993. Low-calorie bulking ingredients: Nutrition and metabolism. *In* Low Calorie Foods and Food Ingredients. R. Khan, Ed.: 51-76. Blackie Academic & Professional. New York.
22. ALLINGHAM, R. P. 1982. Polydextrose—A New Food Ingredient: Technical Aspects. *In* Chemical Foods and Beverages: Recent Developments. G. Charalambous & G. Inglett, Eds.: 293-303. Academic Press. New York.
23. STONE-DORSHOW T. & M. D. LEVITT, 1987. Gaseous response to ingestion of poorly absorbed fructo-oligosaccharide sweetener. Am. J. Clin. Nutr. **46:** 61-65.
24. ASPINALL, G. O. & K. J. CARPENTER. 1984. Structural investigations on the non-starchy polysaccharides of oat bran. Carbohydr. Polym. **4:** 271-278.
25. GIDLEY, M. J., A. J. MCARTHUR & D. R. UNDERWOOD. 1991. ^{13}C-NMR characterization of molecular structure in powder, hydrates and gels of galctomannans and glucomannans. Food Hydrocolloids **5:** 129-140.
26. ENGLYST, H. N., H. W. TROWELL, D. A. T. SOUTHGATE & J. H. CUMMINGS. 1987. Dietary fiber and resistant starch. Am. J. Clin. Nutr. **46:** 873-874.
27. ENGLYST, H. N., S. M. KINGMAN & J. H. CUMMINGS. 1992. Classification and measurement of nutritionally important starch fractions. Eur. J. Clin. Nutr. **46**(Suppl 2): S33-S50.
28. STEPHEN, A. M., A. C. HADDAD & S. F. PHILLIPS. 1983. Passage of carbohydrate into the colon. Direct measurements in humans. Gastroenterology **85:** 589-595.

29. ENGLYST, H. N. & J. H. CUMMINGS. 1985. Digestion of polysaccharides of some cereal foods in the human small intestine. Am. J. Clin. Nutr. **42**: 778-787.
30. ENGLYST, H. N. & J. H. CUMMINGS. 1986. Digestion of the carbohydrates of banana (Musa paradisiaca sapientum) in the small intestine. Am. J. Clin. Nutr. **44**: 42-50.
31. ENGLYST, H. N. & J. H. CUMMINGS. 1987. Digestion of polysaccharides of potato in the small intestine of man. Am. J. Clin. Nutr. **44**: 423-431.
32. ENGLYST, H. N. & H. N. CUMMINGS. 1987. Fermentation in the human large intestine and the available substrates. Am. J. Clin. Nutr. **45**: 1243-1255.
33. ENGLYST, H. N. & G. T. MACFARLANE. 1986. Breakdown of resistant starch and readily digestible starch by the human gut. J. Sci. Food Agric. **37**: 699-706.
34. SCHEPPACH, W. 1994. Effects of short-chain fatty acids on gut morphology and function. Gut **35**(1, suppl.): S35-S38.
35. KENNEDY, J. P. 1991. Structured lipids: Fats of the future. Food Technol. **45**: 76-83.
36. MASCIOLI, E. A., V. K. BABAYAN, B. R. BISTRIAN & G. L. BLACKBURN. 1988. Novel triglycerides for special medical purposes. J. Parenter. Enteral Nutr. **12**: 128S.
37. PETERS, J. C., B. N. HOLCOMBE, L. K. HILLER & D. R. WEBB. 1991. Caprenin 3. Absorption and caloric value in adult humans. J. Am. Coll. Toxicol. **10**: 357-367.
38. SMITH, R. E., J. W. FINLEY & G. A. LEVEILLE. 1994. Overview of SALATRIM, a family of low-calorie fats. J. Agric. Food Chem. **42**: 432-434.
39. KOSMARK, R. 1996. SALATRIM: Properties and applications. Food Technol. **50**: 98-101.
40. FINLEY, J. W., G. A. LEVEILLE, L. P. KLEMANN, J. C. SOURBY, P. H. AYRES & S. APPLETON. 1994. Growth method for estimating the caloric availability of fats and oils. J. Agric. Food Chem. **42**: 489-494.
41. HAYES, J. H., J. W. FINLEY & G. A. LEVEILLE. 1994. *In vivo* metabolism of Salatrim in the rat. J. Ag. Food Chem. **42**: 500-514.
42. FINLEY, J. W., G. A. LEVEILLE, R. M. DIXON, C. G. WALCHAK, J. C. SOURBY, R. E. SMITH, K. D. FRANCIS & M. S. OTTERBURN. 1994. Clinical assessment of Salatrim, a reduced calorie triacylglycerol. J. Ag. Food Chem. **42**: 581-596.
43. SWANSON, B. G., T. T. BOUTTE & C. C. AKOH. 1994. Digestion and absorption of carbohydrate polyesters. *In* Carbohydrate Polyesters as Fat Substitutes. C. C. Akoh & B. G. Swanson, Eds.: 183-196. Marcel Dekker, Inc. New York.
44. MITTENDORFER, B., Y. ZHENG, D. CHINKES & R. R. WOLFE. 1997. Assessment of the caloric value of a fat substitute using a new tracer method. Ann. N. Y. Acad. Sci. This volume.

Regulatory Aspects of the Introduction of New Macronutrient Substitutes

ALAN M. RULIS,[a] LINDA S. PELLICORE, AND
HELEN R. THORSHEIM

Office of Premarket Approval, HFS-200
Center for Food Safety and Applied Nutrition
Food and Drug Administration
200 C St. SW
Washington, D.C. 20204

A new macronutrient substitute may face several possible regulatory hurdles before it can be introduced into the food supply of the United States. These hurdles will be of varying height, depending on several factors, such as the amount of the substance expected to be consumed, the molecular structure of the substance, and the amount of existing information on the substance and its toxicological and nutritional effects.

The approval process at the Food and Drug Administration (FDA) has been in place since 1958 and has resulted in decisions of high integrity and credibility. The FDA has evaluated over 4500 food additive petitions since the beginning of the effort in 1958. Our mandate derives from the Federal Food, Drug, and Cosmetic Act (the Act), wherein section 201(s) defines a food additive as any substance, the intended use of which results or may reasonably be expected to result, directly or indirectly, in its becoming a component or otherwise affecting the characteristics of any food, if such substance is not generally recognized as safe (GRAS).

REGULATORY STATUS

The first issue that must be addressed is whether the macronutrient substitute is a food additive or is GRAS for the intended use. This issue is purely regulatory, but it is important. It determines whether FDA approval must be granted before its use in food can be considered safe. A substance that is intended to be used in food must first obtain FDA's premarket approval unless the intended use is generally recognized as safe by the community of scientific experts qualified to make such determinations. In other words, GRAS substances do not have to undergo FDA's premarket approval process.

There are two means by which a substance can be considered GRAS: either it may be GRAS based on experience from common use in food prior to 1958 or the general recognition of safety may be established by scientific procedures. In both cases there must be common knowledge about the substance throughout the scientific

---

[a] Tel: (202) 418-3100; fax: (202) 418-3131.

community knowledgeable about the safety of food ingredients and consensus that the use is safe. The first basis, common use in food prior to 1958 (the year the Congress enacted the food additives amendment), is the most common means by which substances are considered GRAS. It is important to note, however, that it is the *use* of a substance that is GRAS, not the substance itself. Therefore, a new use of a substance that is GRAS for a different use is not necessarily GRAS.

The second basis for GRAS status is a general recognition of safety established by scientific procedures. FDA's regulations require that all the information critical to a determination that use of a substance is GRAS be published. It is difficult to argue that there is general recognition of safety in the scientific community when the results of critical studies are not widely available. FDA regulations also require that GRAS status be based on the same quantity and quality of scientific evidence as is required to obtain approval as a food additive. In other words, the standard of safety for a GRAS determination, and its scientific basis, must be the same as for the approval of a food additive with comparable exposure and toxicological potential.

If use of a substance is not GRAS, then it must undergo review and approval as a food additive by the FDA prior to its use in food. The remainder of this paper will focus on macronutrient substitutes that would be considered food additives and the premarket approval process that they must undergo before their use can be considered safe. This is the process that additives such as aspartame, polydextrose, and olestra have undergone.

REGULATION OF FOOD ADDITIVES

The primary question that the FDA must consider is whether use of an additive is safe. Section 409 of the Act states that a food additive shall be considered unsafe unless there is a regulation that prescribes the conditions under which such additive may be safely used. The burden of proof of safety is on the petitioner for a new food additive. The FDA reviews data that are conducted and presented to the agency in the form of a petition. We make an independent evaluation of those data and conclude whether or not the petitioner has proven that the use would be safe. If so, we can issue a regulation allowing the safe use of the additive.

Unfortunately, the statute does not define the word "safety." The legislative history of the Act does provide some guidance, however, on what is meant by the term "safe." The concept of safety used in the 1958 legislation involves the question of whether the substance is hazardous to the health of humans or animals. Safety requires proof of a reasonable certainty that no harm will result from the proposed use of the additive. It does not and cannot require proof beyond any possible doubt that no harm will result under any conceivable circumstance. This language, which is from the House of Representatives report of the 85th Congress, has been adopted in our regulations in Title 21 of the Code of Federal Regulations (CFR), Section 170.3.

The safety decision that the FDA makes is not an academic inquiry or a search for complete knowledge on the additive. Nor is it intended to ensure safety with absolute certainty, because that is not possible. In addition, it is not intended to enforce or limit consumer choices among safe foods. That issue is a separate matter that does not fall within the jurisdiction of the Office of Premarket Approval. Although desirability and potential beneficial qualities of additives and the foods in which they are used are interesting and important subjects from a public policy point of view, it is important to note that they are not issues that the Act permits the FDA to consider in its safety evaluation.

What the safety decision does, in fact, do is ensure safety. It is a consensus decision that is reached with uncertainty, but that must, in the end, protect public health. The decision must withstand scientific, procedural, and legal challenge from all sides. The residual uncertainty must not be out of line with what has been previously tolerated in the context of all previous similar safety decisions. Hence, although there is no absolute safety, there has to be a reasonable certainty of no harm from use of the additive in order for the agency to approve its use.

THE ROAD FROM MICROINGREDIENTS TO MACROINGREDIENTS

A food additive petition for microingredients will traditionally have information about the identity and composition of the additive, the proposed use, and quantity to be used. There will be data establishing its intended effect and likely intake scenarios. There will also be analytical methods for quantitatively detecting the additive in food. In addition, there will be full reports and data from safety studies assessing the toxicological properties of the additive. Finally, under the National Environmental Policy Act, the petition will address environmental considerations that would result from approval of the additive. This information allows the FDA to evaluate the safety of the additive at the expected consumption level.

FIGURE 1 illustrates the spectrum of possible exposures to food additives, ranging from very low exposures from additives used in packaging that migrate very little into the food, all the way to ingredients approaching exposures to whole foods. Low exposure at the narrow end of the spectrum in FIGURE 1 allows us to apply a "toxicology-based" review. In this regime, the FDA's approach has been to employ toxicological feeding studies in test animals. In such studies, the test animals are fed much higher doses of the new food additive than humans are expected ever to ingest. In fact, the test doses are administered in amounts sufficiently high to actually cause toxicity, thereby establishing what specific organs are targets for toxic effects from the substance. Multiple dose levels are fed in these studies, to assess whether responses seen can be shown to vary with dose in any way. If any treatment-related effects are observed, then the highest dose observed to cause no adverse effects (the so-called no-observed-adverse-effect level) in the most sensitive species studied is used with appropriate safety factors to derive an acceptable daily intake (ADI) for the additive. This ADI can then be compared to the estimated daily intake (EDI) for humans, which is intended to represent chronic exposure averaged over a lifetime. If the ADI is shown to be above the EDI for persons expected to consume relatively high quantities of the additive (usually the 90th percentile consumers), then the additive can be considered safe for its intended use.

An important consideration with macronutrient substitutes is the expected level of consumption of the additive. In many cases, such as artificial sweeteners, much less of the additive is consumed than of the substance it is replacing (in this case

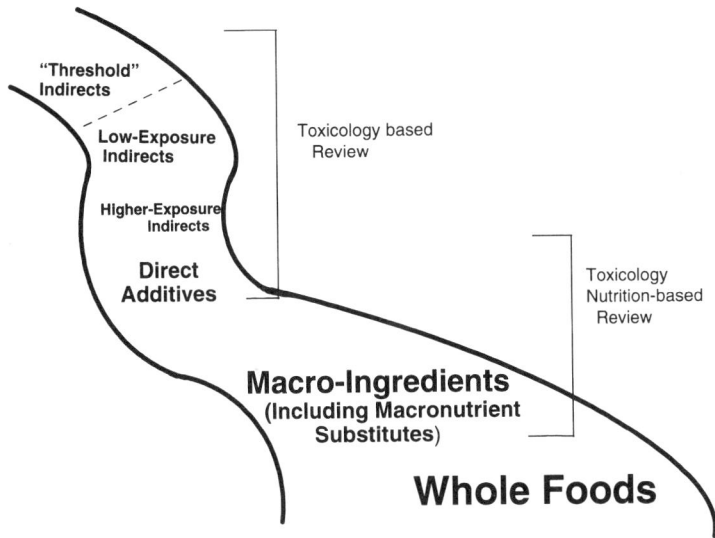

FIGURE 1. Spectrum of food ingredients.

sugar). Therefore, although substituting for a macronutrient, the additive is not itself a macroingredient in food and therefore does not constitute a significant percentage of the diet. In other cases, such as olestra, the additive will be a macroingredient because it will be present in food at levels comparable to the ingredient for which it is substituting. When the additive is not a macroingredient, the food additive approval process is essentially the same as for other additives consumed at low levels, as discussed above.

THE REGULATORY PROCESS FOR MACROINGREDIENTS

When consumption of a macronutrient substitute will be large enough that it will comprise a significant part of the diet, then additional considerations and concerns enter into the food additive review process, and we move into the "toxicology and nutrition-based" regime of FIGURE 1. The FDA has not yet had to consider these issues for many additives; hence the process is still developing.

A major way in which macroingredients differ from typical food additives is that in estimating exposure we need to consider scenarios other than those represented by the lifetime-averaged EDI. We have found it important to also consider some short-term exposure possibilities and to consider whether there will be certain eating scenarios that will cause either higher or lower concern because of possible interactions between the additive and nutrients in the diet. For example, in the case of olestra in savory snacks, it is possible that a significant percentage of nutrient consumption will occur separate from olestra consumption. Hence, by relying, as the FDA did, on studies in which all meals were eaten with olestra, olestra's observed effect on nutrient absorption in those studies likely represented an extreme of what would be experienced in real life. The level of vitamin compensation derived from those studies was determined to be sufficient to encompass a wide range of eating patterns.

As with all food additives, the estimated exposure to, and chemical characteristics of, a macronutrient substitute will determine the level of concern it raises and will therefore determine the level of safety testing that is required. In general, the traditional battery of toxicology tests will need to be performed. If there is reason to be concerned about the effects of the substance on nutrient availability, carefully designed pilot studies should be carried out prior to beginning toxicological studies in order to avoid the possibility that such effects will confound the results of such studies. If necessary, diet formulations should be carefully controlled in such a way as to avoid such problems.

If exposure to the additive is expected to be high, such as with fat replacers, studies in addition to, or sometimes in place of, traditional toxicology studies will be necessary in order to adequately assess the safety of the proposed use. In the case of olestra, more than 150 safety studies were evaluated prior to approval by the agency earlier this year. These data supported the agency's conclusion that olestra is not toxic or carcinogenic, not genotoxic, and not teratogenic. The absorption, distribution, metabolism (including by gastrointestinal (GI) microflora), excretion, and accumulation of the substance in the body should be examined. For example, in the case of olestra, the agency relied on a series of absorption studies conducted with high levels of radiolabeled olestra in rats, guinea pigs, and minipigs to show that nearly all of the ingested olestra was not metabolized or absorbed, but rather remained intact and passed through the GI tract unchanged. Analysis of liver tissue from rats fed olestra for two years showed that olestra does not accumulate in the body. Thus, once the agency determined that the toxicity of olestra was of no concern, because it is not absorbed, the focus shifted to nutritional issues.

Studies assessing the effects of the substance on nutritional status should be considered in certain circumstances, for example, for lipophilic substances that are not absorbed and that can affect the bioavailability of fat-soluble vitamins. Because of the difficulty of designing studies adequate to address both nutritional and toxicological safety simultaneously, separate studies that focus on nutritional effects may be necessary. Alternative (for example, nonrodent) animal models should be considered. Swine are a good choice for nutritional studies, for example, because their GI tracts are similar to those of humans, and they can tolerate diets that, like human diets, contain high levels of fat. Studies must be very carefully designed to ensure that the level of nutrients being fed is accurately measured and is appropriate.

Clinical studies can be extremely valuable in evaluating the nutritional and gastrointestinal effects of an additive and can be useful in evaluating other effects that require questioning of the study subjects, such as the intensity and frequency of gastrointestinal disturbances. (It is difficult to ask a mouse or a pig whether its stomach hurts.) Studies on individuals with compromised bowel integrity (*e.g.,* those with inflammatory bowel diseases) can help to evaluate the possible effects of the substance on the GI tract. If there is some reason to suspect that the ecology or metabolism of GI microflora will be altered by the substance, studies that address the effects of the additive on GI microflora should be considered. In addition, the effect of consumption of the additive on the extent or rate of drug absorption should be investigated if there is a reason to suspect an interaction.

In all safety studies, the material tested should be representative of material to which consumers will be exposed. For this reason, if typical food processing conditions affect the additive in a way that could affect its safety (*e.g.,* by changing the amount or type of impurities), the additive tested for safety should be first subjected to conditions that typically would be used to prepare food with the additive. Because of the novel nature of the studies that may be required, the FDA has been encouraging industry to consult with the agency early during the product development process for guidance on protocols.

One of the mechanisms the agency has used to evaluate macroingredient petitions is through the use of expertise outside of the agency, for example, in other agencies and academia. In this way we have been able to apply as broad a spectrum of experience and knowledge to the problem as possible. In the case of olestra, scientists from the Center for Food Safety and Applied Nutrition (CFSAN) were aided by scientists at the United States Department of Agriculture and the agency's Center for Veterinary Medicine in performing in-depth reviews of the studies submitted in the petition. The agency then brought together senior agency scientists to form a regulatory decision team (RDT), which was responsible for synthesizing the results of all the studies and recommending a decision to the director of the CFSAN. The RDT not only considered the results of the in-depth reviews but also conferred with several outside scientists with expertise in several areas, such as nutrition, pediatric gastroenterology, and colonic function, who had been hired as special government employees to aid the agency in its decision. These consultations were done on a one-on-one basis, with each expert assigned to narrowly defined issues, and were in compliance with the requirements of the Federal Advisory Committee Act. Once these consultations were completed, the RDT put together a final recommendation in a briefing document that was reviewed by a meeting of a special Olestra Working Group and, immediately following, a meeting of the full Food Advisory Committee (FAC). Both the working group and the FAC possessed a wide range of expertise, and presentations to these bodies were made not only by the FDA reviewers and the petitioner but by members of the public as well. We asked the FAC and the working group to assess, in light of the state of the science relative to macro-food ingredients, whether all the issues of public health significance with respect to olestra had been addressed. The FDA's final decision to approve olestra came after listening to the opinions of the working Group and FAC members and considering any comments we had received separately on the petition. The decision was based on a fair evaluation of all the data of record, using the safety standard of reasonable certainty of no harm, and demonstrated the level of scrutiny and diligence that the agency feels is necessary in reviewing petitions for new macroingredients.

In summary, the regulatory safety review of macroingredients differs in several important ways from typical food additives that are not consumed in large amounts. A prime consideration is whether the additive might interact with nutrients and other substances present in the digestive system at the same time. The standard of safety for macroingredients, however, is the same as for any additive: there must be a reasonable certainty of no harm from the intended use of the substance. As always, the FDA makes the safety decision, but because of the difficult issues and controversial nature of the decisions involved with macroingredients, the agency is increasingly using advice from experts in academia and other government agencies to broaden the base of expertise applied to the safety review of such ingredients, to ensure that the agency's decision is scientifically sound and legally defensible.

Energy Balance: Role of Genetics and Activity

F. XAVIER PI-SUNYER [a]

Division of Endocrinology, Diabetes, and Nutrition
St. Luke's-Roosevelt Hospital Center
Columbia University College of Physicians and Surgeons
New York, New York 10025

To maintain a given body weight, energy intake must equal energy expenditure. With an increase in intake, a decrease in expenditure, or a combination of the two, body weight increases. In the United States, the prevalence of obesity is increasing, so that now over one-third of the adult population is overweight.[1] It is likely that the cause of this increase is related to both increased intake and decreased expenditure, which seem to be a common pattern in our lives.[2]

GENETIC PREDISPOSITION VERSUS ENVIRONMENT

Whether obesity is due to a genetic predisposition, or to environmental circumstances, has long been the subject of debate. The preponderance of data suggest that it is a combination of the two. A certain genetic makeup can give an individual a predisposition to obesity, and the appropriate environment can lead to the phenotypic expression of it.[3]

An example of this in a population group are the Pima Indians, who live in Arizona. These individuals were, as far as we know, of normal weight in the 19th century, when they lived as farmers near the Gila River, worked at physical labor, and ate a diet high in complex carbohydrates and low in fat and alcohol. Today, they live a sedentary existence, eat a high-fat and alcohol diet, and have become very obese as a group. The high prevalence of obesity has also led to a high prevalence of diabetes mellitus.[4] These people have the same genetic makeup as their predecessors one hundred years ago. Their genes have not changed, but the environment has been greatly altered, and their biological predisposition to obesity is now well expressed.

That there is a genetic predisposition in certain people and certain groups has been shown by a number of recent studies. Stunkard *et al.*[5] reported on children in Denmark who had been adopted by foster parents and who were weighed as adults, as were their biological parents and their foster parents. The investigators found that the children, as adults, tracked much closer to their biological parents' weights than to their foster parents', suggesting that genetics were more important than environment with regard to their eventual adult weight.

Bouchard *et al.*[6] also showed the importance of genetics in an overfeeding study in a group of identical twins. They fed the twins an extra 1000 kcal per day for a

[a] Tel: (212) 523-4161; fax: (212) 523-4830; e-mail: fxp1@columbia.edu.

period of 3 months and followed the change in their weight and body composition. They found that although all gained weight, the difference in increase was very much closer within twins than between twins, suggesting that the response to overfeeding has a strong genetic component.

In the most recent estimates, it is calculated that between 30 and 40 percent of the variance in weight is genetically determined, whereas the rest is environmentally determined.[7] There have been over 30 suggested loci for genetic influences on body weight, and there have been almost as many for body fat distribution, which is also thought to be influenced by genetics.

BODY WEIGHT REGULATION

Much effort has been expended over the years to try to determine how food intake is regulated. Both short-term and long-term regulation have been postulated. The short-term regulation is thought to occur primarily preabsorptively and regulates the duration and amount of a single meal. The long-term regulation has been postulated to be a feedback signal from body mass or body fat mass to the central nervous system, which acts as a homeostatic signal to maintain weight (or fat) at a certain given level.

Short-term regulation of food intake has been extensively studied in experimental animals and humans using mostly a single meal paradigm. Signals have been postulated to come from stretch, chemical, or osmotic receptors in various parts of the stomach and small intestine. Also, gut peptides, which are released when food hits the gut, such as cholecystokinin, bombesin, neurotensin, and glucagon-like peptide, have been reported to signal the brain through the afferent branch of the vagus nerve, or directly.[8]

Long-term regulation has over the years been postulated to occur from signals emanating from a ''sensor'' of either body weight or body fat.[9] The most commonly postulated marker has been the adipose tissue, but where the signal emanated from and where it was received was unclear. Early studies of brain-lesioned animals showed that lesions of the ventromedial hypothalamus caused obesity[10] and lesions of the ventrolateral hypothalamus caused weight loss.[11] Later studies, which have tried to map particular neural areas, have found this to be a very complex system, with a large number of tracts and areas being involved. There is no doubt, however, that body weight can be manipulated up or down by lesioning or stimulation of certain hypothalamic areas, suggesting that the receptors of whatever signals regulate body weight reside there, or signal-transduction pathways course through there.

The theory of a circulating factor that regulates body weight was strengthened by studies with parabiotic rats. Stimulating the ventromedial hypothalamus of a rat repeatedly makes that rat hyperphagic and obese.[12] Its parabiotic partner, on the other hand, reduces food intake and loses weight. This suggests that a ''satiety'' factor from the fat rat is crossing to the parabiotic partner, inhibiting food intake. Similar experiments with parabiotic animals have been done in which one of the partners has been overfed by tube. Again, the partner stops eating.[13]

Subsequent parabiotic studies were done by Coleman *et al.*[14] at the Jackson Laboratories with obese mice. These investigators joined *ob/ob* mice with normal mice and found that the *ob/ob* mice lost weight although the normal mice did not. They joined *db/db* mice and normal mice and found that the *db/db* mice maintained their obese weight whereas the lean mice lost weight. They then joined *ob/ob* mice to *db/db* mice and found that the *ob/ob* mice lost weight whereas the *db/db* mice stayed obese. They postulated from these experiments that the *ob/ob* mice lacked a "satiety" factor, that *db/db* mice had a defective receptor for the factor, whereas the normal mice had both normal factor and receptor. The factor they called the "*ob* protein."

LEPTIN AS REGULATOR OF BODY WEIGHT

In 1994, the gene for this "*ob* protein" was cloned by Zhang et al.[15] and the *ob* protein identified. It has turned out that Coleman was right. The *ob/ob* animal has a defective gene for the *ob* protein and either does not make it or makes a defective protein; the *db/db* animal has a defective receptor for the *ob* protein. This protein has been named leptin.

With the discovery of leptin, there was great excitement that this was the long-sought peripheral signal that regulates body fat. This was bolstered by the fact that the hyperphagia of the *ob/ob* animal could be reversed with injections of leptin, either intraperitoneally[16-18] or intracerebrally,[19] but the leptin had no effect on the hyperphagia of the *db/db* mouse. In addition, the weight loss that occurred in these animals could not all be accounted for by the decreased food intake, implying that energy expenditure in these animals (which are hypometabolic) had increased.[16]

Subsequent studies have shown that leptin is only expressed in adipose tissue[20,21] and that it is released from the adipocyte into the general circulation. It soon became clear, however, that dietary fat mice had high levels of leptin.[22] When it became possible to measure leptin in humans, it was found that leptin levels correlated well with body mass index and total body fat.[23] Thus, leptin levels were more elevated the fatter a person was. In addition, no evidence of an abnormal or mutated leptin gene producing abnormal leptin (or no leptin at all) has been found in obese humans.[24] This suggests that if leptin is truly a signal that regulates body weight, fat people show a leptin resistance and the problem is in the leptin receptor or a subsequent signal transduction pathway.

Tartaglia et al.[25] then cloned the leptin receptor from the choroid plexus of the mouse. The receptor was subsequently cloned in obese humans and was found to be normal.[26] Thus, if there is a problem in fat people, it must reside beyond the receptor in the signal transduction pathway.

There has been an effort to clarify this pathway. Schwartz et al.[27] have evidence to suggest that leptin decreases neuropeptide Y in the arcuate nucleus of the brain and have suggested that this is one of the pathways by which leptin could decrease food intake. However, more recently, knockout mice with no neuropeptide Y have been found to regulate food intake and body weight adequately, casting doubt on the importance of this pathway.[28] Much more study will be necessary before the importance of the leptin system to body weight regulation is clarified.

Besides leptin and neuropeptide Y, there are many other central nervous neurotransmitters that may be important in food intake. Examples are galanin, polypeptide y

(PPY), corticotropin-releasing hormone (CRH) opioids, and insulin. Most recently, Schwartz et al.[29] have proposed that neuropeptide Y increases food intake and that CRH decreases it, and that a balance between these substances is important in regulating body weight. Although advances have come very fast in the last few years with regard to the central nervous system control of food intake, much work remains to be done.

METABOLIC PREDICTORS OF WEIGHT GAIN

Although clarifying the mechanisms whereby food intake is regulated is very important in deducing the etiology of obesity, there are also mechanisms that are being uncovered with regard to energy expenditure and nutrient partitioning that may be equally important.

There are three predictors of weight gain that have been reported in recent years. They are a low resting energy expenditure, an elevated respiratory quotient (RQ), and insulin sensitivity.

Bogardus et al.,[30] studying the Pima Indians in Arizona, noted that when they measured 24-hour resting energy expenditure in different individuals within and between families, the expenditure values of family members tended to be similar, suggesting a familial pattern. The investigators, having classified individuals as having a low resting metabolic rate, a normal resting metabolic rate, and a high resting metabolic rate, then followed them longitudinally for five years. They found that those persons with a low resting metabolic rate gained more weight over this period of time.[31]

When these studies of resting energy expenditure were done, RQs were also measured while on a standard diet. Again, it was found that RQs showed a familial pattern, with some families having relatively high ones and others relatively low ones.[32] Those individuals with the higher RQs were more likely to gain weight over a five-year period.[32] In a second study, a high fasting RQ was similarly found to be a predictor of weight gain over an average follow-up of ten years in nonobese men.[33] This has bolstered the results of the first study. A person with a higher RQ will preferentially oxidize more carbohydrate than fat. Although the RQ will tend to reflect the food quotient of the diet,[34] given a similar diet, some individuals will vary somewhat with regard to RQ. A person with a higher RQ who preferentially oxidizes more carbohydrate will tend to deposit more fat. It has been postulated that because carbohydrate is deposited as glycogen, the glycogen can act as a satiety signal and inhibit further food intake. Fat, however, is easily deposited in the fat depots, which act as a sink from which few satiety signals emanate, thus not putting a brake on food intake. The net result may be an increase in weight. Although the mechanism outlined is to-date only a hypothesis, it would explain the role of an elevated RQ in weight gain.

The role of insulin sensitivity as a predictor of weight gain has gained considerable credence in the last few years. Again, in the longitudinal studies of the Pima Indians, it has been found that those individuals with the greatest sensitivity are likely to gain the most weight over time.[35] The mechanism proposed for this is that the fat cells of these individuals, by being very insulin sensitive, readily use carbohydrate for fuel in muscle and allow dietary fat to be directly deposited in fat cells, where gradual accretion can occur. This process is abetted by high levels of lipoprotein lipase in the adipose tissue. Lipoprotein lipase hydrolyzes circulating triglycerides to free fatty acids and glycerol and allows the free fatty acids to enter the fat cells and be reconverted to triglycerides and stored.[36] Also, the insulin sensitivity means that lipolysis is easily inhibited by insulin, so that free fatty acids and glycerol are less easily available from fat stores to be used. As an insulin-sensitive individual gains weight and fat, the individual's fat and muscle cells become more insulin resistant, lipoprotein activity decreases, and the accretion of fat slows down and finally stops.

EFFECT OF EXERCISE

The prevalence of obesity among Americans is about double today what it was in 1900. Yet Americans are consuming about 5% fewer calories today than they were then.[37] If they are consuming less and yet increasing in weight, they must be expending less energy. The inactivity is the price of a technologically advanced society with unprecedented mechanical help at our disposal for both work and leisure activities. A humorous but telling small example of energy savings has been reported by the Illinois Bell Telephone Company, which has estimated that in the course of one year an extension telephone saves a person approximately 70 miles of walking. This could be translated to as much as 7,000 to 10,000 kcal/year, which is the caloric equivalent of two to three pounds of fat.[38]

It has been difficult to document the role of inactivity in obesity. The best data is again from the Arizona NIH research group, who studied spontaneous activity of individuals in a room calorimeter during 24-hour energy-expenditure studies. They found that the percentage of time that the subjects were active in the chamber varied widely, from 4.4 to 17.5%.[39] In addition, they found that family membership accounted for 57% of the variance in spontaneous activity.[40] This strongly supports a genetic influence on activity patterns. More recently, these investigators have suggested that activity in these individuals correlates with sympathetic nervous system activity,[41] so that the autonomic nervous system may be involved.

Although generally in free-living studies obese patients tend to be less active than lean patients, it has been very difficult to decipher whether they are obese because they are less active or are less active because they are obese.[42]

Whether exercise causes an inhibition of food intake is unclear. There have been a number of studies, and these have shown differing results.[42] We have done studies comparing lean and obese sedentary women who were asked to exercise on a treadmill to expend extra energy at a caloric level of 10% and 25% of daily caloric expenditure for 19-day periods in a metabolic ward.[43,44] The lean women maintained their weight by appropriately increasing food intake. The obese women did not increase food intake and lost weight. Thus, obese individuals seem to be less sensitive to exercise cues. This could be because there is less inherent physiological drive to replace lost calories in these persons as compared to normal weight persons. This possibility supports a stronger role for food-derived signals than for those from exercise in regulating calorie intake in obese people.

SUMMARY

It is clear from the above discussion that much remains to be learned about both energy intake and energy expenditure. Obesity in humans is not likely to be caused by one gene, as it is in certain rodent models of obesity, such as the *ob/ob* mouse and the *fa/fa* rat. It is likely to be a polygenic condition in which numerous genes interact with each other and the environment to express the obesity phenotype. It is likely that genes that affect energy intake as well as genes that affect energy expenditure are involved. The role of leptin as a putative factor in signaling the extent of the fat mass to the central nervous system and controlling both food intake and energy expenditure is unclear at this time. The genetics of energy expenditure are also not clear at this time. There are mechanisms of nutrient partitioning, such as respiratory quotient and lipoprotein lipase activity, that are being discovered to be important. In addition, insulin sensitivity is likely to play a role in the etiology of obesity. Much more investigation will be required before we have a clearer picture of how the above-named factors interact, what the genetic contribution to this is, and how important each factor is to the overall phenotypic expression of obesity.

REFERENCES

1. KUCZMARSKI, R. H., K. M. FLEGAL, S. M. CAMPBELL & C. L. JOHNSON. 1994. Increasing prevalence of overweight among U.S. adults. The National Health and Nutrition Examination Surveys, 1960-1991. J. Am. Med. Assoc. **272:** 205-211.
2. PI-SUNYER, F. X. 1994. The fattening of America. J. Am. Med. Assoc. **272:** 238-239.
3. STUNKARD, A. J. 1988. The Salmon Lecture. Some perspectives on human obesity: Its cause. Bull. N. Y. Acad. Med. **64:** 902-923.
4. KNOWLER, W. C., D. J. POETTIT, P. J. SAVAGE & P. H. BENNETT. 1981. Diabetes incidence in Pima Indians: Contributions of obesity and parental diabetes. Am. J. Epidemiol **113:** 144-156.
5. STUNKARD, A. J., T. I. A. SORENSEN & C. HANIS. 1986. An adoption study of human obesity. N. Engl. J. Med. **314:** 193-198.
6. BOUCHARD, C. & L. PERUSSE. 1993. Genetics of obesity. Annu. Rev. Nutr. **13:** 1477-1482.
7. BOUCHARD, C., A. TREMBLAY, J. P. DESPRES, A. NADEAU, P. J. LUPIEN, G. THERIAULT, J. DUSSAULT, S. MOORJANI, S. PINAULT & G. FOURNIER. 1990. The response to long-term overfeeding in identical twins. N. Engl. J. Med. **322:** 1477-1482.
8. GIBBS, J. & G. P. SMITH. 1992. Effects of brain-gut peptides on satiety. In Obesity. P. Bjorntorp & B. N. Brodoff, Eds.: 399-410. J.B. Lippincott Co. New York.
9. WEIGLE, D. S. Appetite and the regulation of body composition. 1994. FASEB J. **8:** 302-310.
10. HOEBEL, B. G. & P. TEITLEBAUM. 1966. Weight regulation in normal and hypothalamic hyperphagic rats. J. Comp. Physiol. Psychol. **61:** 189-193.
11. KEESEY, R. E., P. C. BOYLE, J. W. KEMNITZ & J. S. MITCHEL. 1976. The role of the lateral hypothalamus in determining the body weight set-point. *In* Hunger: Basic Mechanisms and Clinical Implications. D. Novin, W. Wywicka & G. Bray, Eds.: 313-326. Raven Press. New York.
12. PARAMESWARAN S. V., A. B. STEFFENS, G. R. HERVEY & L. DE RUITER. 1977. Involvement of a humoral factor in regulation of body weight in parabiotic rats. Am. J. Physiol. **232:** R150-R157.
13. HARRIS, B. S. & R. J. MARTIN. 1984. Specific depletion of body fat in parabiotic partners of tube-fed obese rats. Am. J. Physiol **247:** R380-R386.

14. COLEMAN, D. L. 1973. Effects of parabiosis of obese with diabetic and normal mice. Diabetologia **9:** 294-298.
15. ZHANG, Y., R. PROENCA, M. MAFFEI, M. BARONE, L. LEOPOLD & J. FRIEDMAN. 1994. Positional cloning of the mouse gene and its human homologue. Nature **372:** 425-432.
16. HALAAS J. L., K. S. GAJIWALA, M. MAFFEI, S. L. COHEN, B. T. CHAIT, D. RABINOWITZ, R. L. LALLONE, S. K. BURLEY & J. M. FRIEDMAN. 1995. Weight-reducing effects of the plasma protein encoded by the obese gene. Science **269:** 543-546.
17. PELLEYMOUNTER, M. A., M. J. CULLEN, M. B. BAKER, R. HECHT, D. WINTERS, T. BOONE & F. COLLINS. 1995. Effects of the obese gene product on body weight regulation in *ob/ob* mice. Science **269:** 540-543.
18. STEPHENS, T. W., M. BASINSKI, P. K. BRISTOW, J. M. BUE-VALLESKEY, S. G. BURGETT, L. CRAFT, J. HALE, J. HOFFMAN, H. J. HSIUNG, A. KRIAUSIUNAS, W. MACKELLAR, P. R. ROSTECK JR., B. SCHONER, D. SMITH, F. C. TINSLEY, X-Y. ZHANG & M. HEIMAN. 1995. The role of neuropeptide Y in the antiobesity action of the obese gene product. Nature **377:** 530-532.
19. CAMPFIELD, L. A., F. J. SMITH, Y. GULSEZ, R. DEVOS & P. BURN. 1995. Mouse *Ob* protein: Evidence for a peripheral signal linking adiposity and central neural networks. Science **269:** 5406-549.
20. MAFFEI M., H. FEI, G. H. LEE, C. DANI, P. LEROY, Y. ZHANG, R. PROENCA, R. NEGREL, G. AILHAUD & J. M. FRIEDMAN. 1955. Increased expression in adipocytes of *ob*RNA in mice with lesions of the hypothalamus and with mutations at the *db* locus. Proc. Natl. Acad. Sci. USA **92:** 6957-6950.
21. MASUZAKI, H., Y. OGAWA, N. ISSE, N. SATOH, T. OKAZAKI, M. SHIGEMOTO, K. MORI, N. TQAMURA, K. HOSODA, Y. YOHIMASA, H. JINGAMI, T. KAWADA & K. NAKOA. 1995. Human obese gene expression: Adipocyte-specific expression and regional differences in the adipose tissue. Diabetes **44:** 855-858.
22. FREDERICH, R. C., A. HAMANN, S. ANDERSON, B. LOLLMAN, B. B. LOWELL & J. S. FLIER. 1995. Leptin levels reflect body lipid content in mice. Evidence for diet-induced resistance to leptin action. Nature Med. **1:** 1311-1314.
23. CONSIDINE, R. V., M. K. SINHA, M. L. HEIMAN, A. KRIAUCIUNAS, T. W. STEPHENS, M. R. NYCE, J. P. OHANNESIAN, C. C. MARCO, L. J. MCKEE, T. L. BAUER & J. F. CARO. 1996. Serum immunoreactive-leptin concentrations in normal weight and obese humans. N. Engl. J. Med. **334:** 292-295.
24. CONSIDINE, R. V., E. L. CONSIDINE, C. J. WILLIAMS, M. R. NYCE, S. A. MAGOSIN, T. L. BAUER, E. L. ROSATO, J. COLBERG & J. F. CARO 1995. Evidence against either premature stop codon or the absence of obese gene mRNA in human obesity. J. Clin. Invest. **95:** 2986-2988.
25. TARTAGLIA, L. A., M. DEMBSKI, X. WENG, N. DENG, J. CULPEPPER, R. DEVOS, G. J. RICHARDS, L. A. CAMPFIELD, F. T. CLARK, J. DEEDS, C. MUIR, S. SANKER, A. MORIARTY, K. J. MOORE, J. S. SMUTKO, G. G. MAYS, E. A. WOLF, C. A. MONROE & R. I. TEPPER. 1995. Identification and expression cloning of a leptin receptor, *Ob*-R. Cell **83:** 1263-1271.
26. CONSIDINE, R. V., E. L. CONSIDINE, C. J. WILLIAMS, T. M. HYDE & J. F. CARO. 1996. The hypothalamic leptin receptor in humans: Identification of incidental sequence polymorphisms and absence of the *db/db* mouse and *fa/fa* rat mutations. Diabetes **45:** 992-994.
27. SCHWARTZ, M. W., D. G. BASKIN, T. R. BUKOWSKI, J. L. KUIJPER, D. FOSTER, G. LASSER, D. E. PRUNKARD D., PORTE, JR., S. C. WOODS, R. J. SEELEY & D. S. WEIGLE. 1996. Specificity of leptin action on elevated blood glucose levels and hypothalamic neuropeptide Y gene expression in *ob/ob* mice. Diabetes **45:** 531-535.
28. ERICKSON, J. C., K. E. CLEGG & R. D. PALMITER. 1996. Sensitivity to leptin and susceptibility to seizures of mice lacking neuropeptide Y. Nature **381:** 415-418.

29. SCHWARTZ, M. W., R. J. SEELEY, L. A. CAMPFIELD, P. BURN & D. G. BASKIN. 1996. Identification of targets of leptin action in rat hypothalamus. J. Clin. Invest. **98:** 1101-1106.
30. BOGARDUS, C., S. LILLIOJA, E. RAVUSSIN, W. ABBOTT, J. K. ZAWADSKI, A. YOUNG, W. C. KNOWLER, R. JACOBOWITZ & P. P. MOLL. 1986. Familial dependence of the resting metabolic rate. N. Engl. J. Med. **315:** 96-100.
31. RAVUSSIN, E., S. LILLIOJA, W. C. KNOWLER, L. CHRISTIN, D. FREYMOND, W. G. H. ABBOTT, V. BOYCE, B. V. HOWARD & C. BOGARDUS. 1988. Reduced rate of energy expenditure as a risk factor for body-weight. N. Engl. J. Med. **318:** 467-472.
32. ZURLO, F., S. LILLIOJA, B. L. ESPOSITO DEL PUENTE et al. 1990. Low ratio of fat to carbohydrate oxidation as a predictor of weight gain: Study of 24-hr RQ. **259:** E650-E657.
33. SEIDELL, C. S., D. C. MULLER, J. D. SORKIN & R. ANDRES. 1992. Fasting respiratory exchange ratio and resting metabolic rate as predictors of weight gain: The Baltimore Longitudinal Study on Aging. Int. J. Obesity **16:** 667-674.
34. FLATT, J. P. 1988. Importance of nutrient balance in body weight regulation. Diabetes Metab. Rev. **6:** 571-581.
35. SWINBURN, B. A., B. L. NYOMBA, M. F. SAAD, F. ZURLO, I. RAZ, W. C. KNOWLER, S. LILLIOJA, C. BOGARDUS & E. RAVUSSIN. 1991. Insulin resistance associated with lower rates of weight gain in Pima Indians. J. Clin. Invest. **88:** 168-173.
36. ECKEL, R. H. 1989. Lipoprotein lipase: A multifunctional enzyme relevant to common metabolic diseases. N. Engl. J. Med. **320:** 1060-1068.
37. FRIEND, B. 1974. Changes in nutrients in the U.S. diet caused by alterations in food intake patterns. Prepared for The Changing Food Supply in America Conference, May 22, 1974, sponsored by the Food and Drug Administration.
38. STERN, J. S. 1984. Is obesity a disease of inactivity? In Eating and Its Disorders. A. Stunkard & E. Stellar, Eds.: 131-140. Raven Press. New York.
39. ZURLO F., R. T. FERRARO, A. M. FONTVIELLE, R. RISING, C. BOGARDUS & E. RAVUSSIN. 1992. Spontaneous physical activity and obesity: Cross-sectional and longitudinal studies in Pima Indians. Am. J. Physiol. **263:** E296-E300.
40. RAVUSSIN, E., A. M. FONTVIELLE, B. A. SWINBURN & C. BOGARDUS. 1993. Risk factors for the development of obesity. Ann. N. Y. Acad. Sci. **683:** 141-150.
41. CHRISTIN, L., M. O'CONNEL, C. BOGARDUS, E. DANFORTH JR. & E. RAVUSSIN. 1993. Norepinephrine turnover and energy expenditure in Pima Indian and white men. Metabolism **42:** 723-729.
42. SEGAL, K. & F. X. PI-SUNYER. 1989. Exercise and obesity. Med. Clin. North Am. **73:** 217-236.
43. WOO, R., J. S. GARROW & F. X. PI-SUNYER. 1983. Effect of exercise on spontaneous food intake in obesity. Am. J. Clin. Nutr. **36:** 470-477.
44. WOO, R., J. S. GARROW & F. X. PI-SUNYER. 1985. Effect of increased physical activity on voluntary intake in lean women. Metabolism **34:** 836-841.

Effect of Fat Intake on Energy Balance

P. ANTONIO TATARANNI [a] AND ERIC RAVUSSIN

Clinical Diabetes and Nutrition Section
National Institute of Diabetes and Digestive and Kidney Diseases
National Institutes of Health
Phoenix, Arizona 85016

During the past three decades the prevalence of obesity in the United States and the United Kingdom has dramatically increased.[1,2] This increase seems to be attributable, in part, to environmental factors, such as a high-fat diet and sedentariness, the combination of which has recently been defined as *pathoenvironment*.[3] Epidemiological evidence supports a role of dietary fat in the etiology of obesity. Obesity is less prevalent in countries characterized by a diet with a low fat to energy ratio (China, Japan), and immigrants from these countries increase their body size when exposed to a westernized high-fat alimentary regimen.[4] Within a given population, a number of cross-sectional studies have also shown that obesity is more prevalent among people whose fat intake is high.[5-7] In a large prospective study, the Nurses' Health Study, cross-sectional analyses confirmed a positive association between fat intake and body mass index, but baseline fat intake was not clearly associated with subsequent weight gain.[8] For populations like the Pima Indians of Arizona, the Nauruans of the Pacific Islands, and some African communities who practiced a traditional lifestyle, but who have been abruptly exposed to modern times, living in the *pathoenvironment* has resulted in an unparalleled high prevalence of obesity and noninsulin-dependent diabetes.[9,10]

Because obesity is the result of a positive energy balance, the association between high fat intake and obesity lies in the ability of fat to increase energy intake, reduce energy expenditure, or both. High fat diets have been shown to increase energy intake.[11,12] This seems to be due to the minimal appetite-suppressant effect of fat,[13,14] its high energy density (and the inability of the body to detect changes in the energy density of food),[15,16] and the high palatability and high hedonic attribute of a high-fat diet.[17] By contrast, there is very little evidence of an effect of fat intake on energy expenditure, despite the known low thermic effect of fat.[18] In agreement with others,[19,20] but not all,[21] we found no evidence of a decrease in 24-h energy expenditure in 20 Pima Indians on a high-fat diet compared with a high-carbohydrate diet.[22]

This paper will review the short- and long-term effects of fat intake on energy balance and discuss the possible mechanisms explaining a role of high-fat intake in the etiology of obesity.

---

[a] Address for correspondence: P. Antonio Tataranni, M.D., CDNS, NIH-NIDDK, 4212 N. 16th Street, Room 541-A, Phoenix, AZ 85016. Tel: (602) 200-5301; fax (602) 200-5335; e-mail: q5t@cu.nih.gov.

EFFECT OF FAT INTAKE ON SHORT- AND MIDTERM ENERGY BALANCE

Studies of the effects of dietary fat on substrate utilization and nutrient balance have flourished with the application to human physiology of the indirect calorimetry technique, a noninvasive method to measure energy expenditure and substrate oxidation rates for periods varying from hours (ventilated hood apparatus) to days (respiratory chamber) (for a review on this topic, see ref. 23). Using indirect calorimetry in seven young subjects, Flatt et al. studied substrate oxidation in response to meals with different fat and energy content.[24] Nine hours after a low-fat breakfast, carbohydrate (CHO) and protein intakes were matched by oxidation, whereas fat balance was negative. When approximately 300 kcal of fat (long-chain triglycerides or a combination of long- and medium-chain triglycerides) was added to the breakfast, CHO and protein balances were again established after 9 h, whereas fat balance was positive. The fact that fat oxidation was not influenced by the fat content of the meal was then reproduced by Schutz et al.[25] These authors studied seven young subjects for two days in a respiratory chamber: on the first day subjects were fed a weight maintenance diet, whereas on the second day approximately 100 g of fat was added to the diet. The additional amount of fat in the diet failed to increase 24-h energy expenditure and did not promote fat oxidation resulting in positive fat and energy balance. Furthermore, a close correlation between overall daily energy balance and fat balance was observed. Thomas et al. studied the influence of dietary composition on substrate oxidation and body weight in a group of 11 lean and 10 obese subjects fed a high-carbohydrate or a high-fat diet for one week each.[26] All subjects ate more when fed a high-fat diet, thus conforming that high-fat diets tend to promote overeating and weight gain. Daily energy expenditure was not different on either diet, and CHO and protein oxidation rates matched their respective intakes after one week. Fat balance was achieved on the high CHO diet, but on day 7 of the high-fat diet, fat intake and oxidation were unrelated. In response to the high-fat diet, a tendency towards an increased fat oxidation was observed in lean but not obese subjects. Both groups were, however, in positive fat and energy balance, the more positive energy balance being observed in the obese group. Together these studies indicate that fat intake does not affect fat oxidation in the short term (hours or days) and over a more prolonged period of observation (week). Also, differences in the ability to respond to an overload of dietary fat seem to occur (lean vs. obese subjects). Recently Jebb et al.[27] continuously measured energy metabolism for 12 days in six lean men living in a respiratory chamber while subjected to overfeeding (+33% of energy requirements) and underfeeding (−67% of energy requirements). They observed that even after 12 days of such extreme nutritional manipulations, CHO and protein intakes continued to exert direct autoregulatory feedback on their oxidation rates. By contrast, fat oxidation was not sensitive to dietary fat intake and was inversely related to the oxidation of the other substrates. Furthermore, changes in fat balance accounted for 74% and 84% of the energy imbalance during overfeeding and underfeeding, respectively. This study clearly indicates that metabolic fuel selection in the human body is dominated by an oxidative hierarchy, that is, the need to maintain CHO and protein balances, which in turn induces inhibition of fat oxidation during energy surplus. The macronutrient oxidative hierarchy is partly dictated by the limited size of the glycogen stores and the tight control of nitrogen balance. Although protein stores can increase in size in response to such growth stimuli as growth hormones androgens, physical training, and weight gain, they do not increase in response to increased intake of dietary protein. Instead, protein balance is achieved on a day-to-day basis in ways that are not completely understood. Therefore, because the body has limited capacity for carbohydrate storage and tightly regulates protein balance, these two nutrients are oxidized in proportion to their intakes. Also, because there is a ceiling to adaptive changes in energy expenditure, an increased oxidation of CHO and protein leads to decreased fat oxidation. The oxidative hierarchy is evident only under condition of energy surplus, inasmuch as isoenergetic high-fat diets have no major impact on energy expenditure and substrate oxidation in humans.[22]

EFFECT OF FAT INTAKE ON LONG-TERM ENERGY BALANCE

Because fat intake does not stimulate fat oxidation in the short and midterm, excess dietary fat intake results in deposition of triglycerides in the adipose tissue until a new equilibrium between fat intake and oxidation is reached. We[28] and others[29] have reported a positive correlation between the degree of adiposity and fat oxidation. From cross-sectional observations, Schutz et al. estimated that a change of 10 kg in the fat mass induces a change of about 20 g/d in fat oxidation in resting conditions.[30] Longitudinal studies have also confirmed that the rate of lipid oxidation increases as fat mass increases.[28] Therefore, the increased fat oxidation associated with the enlargement of the fat mass represents a means by which the body reequilibrates fat balance, thus protecting itself from a continuing expansion of the fat depots. The higher fat oxidation associated with greater adiposity has been attributed to a larger availability of tissue substrates (nonesterified fatty acids and triglycerides)[31] and a higher degree of insulin resistance.[32] Hyperlipidemia and insulin resistance are possibly linked by a cause and effect relationship (Randle Cycle[33]) and ultimately lead to diabetes.[34,35] Although obesity can be regarded as the general mechanism to compensate for increased fat intake, there are interindividual differences in this response.

VARIABILITY OF THE METABOLIC RESPONSE TO FAT INTAKE: ROLE OF GENETICS

Several lines of evidence indicate that some individuals respond with larger weight gain than others when exposed to an increased dietary fat content. Thomas et al.[26] observed that whereas lean subjects tended to increase their lipid oxidation rates after seven days on a high-fat diet, obese subjects failed to do so. Raben et al.[36] have recently shown that, independent of energy balance, a 50% increase in fat intake resulted in preferential fat storage in postobese women as compared to controls, because of a failure to increase fat oxidation appropriately. This obesity-promoting effect of dietary fat seems to be more evident in children with a familial history of obesity, thus pointing out the possibility of a genetically inherited metabolic deficiency in the control of fat balance.[37] The 24-h respiratory quotient (RQ, an index of carbohydrate-to-fat oxidation rates) has been shown to aggregate in families, and interindividual differences in RQ explain some of the variance of body weight gain over time.[28] In 111 Pima Indians followed for 1-4 years, those with a high RQ (≤ 90th percentile), that is, a low fat oxidation rate, had a 2.6 times greater risk of gaining ≥ 10 kg of body weight than those with a low RQ (≤ 10th percentile). Studies in Caucasians have confirmed that a high RQ is a predictor of body weight gain[38] or relapse after weight loss.[39-41]

Taken together these studies indicate that some individuals are characterized by low fat oxidation rates and/or by an inability to increase fat oxidation in response to nutritional challenges. These metabolic characteristics represent a risk factor for body weight gain and seem to be genetically inherited. Genetics may influence nutrient partitioning by underlying the activity of key enzymes of intermediate metabolism such as lipoprotein lipase (LPL), β-hydroxyl acyl CoA dehydrogenase (β-OAC), and acetyl CoA carboxylase (ACC). LPL plays a pivotal role in partitioning lipoprotein-borne triglycerides to adipose (storage) and muscle (mostly oxidation) tissues.[42] At rest, fatty acid oxidation accounts for 80% of muscle substrate oxidation.[43] Muscle LPL is the rate-limiting enzyme hydrolyzing lipoprotein-borne triglycerides to glycerol and fatty acids, which in turn enter the tissue through the endothelia-luminal interfaces of the capillaries.[44] Ferraro et al.[45] found an inverse correlation between muscle LPL activity and RQ in 16 Pima Indians and concluded that some of the interindividual differences in substrate oxidation are associated with differences in muscle LPL activity. β-OAC, another muscle key enzyme in fatty acid beta oxidation, has been found to be related to whole body fat utilization. In a study of 14 Pima Indians, Zurlo et al.[46] observed a negative correlation between RQ and the activity of muscle β-OAC and concluded that a reduced capacity for fat oxidation in the skeletal muscle is accompanied by a lower fat-to-carbohydrate oxidation rate in the whole body. It has recently been suggested that malonyl CoA is a component of a fuel-sensing and signaling mechanism that responds to change in fuel availability.[47,48] The entry of acyl CoA (derived from circulating free fatty acids or endogenous complex lipids) in the mitochondria, where it is oxidized to acetyl CoA, is controlled by malonyl CoA (derived from glucose or other fuels) through its inhibitory effect on carnitine palmitoyl transferase 1. ACC, which synthesizes malonyl CoA, may therefore represent a key enzyme in the regulation of nutrient partitioning and underlie some of the differences in lipid metabolism observed among individuals.

CONCLUSION

When energy is in excess, the human body processes nutrients according to an oxidative hierarchy. Excessive CHO and protein intakes are disposed of by increased oxidation. By contrast, excess fat intake does not promote its own oxidation in the short and midterm. This leads, in the long term, to an increase in fat stores. Although increased adiposity represents the common response to increased fat intake, there are interindividual differences in lipid oxidation (probably genetically determined) protecting from or predisposing to obesity. Genetic studies will allow us to understand the molecular basis of such differences and help design better treatments for obesity and its complications.

SUMMARY

Most epidemiological studies indicate that obesity is more prevalent in populations consuming high fat diets. Furthermore, changes from a traditional to a westernized life style, characterized by a high-fat diet and decreased physical activity, result in dramatic increases in the prevalence and incidence of obesity in Native Americans, Pacific Islanders, and African populations. A possible explanation for the epidemic of obesity in response to high-fat intake can be found in the "oxidative hierarchy" that regulates macronutrient balance in the human body. Although carbohydrate and protein balances seem promptly regulated, fat balance is not. Short and midterm studies show that, unlike carbohydrate and protein intake, fat intake does not promote fat oxidation. Thus, "excess" fat intake results in fat deposition. As fat mass increases, so does fat oxidation, and a new equilibrium is reached when fat oxidation matches fat intake. However, there are large interindividual differences in this compensatory response to increased fat intake. Substrate oxidation is a familial trait, and individuals with a low fat-to-carbohydrate oxidation ratio are more prone to develop obesity than those with a high fat-to-carbohydrate oxidation ratio. Genetics may influence nutrient partitioning by influencing the activity of key enzymes of intermediate metabolism, such as lipoprotein lipase, β-hydroxyl acyl CoA dehydrogenase, and acetyl CoA carboxylase.

REFERENCES

1. KUCZMARSKY, R. J., K. M. FEGAL, S. M. CAMPBELL & C. L. JOHNSON. 1994. Increasing prevalence of overweight among US adults. The National Health and Nutrition Examination Survey 1960 to 1991. J. Am. Med. Assoc. **272:** 205-11.
2. WHITE, A., G. NICOLAAS, K. FOSTER, F. BROWNE & S. CAREY. 1993. Health survey for England 1991; A survey carried out by the Social Survey Division of the OPCS on behalf of the Department of Health. HMSO (Series HS; no 11).
3. RAVUSSIN, E. 1995. Obesity in Britain: Rising trend may be due to 'pathoenvironment.' Lancet **311:** 1569.
4. CURB, J. D. & E. B. MARCUS. 1991. Body fat and obesity in Japanese Americans. Am. J. Clin. Nutr. **53:** 1552S-1555S.
5. ROMIEU, I., W. C. WILLET, M. J. STAMPFER, G. A. COLDITZ, L. SAMPSON, B. ROSNER, C. H. HENNEKENS & F. E. SPEIZER. 1988. Energy intake and other determinants of relative weight. Am. J. Clin. Nutr. **47:** 406-12.
6. DREON, D. M., B. FREY-HEWITT, N. HELLSWORTH, P. T. WILLIAMS, R. B. TERRY & P. D. WOOD. 1988. Dietary fat: Carbohydrate ratio and obesity in middle-aged men. Am. J. Clin. Nutr. **47:** 995-1000.
7. LARSON, D. E., P. A. TATARANNI, R. T. FERRARO & E. RAVUSSIN. 1995. Ad libitum food intake on a 'cafeteria diet' in Native American women: Relations with body composition and 24-h energy expenditure. Am. J. Clin. Nutr. **62:** 911-7.
8. COLDITZ, G. A., W. C. WILLET, M. J. STAMPFER, S. J. LONDON, M. R. SEGAL & F. E. SPEIZER. 1990. Patterns of weight change and their relation to diet in a cohort of healthy women. Am. J. Clin. Nutr. **51:** 1100-1105.
9. KNOWLER, W. C., D. J. PETTITT, M. F. SAAD et al. 1991. Obesity in the Pima Indians: Its magnitude and relationship with diabetes. Am. J. Clin. Nutr. **53:** 1543S-1551S.
10. TAYLOR, R., J. BADCOCK, H. KING et al. 1992. Dietary intake, exercise, obesity and noncommunicable disease in rural and urban populations of three Pacific Islands countries. Am. J. Clin. Nutr. **11:** 283-293.

11. LISSNER, L., D. A. LEVITSKY, B. J. STRUPP, H. J. KALKWARF & D. A. ROE. 1987. Dietary fat and the regulation of energy intake in human subjects. Am. J. Clin. Nutr. **46:** 886-892.
12. TREMBLAY, A., G. PLOURDE, J. P. DESPRES & C. BOUCHARD. 1989. Impact of dietary fat content and fat oxidation on energy intake in humans. Am. J. Clin. Nutr. **49:** 799-805.
13. LAWTON, C. L., V. J. BURLEY, J. K. WALES & J. E. BLUNDELL. 1993. Dietary fat and appetite control in obese subjects: Weak effects on satiation and satiety. Int. J. Obesity **17:** 409-416.
14. COTTON, J. R., V. J. BURLEY, J. A. WESTSTRATE & J. E. BLUNDELL. 1994. Dietary fat and appetite: Similarities and differences in the satiating effect of meals supplemented with either fat or carbohydrate. J. Hum. Nutr. Diet. **7:** 11-24.
15. CAMPBELL, R. G., S. A. HASHIM & T. B. VAN ITALLIE. 1971. Studies of food intake regulation in man. Responses to variation in nutritive density in lean and obese subjects. N. Engl. J. Med. **285:** 1402-1407.
16. POPPITT, S. D. 1995. Energy density of diets and obesity. Int. J. Obesity **19:** 20S-26S.
17. DRENOWSKY, A., D. RISKEY & J. A. DESOR. 1982. Feeling fat yet unconcerned: Self reported overweight and the restraint scale. Appetite **3:** 273-279.
18. FLATT, J. P. 1988. The biochemistry of energy expenditure. In Recent Advances in Obesity Research, G. A. Bray Ed., Vol II: 211-228. Newman. London.
19. LEAN, M. E. J. & W. P. T. JAMES. 1988. Metabolic effect of isoenergetic nutrient exchange over 24-h in relation to obesity in women. Int. J. Obesity **12:** 15-27.
20. MC NEILL, G., A. C. BRUCE, A. RALPH & W. P. T. JAMES. 1988. Interindividual differences in fasting nutrient oxidation and the influence of diet composition. Int. J. Obesity **12:** 455-463.
21. HURNI, M., B. BURNAND, P. PITTETT & E. JEQUIER. 1982. Metabolic effects of a mixed and a high-carbohydrate diet in man, measured over 24-h in a respiratory chamber. Br. J. Nutr. **47:** 33-43
22. ABBOTT, W. G. H., B. V. HOWARD, G. RUOTOLO & E. RAVUSSIN. 1990. Energy expenditure in humans: Effects of dietary fat and carbohydrate. Am. J. Physiol. **258:** E347-351.
23. JÉQUIER, E., K. ACHESON & Y. SCHUTZ. 1987. Assessment of energy expenditure and fuel utilization in man. Annu. Rev. Nutr. **7:** 187-208.
24. FLATT, J. P., E. RAVUSSIN, K. ACHESON & E. JEQUIER. 1985. Effects of dietary fat on postprandial substrate oxidation and carbohydrate and fat balances. J. Clin. Invest. **76:** 1019-1024.
25. SCHUTZ, Y, J. P. FLATT & E. JEQUIER. 1989. Failure of dietary fat intake to promote fat oxidation: A factor favoring the development of obesity. Am. J. Clin. Nutr. **50:** 307-314.
26. THOMAS, C. D., J. C. PETERS, G. W. REED, N. N. ABUMRAD, M. SUN & J. O. HILL. 1992. Nutrient balance and energy expenditure during ad libitum feeding of high fat and high-carbohydrate diets in humans. Am. J. Clin. Nutr. **55:** 934-942.
27. JEBB, S. A., A. PRENTICE, G. R. GOLDBERG, P. R. MURGATROYD, A. E. BLACK & W. A. COWARD. 1996. Changes in macronutrient balance during over- and underfeeding assessed by 12-d continuous whole-body calorimetry. Am. J. Clin. Nutr. **64:** 259-266.
28. ZURLO, F., S. LILLIOJA, A. ESPOSITO-DEL PUENTE, B. NYOMBA, I. RAZ, M. SAAD, B. A. SWINBURN, W. C. KNOWLER, C. BOGARDUS & E. RAVUSSIN. 1990. Low ratio of fat to carbohydrate oxidation as predictor of weight gain: Study of 24-h RQ. Am. J. Physiol. **259:** E650-657.
29. ASTRUP, A., B. BUEMANN, P. WESTERN, S. TOUBRO, A. RABEN & N. J. CHRISTENSEN. 1994. Obesity as an adaptation to high-fat diet: Evidence from a cross-sectional study. Am. J. Clin. Nutr. **59:** 350-355.
30. SCHUTZ, Y., A. TREMBLAY, R. L. WEINSIER & K. M. NELSON. 1992. Role of fat oxidation in long-term stabilization of body weight in obese women. Am. J. Clin. Nutr. **74:** 279-286.
31. BONADONNA, R. C., L. C. GROO, K. ZYCH, M. SHANK & R. A. DE FRONZO. 1990. Dose-dependent effect of insulin on plasma free-fatty acid turnover and oxidation in humans. Am. J. Physiol. **22:** E736-750.

32. SWINBURN, B. A., B. L. NYOMBA, M. F. SAAD et al. 1991. Insulin resistance associated with lower rates of weight gain in Pima Indians. J. Clin. Invest. **88:** 168-173.
33. RANDLE, P. J., C. N. HALES, P. B. GARLAND & E. A. NEWSHOLME. 1963. The glucose fatty-acid cycle. Its role in insulin insensitivity and the metabolic disturbances of diabetes mellitus. Lancet **1:** 785-789.
34. LILLIOJA, S., D. MOTT, M. SPRAUL et al. 1993. Insulin resistance as a precursor of non-insulin dependent diabetes mellitus. Prospective studies in Pima Indians. N. Engl. J. Med. **329:** 1988-1992.
35. PAOLISSO, G., P. A. TATARANNI, J. E. FOLEY, C. BOGARDUS, B. V. HOWARD & E. RAVUSSIN. 1995. A high concentration of fasting plasma non-esterified fatty acids is a risk factor for the development of NIDDM. Diabetologia **38:** 1213-1217.
36. RABEN, A., H. B. ANDERSEN, N. J. CHRISTENSEN, J. MADSEN, J. J. HOLST & A. ASTRUP. 1994. Evidence for abnormal postprandial response to a high-fat meal in women predisposed to obesity. Am. J. Physiol. **267:** E549-559.
37. ECK, L. H. , R. C. KLESGES, C. L. HANSON & D. SLAWSON. 1992. Children at familial risk of obesity: An examination of dietary intake, physical activity and weight status. Int. J. Obesity **16:** 71-78.
38. SEIDELL, J. C., D. C. MULLER, J. D. SORKIN & R. ANDRES. 1992. Fasting respiratory exchange ratio and resting metabolic rate as predictors of weight gain: The Baltimore Longitudinal Study on Aging. Int. J. Obesity **16:** 667-674.
39. FROIDEVAUX, F., Y. SCHUTZ, L. CHRISTIN & E. JÉQUIER. 1993. Energy expenditure in obese women before and during weight loss, after refeeding, and in the weight-relapse period. Am. J. Clin. Nutr. **57:** 35-42.
40. LARSON, D. E., R. T. FERRARO, D. S. ROBERTSON & E. RAVUSSIN 1995. Energy metabolism in weight-stable postobese individuals. Am. J. Clin. Nutr. **62:** 735-739.
41. TATARANNI, P. A., G. MINGRONE, C. A. RAGUSO, A. DE GAETANO, R. M. TACCHINO, M. CASTAGNETO & A. V. GRECO. 1996. Twenty-four-hour energy and nutrient balance in weight stable postobese patients after biliopancreatic diversion. Nutrition **12:** 239-244.
42. ECKEL, R. H. 1989. Lipoprotein lipase: A multi-functional enzyme relevant to common metabolic disorders. N. Engl. J. Med. **320:** 1060-1068.
43. ANDRES, R., G. CADER & K. L. ZIERLER. 1956. The quantitatively minor role of carbohydrates in the oxidative metabolism by skeletal muscle in intact man in the basal state. Measurements of oxygen and glucose uptake and carbon dioxide and lactate production from the forearm. J. Clin. Invest. **35:** 671-682.
44. BORENSZTAIN, J. 1987. Heart and skeletal muscle lipoprotein lipase. *In* Lipoprotein Lipase. J. Borensztain, Ed.: 133-148. Evener. Chicago.
45. FERRARO, R. T., R. H. ECKEL, D. E. LARSON, A. M. FONTVIEILLE, R. RISING, D. R. JENSEN & E. RAVUSSIN. 1993. Relationship between skeletal muscle lipoprotein lipase activity and 24-hour macronutrient oxidation. J. Clin. Invest. **92:** 441-445.
46. ZURLO, F., N. M. PATTI, R. M. CHOKSI, S. SESODIA & E. RAVUSSIN. 1994. Whole-body energy metabolism and skeletal muscle biochemical characteristics. Metabolism **43:** 481-486.
47. ASISH, K. S., T. G. KUROWSKI & N. B. RUDERMAN. 1995. A malonyl-CoA fuel-sensing mechanism in muscle: Effects of insulin, glucose, and denervation. Am. J. Physiol. **269:** E283-289.
48. PRENTKI, M. & B. E. CORKEY. 1996. Are the β-cell signaling molecules malonyl-CoA and cytosolic long-chain acyl-CoA implicated in multiple tissue defects of obesity and NIDDM? Diabetes **45:** 273-283.

Carbohydrates and Energy Balance

R. JAMES STUBBS,[a,c] A. M. PRENTICE,[b,d] AND
W. P. T. JAMES [a]

[a]Rowett Research Institute
Human Nutrition Unit
Greenburn Road
Bucksburn, Aberdeen, Scotland, AB21 9SB

[b]The Dunn Clinical Nutrition Centre
Hills Road
Cambridge, England, CB2 2DH

INTRODUCTION

In the late 1990s there is perhaps greater interest and concern about the composition of the diet we eat and its effects on the health and well-being of the public at large than at any time this century. There is widespread interest and concern about the potentially detrimental effects of many Western diets that are now linked to a number of major diseases that are the principal causes of mortality in both developed and developing countries. The composition of the diet is heavily involved in the development of coronary heart disease, may account for perhaps 30% of all adult cancers, and is now heavily implicated in the current pandemic of diabetes mellitus and obesity.[1,2] In many Western countries 35–50% of all adults are classified as either overweight (BMI 25-29) or obese (BMI ≥30).[3]

Recently, attention has focused on the possible ways in which macronutrients may affect energy balance (EB) and other aspects of health. There is concern that secular changes in the macronutrient composition of the diet may contribute to the increased prevalence of overweight and obese people in developed and developing countries.[4] Macronutrients can exert two major effects on EB in humans: (1) absorbed macronutrients influence the fuel mix oxidized, which summate to determine energy expenditure (EE); (2) macronutrients can affect the amount of total energy eaten. The metabolic fate of a recently ingested macronutrient, and the efficiency of its utilization, is dependent on which nutrient it is and on the presence or absence of other macronutrients in the diet. The influence of macronutrients on voluntary food intake may or may not also relate to their oxidation and storage, so the effects of macronutrient composition on energy balance may be quite complex. This paper, therefore, focuses specifically on the effects of one particular macronutrient, carbohydrate (CHO), on human EB. The intention is to discuss current, and therefore usually contentious, issues in relation to CHOs and EB. Relationships between the effects of CHO and other macronutrients will only be discussed where appropriate.

---

[c]Tel: +44 1224 712751; fax: +44 1224 716622; e-mail: J. Stubbs@rri.sari.ac.uk.
[d]Tel: +44 1223 415695.

TABLE 1. The Heat of Combustion of Average Dietary Proteins, Carbohydrates, and Alcohol

	kJ/g
Conventional food fats	−37.96–40.09
Conventional food protein	−23.61
Conventional food protein[a] (biological oxidation)	−19.68
Conventional food carbohydrate	−17.5
Ethanol	−29.67

[a] Note that the enthalpy of biological oxidation of dietary protein is dependent on the end products of metabolism, inasmuch as this macronutrient is not completely oxidized in the body. Livesey and Elia have assumed an average value for dietary protein when the end products of its metabolism are urea, ammonia, and creatinine in the nitrogen ratio of 90:5:5. This value is intermediate between the enthalpy of combustion and the metabolizable energy value.[5]

THE ENERGY VALUE OF CARBOHYDRATES

Energy Value of Carbohydrates and Other Macronutrients

To appreciate the energy value of a nutrient and its impact on EB it is important to distinguish between its chemical energy, the energy that the organism derives from that nutrient when it is ingested in food, and the efficiency with which the nutrient is oxidized or stored.

Enthalpy of Combustion (ΔHc)

The ΔHc values of protein, CHO, fat, and alcohol are given in TABLE 1. These values represent the chemical energy contained in these compounds and therefore the energy that is liberated upon complete combustion, or complete biological oxidation by the body.[5] CHO has theoretically the lowest energy density of all of the macronutrients (TABLE 1) in pure chemical terms. This statement, however, assumes that (1) each of the macronutrients is completely digested, and (2) that each of the macronutrients is completely oxidized in the body. Neither of these assumptions is entirely correct. Parenthetically, different proteins differ in composition to a greater extent than other macronutrients, and so their heat of combustion varies considerably, ranging between 17.43–21.15 kJ/g for conventional food proteins and between 17.22–25.98 kJ/g for artificial amino acid mixtures. Dietary intake calculations assume an average protein composition consistent with a Western diet.[5] Because the bioenergetics of biological oxidation are the same as those of combustion (Hess's law; laws of thermodynamics), the ΔHc of the dietary macronutrients should be used when estimating the EE in the physiological oxidation of these metabolic fuels.[5]

TABLE 2. Enthalpy of Combustion of Different Dietary Carbohydrates[5]

	Heat of combustion kJ/g (kcal/g)
Starch	−17.48
Glycogen	−17.52
Sucrose	−16.48
Maltose	−16.49
Lactose	−16.50
Glucose	−15.56
Galactose	−15.56
Fructose	−15.61
Glycerol	−18.03
Xylitol	−16.96
Sorbitol	−16.71
Maltitol	−16.98
Lactitol	−16.98

Do all CHOs have the same gross energy (GE) or ΔHc? TABLE 2 illustrates that they do not. First, the GE per gram of CHO will vary with the chain length of the CHO. This is because di-, tri-, oligo- and polysaccharides are formed by condensation of monosaccharides. For every glycosidic bond formed, a water molecule is lost, and the energy density of the CHO rises. Thus, whereas the ΔHc of glucose is 15.7 kJ/g, that of starch or glycogen is 17.2 kJ/g. Use of the wrong coefficient to estimate glucose oxidation when glycogen is the major source of oxidizable CHO (i.e., fasting) can lead to errors of 10% in estimating the CHO contribution to total EE.[5] The chemical structure of CHOs will also influence the ΔHc of CHO. However, glucose and its derivatives form the bulk of human CHO consumption, and so differences due to chemical composition are unlikely to be large in free-living subjects. When calculating CHO energy derived from dietary intakes, total available CHOs (free sugars: glucose, fructose, galactose, sucrose, maltose, lactose, and oligosaccharides (OS)) and available complex CHOs (dextrins, starch, and glycogen) are often expressed as monosaccharide equivalents. It is important to note that in estimating nutrient intakes from food tables, CHO values expressed as monosaccharide equivalents can exceed 100 g per 100 g of food because the hydrolysis of di- and polysaccharides adds water to each hexose unit. Thus 100 g of starch will hydrolyze to give 110 g of monosaccharide.[6]

Metabolizable Energy (ME) of Carbohydrates

The assumption that each of the dietary macronutrients are completely digested has been questioned in numerous metabolic balance studies in farm animals and subsequently in humans. The first human studies were carried out by Rubner[7] and Atwater.[8,9] More recently Paul and Southgate[10] have reassessed these values based

TABLE 3. Rounded Metabolizable Energy Values for Common Dietary Protein, Carbohydrate, Fats, and Alcohol[6]

Conventional food fats	37
Conventional food protein	17
Conventional food carbohydrate	16
Ethanol	29

on ongoing theoretical considerations and practical results. TABLE 3 gives the *rounded* ME values for the dietary macronutrients. ME is the difference between the gross energy of the food ingested and that which is voided in feces, urinary losses for carbohydrate being essentially nil. This represents the energy available to the organism subsequent to ingestion and is naturally lower than GE. When calculating energy intakes (EIs) it is essential to use ME values and not GE (ΔHc) values, as in the case for estimating fuel oxidation.[11]

Blaxter[12] (pp. 27-34) has emphasized the limitations of using *average* ME values that are commonly used for human nutrients and foods. He notes that the ME value of a nutrient is often specific to a food and its mode of preparation, and that the commonly used approach of using a rounded figure predicates that the ME factors for protein, fat, and CHO are constant and completely independent. They are not. For example, certain unavailable complex CHOs (UCC) decrease the apparent digestion of fat.[12] Blaxter also notes that until recently these values assumed that UCC had zero nutritive value. Blaxter[12] notes as well that Atwater's original approach was to derive numerous food-specific factors. Although many would find this approach overly complex, the contrary practice of assuming constancy of ME coefficients as approximations has undoubtedly introduced significant errors into human studies that attempt to estimate nutrient value and EIs from foods. Blaxter's comparison of American and UK reference values (p. 31) for the ME of some common fresh foods indicates the extent to which differences can arise through the use of different average ME values.[12] Differences can range from zero for polished rice to over 100% for some fruits. Bearing these caveats in mind, it is apparent from TABLES 1 and 2 that, when using average values, the ME values of CHOs are lower than fats and alcohol and are lower than "average" protein. With the exception of proteins, all of the macronutrients can be completely metabolized to carbon dioxide and water with its attendant liberation of energy. Protein is incompletely oxidized due to deamination and ureogenesis. Additional corrections have to be made to account for the urinary output of urea plus other quantitatively minor nitrogenous products that are also excreted.[5]

CHOs vary in their digestibility and hence ME values. There is considerable confusion in the literature relating to the functional terminology of CHO fractions that are digested in the small and large intestine and those that are not.[13] Livesey notes that "variation in the availability of dietary energy has been related formally to the occurrence, utilization and effects of those dietary CHOs which escape small intestinal digestion"[14]—so-called UCC.[15] Previous estimates gave a value of zero for this undigested component of the diet.[10] Recent extensive analyses by Livesey[13,14] and others[15] have, however, led to different conclusions, and it is recommended that these texts are consulted for a comprehensive treatment of this subject. Livesey's examination of over 30 diets with UCC contents ranging from 3–97 g/d indicated a value for ΔHc of 17 kJ/g, a digestibility of 0.7, and a conversion efficiency of 0.3 kJ fecal bacterial energy per kJ CHO fermented, giving an ME value of 8.4 kJ/g for mixed diets. This implies that 50% of the energy in UCC is available to the humans after the process of fermentation and short-chain fatty acid absorption.[14] The factorial calculation by which these values are obtained is given by Livesey.[13] Other factors, such as microwave cooking (which will increase the number of β linkages), can affect the digestibility of available complex CHOs (Cummings, personal communication). Once digested and absorbed, it is apparent that the different macronutrients are given differing priorities in their flux through oxidative and storage pathways.

THE PHYSIOLOGICAL ROLE OF CARBOHYDRATES IN NUTRIENT BALANCE REGULATION

The Nutrient Balance Concept

Macronutrients are not physiologically treated as a single interconvertible energy currency. Protein-energy interactions have long been recognized as functionally important,[16–18] and this has led to the World Health Organization to make not only separate recommendations for protein and energy requirements but also for protein at different levels of energy intake.[19] For humans feeding on Western diets (which at 37–42% fat (as a proportion of energy intake) are high in fat), *de novo* lipogenesis is quantitatively small, and so the balance of each macronutrient appears to be regulated separately.[20] These observations have given rise to the nutrient balance concept,[20] which is based on the following logic. Once body size, its tissue composition, and the level of a person's physical activity have been taken into account, the energy requirements of the human body are largely predictable and remarkably constant. Four recent overfeeding studies, which have measured meticulously the components of the EB equation, suggest that there is little scope to dissipate excess EI by increasing the rate of metabolism (EE).[21–24] However, macronutrient metabolism does not show such inflexibility. The profile of metabolic fuels being used by the body changes with the composition of the diet, nutrient, and energy requirements and with the level of EI. The storage capacity for protein and CHO is limited, and converting these nutrients to a more readily stored form is energetically expensive.[25] It appears that, under Western dietary conditions at least, the net interconvertibility of protein, CHO, and fat is fairly limited.[20] This does not mean that tissue-specific nutrient interconversions cannot occur. In some tissues, individual amino acids can be converted to glucose and fat, and alcohol and glucose to fat (*e.g.*, liver). Whole-body *de novo* lipogenesis can be readily invoked under conditions of very high carbohydrate (HC) diets, with massive CHO overfeeding,[26] or by using mixed hypercaloric nasogastric or parenteral feeding regimes.[27] It is incorrect to state that net *de novo* lipogenesis is quantitatively unimportant in humans; it is more accurate to state that on Western diets *de novo* lipogenesis appears to make a small contribution to total fat storage.[28]

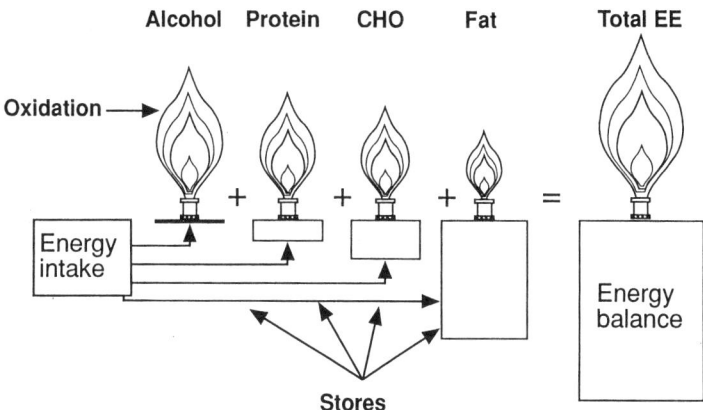

FIGURE 1. A schematic representation of energy balance at the level of nutrient balance. The large flame represents total energy expenditure, which is contributed to by the energy expended in the oxidation of the metabolic fuels. The height of the small flames represents the relative (not to scale) tendency to oxidize each nutrient, subsequent to its ingestion. The size of the fuel store underneath each flame represents the relative storage capacity (not to scale) of the body for each macronutrient. The extent to which macronutrients can be stored varies from virtually zero for alcohol to very large for fat, and this is inversely proportional to their rates of obligatory oxidative disposal subsequent to ingestion. Thus, there is a hierarchy in the extent to which recently ingested nutrients are oxidized.

The above physiological constraints influence the metabolic fate of ingested macronutrients. A positive balance of protein will lead to rapid increase in the oxidation of a high proportion of the amount ingested, the percentage depending on the body's requirements for specific amino acids and the extent to which the enzymes responsible for transamination, deamination, and ureogenesis have been induced. Similarly, as CHO intake increases, more of it is oxidized. Because there is a "ceiling" on adaptive changes in EE, an increased oxidation of protein and CHO will lead to a decreased oxidation of fat. Conversely, fat (long-chain triglyceride) intake does not promote fat oxidation and leads to fat storage.[20,29] Indeed the contribution of fat oxidation to total EE appears to be primarily determined by the amount of protein and CHO being oxidized.[20,29] Alcohol cannot be stored and is disposed of by obligatory oxidation, ultimately at the expense of fat oxidation, so this too promotes fat storage.[30] From a metabolic viewpoint, the human body is analogous to an engine that continually runs (EE) but has a specific order in which it burns up certain fuels (the macronutrients); this seems to relate to the poor ability to store an excess intake of some fuels (alcohol < protein < CHO) in preference to others (long-chain triglycerides). There is thus a hierarchy in the immediacy with which recently ingested macronutrients are metabolized. FIGURE 1 illustrates the ordering of oxidation and storage in the nutrient balance concept. Another way to phrase these concepts is to consider a hierarchy in the extent to which nutrient balance is regulated by oxidative disposal.[20,29,31]

Physiological Regulation of Carbohydrate Balance

The tight physiological regulation of whole-body CHO balance has mainly been revealed by a series of experiments conducted at the Institute of Physiology in Lausanne, Switzerland (see reference 20 for a review), where it has been shown that as CHO intake increases it becomes the preferred metabolic fuel; as CHO intake decreases, it is the conserved metabolic fuel. This has been demonstrated by the following work: (a) After a 480 g load of CHO, net fat synthesis did not exceed oxidation.[32] Because EE was not greatly elevated by the ingested nutrients, this large intake of CHO stimulated CHO oxidation and decreased fat oxidation. (b) Acheson *et al.*[26] examined the mechanism by which a very large CHO intake is disposed of during seven days of massive, progressive CHO overfeeding. Glycogen stores were initially depleted over three days by a high-fat (HF) diet (15% protein, 75% fat, and 10% CHO), with total intake decreasing from 8.35 MJ to 5.7 MJ and by exercise. CHO overfeeding was then achieved by feeding subjects 15.25 MJ on the first day, increasing to 20.64 MJ on the final day (11% protein, 3% fat, and 86% CHO). CHO stores were initially saturated, and maximal rates of CHO oxidation were reached before net lipogenesis was substantially invoked. This took two to three days of massive CHO overfeeding and an estimated addition of 500 g to glycogen stores; then *de novo* lipogenesis was inferred from respiratory exchange. Parenthetically, this suggests that studies seeking to examine evidence of net *de novo* lipogenesis in humans should exceed three to four days inasmuch as it can take up to three days for net lipid synthesis to exceed net lipid oxidation. The high rates of CHO oxidation in this study, together with high levels of *de novo* lipogenesis, induced a 27% increase in EE—one of the highest recorded examples of diet-induced thermogenesis. Some of this increase in energy expenditure might, in theory, be accounted for by the generation of what is, in effect, a futile cycle, whereby CHO is converted to fatty acids, but where other fatty acids are also oxidized. This is perceived in calorimetric gas exchange terms as simply carbohydrate oxidation but with a high total oxygen consumption and carbon dioxide output. Nevertheless, Acheson *et al.*[26] concluded that under normal western diet conditions *de novo* fatty acid synthesis is a quantitatively insignificant pathway in the human organism. This conclusion has recently been supported by metabolic tracer studies by Hellerstein *et al.*[28] who used isotope analyses of very low-density lipoproteins in conjunction with a xenobiotic probe for sampling the cytosolic acetyl CoA pool and thereby calculating the usual rate of acetyl CoA to fatty acid synthesis in humans using C^{13} acetate.

Randle[33] has also shown how CHO oxidation is spared by increased fat oxidation, when circulating nonesterified fatty acids increase. This usually occurs when the level of dietary energy and CHO decrease. Under conditions of adequate CHO stores, the ingestion of a HF diet that contains a substantial amount of CHO will lead to a situation where the CHO is given priority in terms of oxidation over fat, even after a single meal of 3.59 MJ, as demonstrated by Flatt *et al.*[34] Thus, over a period of 9 hours, rates of fat and CHO oxidation were not affected by the fat content of a meal. It can be concluded from this and the other Lausanne studies that, in the absence of alcohol or inordinately high loads of protein, the main factor determining the oxidized fuel mix after a meal is the amount of CHO ingested. As CHO ingestion and hence stores decrease, fat oxidation will increase, by default, to meet the energy requirements of the organism. The Randle glucose-alanine and Cori cycles ensure that the basal requirement for glucose oxidation is satisfied under all but the most extreme conditions of CHO deprivation.

In general, increased CHO intake increases the rate of its own oxidation and storage. Because adaptive thermogenesis appears very limited, this elevated rate of CHO oxidation will suppress fat oxidation and promote fat storage. A decreased CHO intake invokes increased fat oxidation to meet energy requirements.

Because physiological studies show that excess energy taken in as either alcohol or fat promotes fat storage, it has been suggested that consuming a high proportion of EI as fat and alcohol predisposes individuals to dietary-induced obesity. It has also been implied that, because sugars and other CHOs do not induce significant degrees of *de novo* lipogenesis in humans feeding on a Western diet, HC intakes are less likely to predispose people to fat storage and weight gain. The above discussion indicates that this argument is in itself erroneous. Excess energy, taken in the form of any nutrient, will ultimately promote fat storage[35] unless dietary macronutrients differentially affect subsequent appetite and/or obligatory thermogenesis.

Is the total EE influenced by diet composition? CHO oxidation contributes more to postprandial EE than fat because CHO is the major fuel being oxidized in the postprandial period,[34] and the energy used for glycogen storage exceeds any immediate small cost of fat absorption with later peripheral storage (see below). However, as the postprandial rise in CHO oxidation diminishes, fat oxidation makes a greater contribution to EE. In order to assess the importance of macronutrient-based thermogenic responses for EB, it is important to consider the effect of different nutrients on EE over periods of at least 24 hours. When the fat to CHO balance of subjects is grossly perturbed at maintenance levels, over one[29,36] or two days,[37] 24-hour EE is very similar. Leibel *et al.*[38] have carefully examined whether extreme changes in the fat to CHO ratio of the diet influence maintenance energy requirements over much longer periods. Isoenergetic liquid diets contain different percentages of EI as CHO (low 15%, intermediate 40 or 45%, high 75, 80, or 85%); a constant 15% of energy as protein and the balance as fat were fed to 16 subjects over 15 to 56 days. Extreme variations in the fat to CHO ratio of the diet produced no detectable evidence of significant variation in energy requirements as a function of the dietary fat to CHO ratio. Thus, whatever the theoretical subtleties of the different routes for processing the different macronutrients when normal subjects are fed to EB, the fat to CHO ratio of the diet does not exert quantitatively discernible effects on energy requirements.

The Energy Cost of Nutrient Storage

Protein ingestion induces the largest obligatory metabolic rise in EE due to the energetic costs of protein synthesis, gluconeogenesis, and ureogenesis, which amount to ~0.25 MJ per MJ of ingested protein.[25] The energetic cost of converting glucose to glycogen is estimated at ~0.05 MJ per MJ of ingested CHO, whereas the corresponding cost for *de novo* lipogenesis from CHO amounts to ~0.24 MJ per MJ of ingested CHO.[25] The cost of fat storage from dietary fat amounts to ~0.02 MJ per MJ of ingested fat, because this process does not require substantial metabolic interconversion of nutrients.[25] When EB is perturbed, fat and CHO may exert different effects on EB due to differences in the energetic efficiency of their handling. Two studies have shed some light on this issue. McNeill et al.[39] compared the effects of over- and underfeeding fat and CHO by 40% of energy requirements over seven days. Body weight was increased by 1.35 kg over a week when subjects were overfed, as opposed to a gain of 0.84 kg when the same excess was given as fat. When subjects were underfed they lost 1.70 kg when the energy was removed as CHO, compared to a loss of 0.72 kg when the energy deficit was derived from fat. The authors argued that these differences could be accounted for by changes in CHO stores. Indeed, CHO is stored with water in a ratio of 1 : 3, and so a net change of CHO stores amounting to 330 g should lead an attendant change in body weight (due to water) of around 1 kg. Under these conditions body weight is not a good proxy for changes in EB.

Horton et al.[40] have examined this issue with a greater degree of resolution. They overfed nine lean and seven obese subjects for 14 days by 50% of maintenance energy requirements as CHO or fat. In this study, each subject resided in a whole-body indirect calorimeter for days 0, 1, 7, and 14. The amount and composition of energy stored could then be estimated from nutrient and EB estimates in the calorimeter. CHO overfeeding produced progressive increases in CHO oxidation and 24-hour EE, giving an overall energetic efficiency of CHO storage of 75-85%. Fat overfeeding did not greatly elevate fat oxidation or EE, giving an efficiency of storage of 90-95%. These findings are in good agreement with Flatt's initial theoretical estimates.[25]

Does the composition of the diet differentially influence EB during weight loss? James et al.[41] have reviewed the metabolic responses to semistarvation. They discuss several studies that have examined this issue and note that the metabolic response (independent of tissue loss) to semistarvation is very limited. Two recent studies that have compared the effects of high-protein (HP), HF, and HC weight-reducing diets (4.2 MJ/d) on either resting EE,[42] or on subjective appetite (Stubbs et al., unpublished) found no difference in weight loss over two weeks per dietary treatment. The Whitehead study[42] found that the HP diet tended to preserve lean body mass and so limit the decrease in EE associated with the loss of lean body mass during dieting. There was, however, no detectable difference between the HC and HF diets.

We may conclude that the principal changes in the energy available from carbohydrates relate to the ΔHc differences due to the chain length of common dietary CHOs that can be appreciated by expressing CHOs of differing chain lengths as monosaccharide equivalents. Differences in available dietary energy, expressed in terms of ME, can be largely related to the occurrence, utilization, and effects of those dietary CHOs that escape small intestinal digestion.[13] Currently, habitual Western diets differ by no more than 5% with regard to available carbohydrate, although, theoretically, this value could be greater on diets containing extreme amounts of UCCs. CHO is less efficiently stored as body fat than dietary fat, but these differences are only apparent during quite extreme overfeeding with HC diets and are less apparent during moderate overfeeding on Western-type diets. Because CHO shows enhanced thermogenesis when being converted to fat, this does not mean that an excess CHO intake is less likely to promote fat storage. Rather it means that an excess CHO intake is less likely to promote *de novo* lipogenesis. The relative inefficiency of conversion of CHO to fat is therefore not likely to have a large impact on EB when subjects overfeed on Western diets, because *de novo* lipogenesis is relatively rare under these conditions and the body under such feeding conditions stores the available dietary fat in preference to having a less efficient mix of carbohydrate to fat synthesis with continued fatty acid oxidation.

Thus, it can be appreciated that CHOs are unlikely to produce large, significant changes in EB through changes in either efficiency of digestion (~5% of EI) or metabolic utilization (~5% of EE), except under more extreme conditions than those usually encountered on Western diets. It is theoretically possible that small secular changes in the mix of carbohydrates could, over longer periods, influence overall EB[20] in populations, but overweight and obesity appear to be increasing in prevalence at a faster rate and to a greater extent than can be accounted for by these subtleties in CHO processing.

If the total level of EE is not greatly influenced by the nutrient composition of the diet (except under extreme conditions of overfeeding or of diet composition), then any large diet-induced changes in nutrient balance can only significantly influence EB if fat, protein, CHO, and alcohol have different effects on appetite, or differing satiating efficiencies. (The relative satiating efficiency of a macronutrient (per unit time) would be the extent to which each MJ of positive nutrient balance suppresses subsequent EI compared to other macronutrients.) This is best illustrated by a hypothetical example. If EI is regulated regardless of diet composition on the basis of some feedback mechanism linked to EB (energostatic regulation), then an excess EI as fat would lead to a positive fat (and hence energy) balance. Then the energy-based control of feeding would suppress subsequent EI, however, leading to the mobilization and oxidation of the recently stored fat load, thus restoring EB. The same argument can be made for each of the macronutrients. It is therefore important to consider whether protein, CHO, fat, and alcohol have different effects on EI.

CARBOHYDRATES AND APPETITE

Carbohydrate-based Models of Feeding

CHOs have always had a special place in the minds of theorists concerned with the role of diet composition in producing physiological signals that may influence feeding behavior. Mayer initially suggested that EB regulation occurred predominantly through short-term "glucostatic" responses that could be corrected by longer-term "lipostatic" regulation, should short-term regulation be sufficiently perturbed.[43] Mayer argued that the "central role of CHOs in the economy of the central nervous system, the lack of its storage, its preferential utilization, the thoroughness of its regulation, and its role in turn as the central regulator of overall metabolism" were potent arguments for the role of CHO as the key factor that "can successfully be integrated with energy metabolism and its components." In 1963 Russek postulated the presence of glucose receptors in the liver and formulated the hepatostatic theory of EB regulation.[44] Flatt extended these models in 1985 and evolved the glycogenostatic model of appetite regulation, which is based on the logic relating to nutrient balance discussed above.[45] These models are depicted in FIGURE 2.

Dietary CHOs have also been viewed as being central to nutrient selection models through their putative effects on the synthesis of the neurotransmitter, serotonin (5-

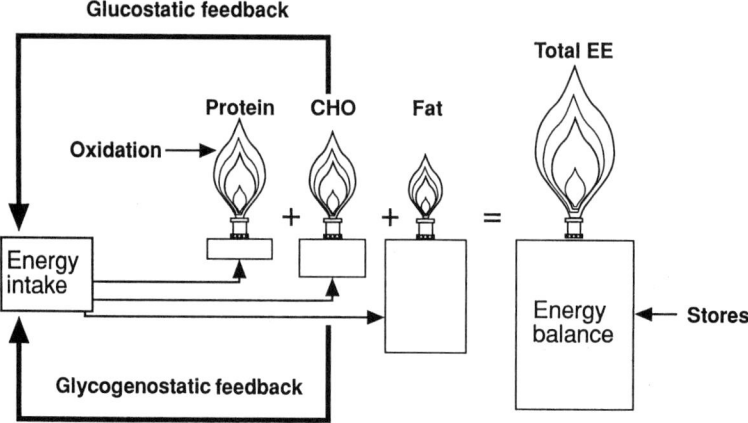

FIGURE 2. The glucostatic and glycogenostatic models of energy intake regulation in which changes in peripheral glucose utilization (glucostatic) or carbohydrate stores (glycogenostatic) are proposed to exert negative feedback on subsequent energy intake.

HT). It was hypothesized that dietary-induced biochemical oscillations in the ratio of plasma tryptophan to plasma levels of the large neutral amino acid (LNAA) directly influenced tryptophan transport and its availability for 5-HT synthesis and therefore for serotoninergic activity. This activity, in turn, was supposed to influence directly a behavioral alternation in the selection of protein rather than carbohydrate.[46] Brain serotonin synthesis does seem to be affected by the uptake of its precursor, tryptophan, across the blood brain barrier, and the LNAAs do compete with tryptophan for uptake by the transporter that traverses the blood-brain barrier. It was also proposed that a CHO meal stimulated insulin release, which would increase the ratio of tryptophan: LNAAs in the blood by lowering the plasma concentrations of the other LNAAs, most notably leucine, isoleucine, and valine. The resultant elevation in brain serotonin levels was then perceived to decrease CHO selection. As CHO intake fell, the rate of tryptophan uptake into the brain would also fall and the cycle would begin again. Conversely, protein intake might increase the ratio of large neutral amino acids to tryptophan, reversing this mechanism and so increasing CHO selection. Fernstrom[47] has reviewed this model, and he, with others, have concluded that the system does not operate as a mechanism for diet selection, although the importance of the serotonin system as a central mechanism influencing feeding behavior remains undiminished.[48] The detailed reasoning for these conclusions can be found in Fernstrom[47] and associated discussion papers.

The remaining CHO-based models of feeding have recently attracted more interest. Mayer, Russek, and Flatt's models of CHO control predict broadly similar effects on feeding behavior: (1) CHO-stores or metabolism exert a negative feedback on EI; (2) because of this feedback, diets high in fat but low in CHO will promote excess EIs; (3) manipulating CHO status, that is, oxidation or CHO stores, will reciprocally influence EI; and (4) excess *ad libitum* EIs on HC diets should be very difficult to achieve without a conscious effort, due to the strength of putative negative feedback arising from CHO status. The key question in relation to these models is whether they are useful. Is there evidence that glucostatic or glycogenostatic mechanisms exert a large enough influence on feeding behavior to be quantitatively important in the laboratory and in real life? To support these mechanisms, studies should demonstrate a high probability that changes in CHO status will exert predictable effects on feeding behavior that are consistent with the predictions of these models. CHO-based models of EB regulation are intuitively attractive because the predictions of these models appear to be consistent with the role of fat as a risk factor for weight gain,[49] because these predictions are testable, and because the predictions of these models offer a potential means of manipulating energy balance.

Do Carbohydrate Stores/Metabolism Exert Powerful Negative Feedback on EI?

Epidemiological studies suggest that body mass index (BMI) is inversely associated with CHO intake and directly associated with fat intake. Unfortunately, in a number of these studies, BMI is also inversely associated with EI.[30,50] This may relate to preferential underreporting in the obese.[49] This confounder weakens the conclusions from cross-sectional studies. However, longitudinal studies suggest that increased fat intake is a risk factor for subsequent weight gain.[48]

More tightly controlled laboratory studies have demonstrated that increasing the energy density of the diet by covertly adding fat has led to increasing energy intake but not to increasing the amount of food ingested (*e.g.,* refs 51 and 52). Conversely, decreasing dietary energy density by removing the dietary fat has led to lower levels of EI.[53] These data implicate excess fat intake as a risk factor for weight gain but do not necessarily suggest that the body is totally blind to fat, from a regulatory perspective. Indeed, deliberate reductions in energy intake from either fat or CHO are both compensated for by a nonspecific increase in EI on a day-to-day or a meal-to-meal basis, when subjects are allowed to select from a variety of familiar foods (see ref. 31 for a review). In our own studies, conducted over a week, to assess the impact of CHO oxidation or balance changes in the effects of HF diets on EI, we fed six men *ad libitum* on covertly manipulated low-fat (LF), medium-fat (MF) or HF diets where energy density was selectively increased with fat while they occupied a large calorimetric chamber.[52] As the fat content of the diet increased, the total weight of food eaten stayed the same, so EI increased, leading to a progressively positive EB. The relationship between the changes in actual, cumulative nutrient balance over time and the subsequent day's EI was examined to assess possible feedback from macronutrient balances on EI. The previous day's cumulative balance of CHO and protein was negatively related to the subsequent day's EI (and balance), or to a change in these variables, but there was no apparent suppression of intake in relation to the previous day's cumulative fat balance. The effect of a positive protein balance was greater than that for CHO storage. The oxidation of all of the macronutrients predicted a reduction in the subsequent day's EB, but this effect was again hierarchical, with protein oxidation exerting a stronger predicted fall in intake than CHO, which, in turn, exerted a marginally stronger effect than fat. These

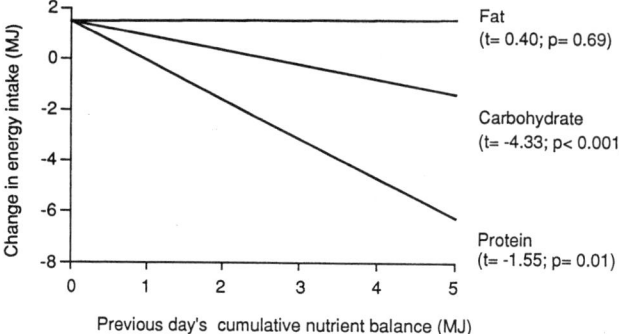

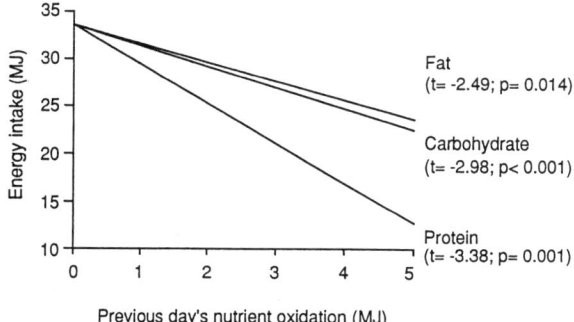

FIGURE 3. Regression plots of change in energy intake (MJ) against the previous day's cumulative balance (MJ) of protein, carbohydrate, and fat (top panel). Subsequent delta EI = 1.49 + 0.02 (cumulative fat balance) − 0.57 (cumulative CHO balance) − 1.55 (cumulative protein balance). Regression plots of change in energy intake (MJ) against the previous day's cumulative oxidation (MJ) of protein, carbohydrate, and fat (bottom panel). Subsequent EI = 33.56 − 1.99 (fat oxidation) − 2.23 (CHO oxidation) − 4.17 (protein oxidation).

relationships are illustrated in FIGURE 3. Thus the previous day's cumulative stores *and* the oxidation of protein and CHO were negatively related to subsequent EI. Importantly, although fat oxidation seemed to predict, to a modest extent, the subsequent day's EI, alterations in fat stores did not show any effect on the subsequent day's EI. These data suggest that it is the component of obligatory oxidative disposal that underlies the potentially suppressive effects that protein and CHO, but not fat balance, exert on subsequent EI.[52] This interpretation is depicted in FIGURE 4. Another study compared *isoenergetically* dense diets of protein, CHO, and fat over the course of a day and found the HP diet to be the most satiating and HC foods to be more satiating than HF foods but only for the first hour after each ingestive event.[54] These findings support the relationships shown in our larger study.[52]

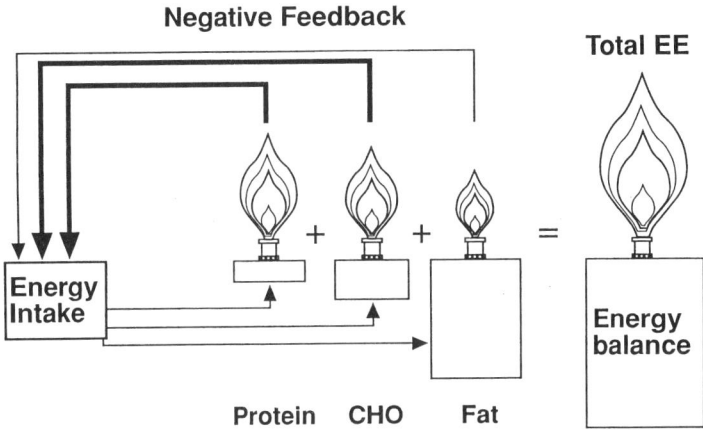

FIGURE 4. The "hierarchical oxidation hypothesis," whereby the regulation of nutrient balance by obligatory oxidative disposal of protein and carbohydrate, but not fat, correlates with satiety.

CHO-based models of feeding predict that excess EIs occur on HF diets, not because they are energy dense, but because the negative feedback from CHO oxidation or stores is diminished and subjects are actively increasing EI to optimize CHO status. It is apparent that excess EI on HF, energy-dense diets is a passive process, inasmuch as subjects eat similar amounts of food and fail to decrease intake in response to the increased energy density of the diet. At very-high energy densities food intake will decrease but not enough to prevent excess EI.[55] Two studies have examined the effects of allowing subjects to feed *ad libitum* on HF and LF isoenergetically dense diets. One study was conducted in women[56] (dietary energy density was 4.2 kJ/g) and one in men[57] (energy density was 4.8 kJ/g). In both studies subjects ate near-identical amounts of food and hence energy, regardless of diet composition. There was no evidence of excess EIs or weight gain in either study. These data cast doubt on the notion that increases in CHO oxidation and/or storage *per se* are the major factors that exert powerful, unconditioned, negative feedback on food or EI.

CHO-based models of feeding also predict that manipulation of CHO status (oxidation or stores) will reciprocally influence EI. Two studies have examined this issue in detail. In the first of these studies, the effect of altering CHO balance on day-to-day food intake was examined.[36] Nine men were each studied twice, during which time they were housed in an indirect calorimeter for 48 hours. CHO stores were depleted over the first 24 hours to create a difference of 2.45 ± 0.67 MJ, compared with a control (MF) diet, while controlling EB. *Ad libitum* food intake was assessed over the subsequent 24 hours. The CHO "depletion" was achieved using a very HF (85% of energy), low CHO (3% of energy) diet. This extreme dietary manipulation did not affect the subsequent day's *ad libitum* EI, compared with the control. Instead, CHO balance was reestablished by directing more dietary CHO towards storage and by maintaining high rates of fat oxidation throughout the *ad libitum* day. Thus, plasticity in fuel utilization, not appetite, was the primary mechanism for reestablishing nutrient balance.

A subsequent follow-up study extended this investigation in six men who were each studied three times in five-day experiments.[37] They received either an HC diet, providing 79% of EI; a medium CHO (MC) diet, comprising 48% of EI; or a low CHO (LC) diet, which provided only 9% of EI, over 48 hours, after two days on a maintenance diet. The impact of these manipulations on food intake throughout the fifth day was examined. EB proved to be similar on each treatment, and, despite a difference in CHO balance of 4.99 MJ between the HC and LC diet, by the morning of the fifth day, there was no significant effect on EI during that day. Again, CHO balance was reestablished by an autoregulatory change in CHO oxidation rather than by altered food intake. Thus, large changes in nutrient balance had relatively little effect on subsequent EI when fat and CHO balance, but not EB, was perturbed.

There are, of course, some limitations to these studies. They do not address the issue of food or nutrient selection, because subjects were only able to increase or decrease the amount but not the composition of foods they chose to eat. These studies also uncouple learned behavioral responses from the physiological signals produced by large dietary manipulations. Clearly CHO oxidation is associated with satiety.[38,58-63] However, taken together, this series of studies does suggest that in the short-to-medium term, neither dietary-induced increases in CHO stores nor oxidation *per se* exert powerful unconditioned negative feedback on EI to the extent that increasing CHO ingestion *per se* will induce weight loss. However, decreasing the fat content of the diet is usually attended by a decrease in dietary energy density, which can lead to relatively modest, but prolonged, decreases in EI.[51-53]

CHO-based models of feeding predict that excess EIs on HC diets are unlikely to occur. In a recent study (in press) at the Rowett Research Institute, this prediction was tested. Six normal-weight men were each studied twice during 14 days. After a preliminary two-day period with intakes for maintenance set at 1.6 times their basal metabolic rate, they had *ad libitum* access throughout the next 14 days to one of two covertly manipulated diets. The fat, CHO, and protein in each diet, expressed in terms of energy, were in the proportions of 22:65:13 on the low-energy density (LED) diet, which was set at a density of 348 kJ/100 g. The high-energy density (HED) diet (617 kJ/100 g) had similar macronutrient proportions. Subjects could change the amount but not the composition of the foods they chose. EIs were 8.56 and 14.56 MJ/d, leading to weight gain or loss on the LED and HED diets, respectively (FIG. 5). Intake was not influenced by perceived pleasantness of the diets. However, subjects felt significantly more hungry on the LED diet than on the HED diet, as judged by a linear hunger scale [30.4 mm vs. 25.7 mm (F (1, 160) 30.28; $p < 0.001$)]. In a previous study where subjects consumed excess EIs on HF, HED diets, there was no detectable difference in subjective hunger between dietary treatments.[38] These data suggest that excess EIs are possible on HC, HED diets in *ad libitum* feeding subjects, where conditions preclude diet selection. We interpret the difference in hunger between the diets as being due to an increase in hunger to above-normal levels, only when CHO depletion and a negative energy balance coincided (FIG. 6).

It is known that changes (particularly decrements) in both CHO and fat metabolism do influence feeding behavior in rodents and also in humans. Thus, a small (6–12%) drop in plasma glucose predicts meal initiation in rodents[58] and humans.[59] In rodents

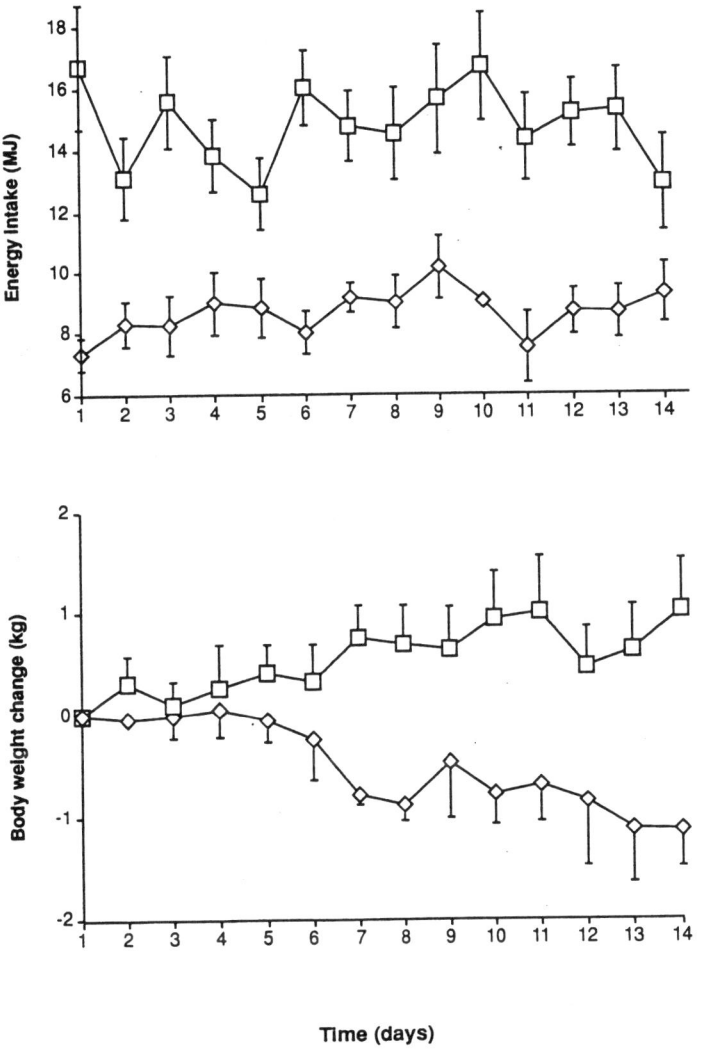

FIGURE 5. Energy intake and change in body weight of six men who fed *ad libitum* on low and medium energy density/high energy density diets for two weeks per treatment. □, high-energy density; ◇, low-energy density.

a small infusion of glucose, which blocks this drop, also delays feeding by up to three hours. Pharmacological inhibition of glucose and fat oxidation also increases feeding in rats.[60] Postprandial CHO oxidation correlates negatively with hunger in humans.[61] Parenteral infusions of amino acids, glucose, or lipid in rats lead to changes in intake that lend towards caloric compensation. However, the degree of caloric

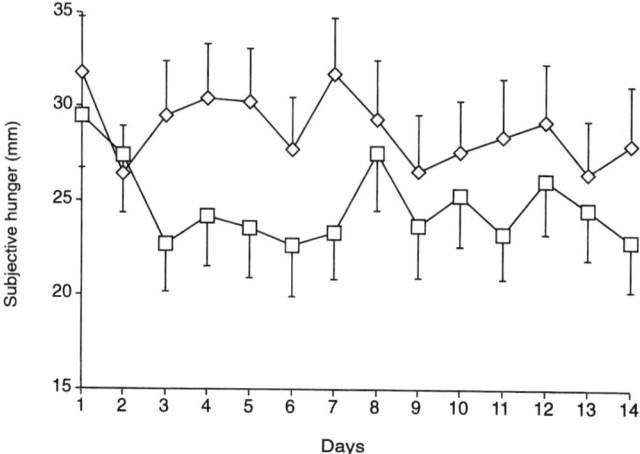

FIGURE 6. Mean daily subjective hunger (expressed as mm along a 100-mm scale) for 6 men feeding ad libitum on the HC diets that were HED or LED. □, high-energy density; ◇, low-energy density.

compensation was only complete when amino acids were infused, whereas around 70% compensation occurred with glucose and less than 50% when fat was infused.[62] Similar effects have been found in one study in humans.[63] There is also new evidence that suggests that the central nervous system monitors CHO and fat oxidation separately but that these signals are integrated in a way that allows the animals to take account of overall fuel status, at least in relation to glucoprivic and lipoprivic rodent-based feeding models.[64] Thus, although there is evidence that decrements in fat and CHO intake and oxidation are well detected and compensated for, the evidence suggests that increments in fat and CHO intake induce less compensation than decrements in intake.

The Concept of a Hierarchy in the Satiating Efficiency of the Dietary Macronutrients

Both the physiological and behavioral literature support the concept of a hierarchy in the satiating efficiency of the macronutrients: that per MJ of energy ingested, protein is more satiating than CHO, which is more satiating than fat under ecological conditions where fat contributes disproportionately to the energy density of the diet. CHO therefore sits in the middle of this hierarchy. When different macronutrients are ingested at the same level of energy density in the diet, protein is by far the most persistently satiating macronutrient, whereas CHO is more satiating than fat but only in the short term. Isoenergetically dense HC and HF diets seem to exert similar effects on appetite over 24 hours[54] and EI over two weeks.[56,57] Energy derived from alcohol appears to completely bypass the appetite control.[31] This is not surprising inasmuch as alcohol is also a physiological depressant, and this effect may override or cancel any satiating potential from its energy content. A recent meta-analysis by Mattes suggests that alcohol produces countercompensatory increases in EI.[65]

The differential influences that macronutrients exert on satiety and EI may operate through a number of sequential mechanisms. This has been set out conceptually by Blundell as a "satiety cascade." This hierarchy in the satiating efficiency of the macronutrients is apparent at the level of nutrient balance regulation[52] and at the level of postabsorptive metabolism.[62,63] It would appear that those nutrients most readily oxidized (parenthetically the most thermogenic) are the most satiating. In general, thermogenesis also correlates with sympathetic activity (Stock, personal communication).

The Influence of Dietary Energy Density versus Macronutrient Composition on Feeding Behavior

The above discussions illustrate the following points. When studied in the laboratory setting, an individual exhibits a strong tendency to eat a similar amount of food from day-to-day, unless a large dietary-induced physiological effect influences intake. Covertly increasing the energy density of the diet using predominantly fat,[52,53] or CHO does not affect food intakes, so there is a general failure to compensate for the change in dietary energy density, at least over a two-week period and when subjects are able to vary the amount but not the composition of their foods. This might imply that EI is simply not regulated at all and that the best way to lose weight would be to consume large amounts of a bulky inert material! However, it must be recognized that some aspect of the experimental environment produces this characteristic behavior. Why should weight and volume appear as such important features of food intake regulation? Blundell[66] argues that every individual has acquired, through a learned process, experience of food seeking and consumption, so that the weight and volume of food will have become associated with its energy value and nutrient composition. He argues that the weight and volume of food consumed reflect the outcome of learned cues with high functional validity and that these cues correlate well with more physiological cues, such as hormone release and energy repletion, which are experienced during the postprandial phase. Thus, food weights and volumes often appear to be the important variables that are monitored subconsciously, given the inability to sense visually or by gastric filling the energy or nutrient content of the food. Unless the nutrient or energy content of the diet produces a large and unlearned, that is, unconditioned, influence that overrides the learned experience, then, during the course of a study, the individual is likely to continue to respond as they would in everyday life. This does not mean that weight is fundamentally more important than energy content. Indeed, in one study by Kendall et al.,[53] subjects were given medium or LF foods to eat for 11 weeks. The LF foods were lower in energy density than the MF foods. Subjects gradually increased their EI on the LF diet in a manner that partially compensated for the low energy intake over the 11 weeks. This suggests that they were gradually changing their perception of weight and volume cues, according to the physical and nutritional properties of the diet. In the case of very LED diets, it may take considerable time to adapt and take greater amounts of food to meet their energy requirements. This does not mean that subjects cannot detect changes in hunger in response to changes in nutrient and energy status, as already noted. Under conditions where the only possible response to covertly manipulated diets is physically to alter the amount eaten, then subjects may not readily compensate. In real life, subjects are able freely to alter both the amount and nature of their food and may respond more rapidly and accurately by selecting foods that differ in composition and energy density. In studies where the energy and nutrient content of diets is surreptitiously manipulated and subjects have *ad libitum* access to a variety of familiar food items, caloric compensation is both more accurate and rapid (see ref. 31 for a review).

Types of Carbohydrates and Appetite

A number of studies have compared the satiating effects of preloads containing different hexoses and found relatively few differences between them in terms of appetite responses. However, it is unclear whether this uniform response relates to the constraints of the preloading method or whether the monosaccharides simply have similar satiating efficiencies. There is some evidence that starches produce a more blunted, yet prolonged influence on satiety than do mono- and disaccharides. However, these effects seem relatively modest, and to date there is little published data to suggest that sugars and starches exert large differential effects on intake. One interesting and important exception to this is the finding that calories contained in drinks appear to be poorly compensated for. In 1955 Fryer supplemented the diet of college students with a HC drink containing 1.8 MJ. Compensation was incomplete (~50%) after eight weeks.[67] Mattes has recently conducted a meta-analysis of feeding responses to either liquid or solid manipulations of the nutrient and energy content of the diet. The analysis suggests that the physical state of ingested CHO intake may be important in influencing subsequent caloric compensation. The reasons for this are at present unclear, but may relate to the rate, timing, and density at which the energy is ingested. There may be a threshold in these parameters, below which energy is poorly detected.

Most work on the effects of different CHOs on EI has been done with UCC or fiber. The time-energy displacement concept has been invoked to suggest that the addition of UCCs to the diet enhances satiation and limits meal sizes. This effect is apparent in some of the studies discussed above, and the phenomenon has been used to limit weight gain in farm animals on single feeds.

In all, over 50 studies have been conducted that have examined the effects of dietary fiber on food intake and body weight.[68] These have been extensively covered in four recent reviews,[68-71] to which the reader is referred for a detailed discussion of this issue. In summary, various loads of UCC or fiber at one meal have been shown to decrease both hunger and EI at the next meal, but the effects are relatively modest. Levine and Billington note that 26 of 38 long-term studies have examined the effects of increased UCC ingestion on body weight. The results of this seemingly large number of trials are equivocal because of the different forms of fiber used, the different vehicles chosen (*i.e.,* ranging from real foods to tablet formulations), different subject populations, and the varying degrees of experimental control, ranging from overt to double-blind manipulations. The conclusion seems to be that supplementing the diet with tolerable levels of extracted UCC appears to have, at best, modest effects in decreasing body weight over several months or more. However, fiber-rich bulky diets of low-energy density may have different effects, and the reader should consider the methodological issues detailed in a number of references[68–71] before drawing firm conclusions.

SWEETNESS AND ENERGY BALANCE

For the last decade there has been a healthy controversy raging about the role of sweetness, sucrose and artificial sweeteners[72,73] in maintaining energy balance. The key issue relates to what effects sweetness, plus or minus CHO energy, has on appetite and EB. There are three main hypotheses: (1) adding sweetness without calories to foods leads to lower levels of EI than when sweetness with calories are added; (2) sweetness without calories leads to a cephalic phase stimulation to eat; and (3) ingestion of sugars (sweetness with calories) correlates with thinness and lowers fat intake, which is itself the reason for the lower body weight. These stark alternatives have probably been interpreted too rigorously because the effects of these factors on appetite and EI are likely to be influenced by the conditions under which they are assessed.

There is little doubt that most animals display a preference for sweetness at a very early age, and that sweetness is a factor favoring the selection and subsequent ingestion of sweet foods. Conversely, different people exhibit markedly different preferences for sweetness intensities, and so simply adding sweetness to foods will not stimulate everyone to eat. Assuming that sweetness does in general stimulate the selection and consumption of these foods, the next question relates to whether sweetness with or without calories differentially affects appetite and EI.

Does Sweetness without Calories Lead to Lower Levels of EI and Body Weight than Sweetness with Calories?

Despite the common assumption that replacing dietary sugars with intense sweeteners will promote a more negative EB, there is a remarkable paucity of data to demonstrate this effect. The work of Porikos *et al.* is unusual because subjects were already in a positive EB on the control diets (probably due to the sumptuous mode of food presentation) and were then in approximate EB on the LED, aspartame-enriched foods.[74] There is certainly little epidemiological evidence to suggest that artificial sweetener consumption correlates with lower BMIs, or that increased artificial sweetener consumption in the population has contributed to any reduction in the prevalence of overweight or obese people. Statistical modeling of feeding responses to intense sweeteners suggests that energy compensation when sweeteners are substituted for sugars will occur in the population.

A problem with the majority of laboratory studies that examine the effect of sweetness, sugars, and artificial sweeteners is that many are short term and therefore do not address the issue of EB (see Anderson [73]). It is also possible that covert replacement of sugars with artificial sweeteners is more likely to decrease EI if subjects can only alter the amount they eat of a diet of fixed composition rather than having access to a variety of familiar foods.

Does Sweetness without Calories Lead to a Cephalic-phase Stimulation to Eat?

Most authors seem to be in agreement that the purely postingestive effects of aspartame do not stimulate intake.[73,74] Blundell and Hill initially reported that artificially sweetened drinks can actually stimulate appetite. They suggested that sweetness without calories provides a sensory cue for CHO calories, which leads to cephalic-phase physiological changes that anticipate EI.[75] They note that intense sweeteners have only been found to stimulate intake when a food has been sweetened with intense sweeteners or when a less sweet food has been compared with an isoenergetically equivalent food to which sweetness has been added (their "additive principle") and not when two foods of differing energy density but the same level of sweetness are compared: This they call the "substitutive principle." Again, this area is bedeviled by methodological controversies, such as the appropriate drink vehicle for the sweetener (water or a familiar soft drink), the time course of the experiment, and the subjects used. Blundell and Rogers argue that the strongest experimental designs contain tests of both the additive and substitutive principle.[75] No long-term studies that address energy balance have yet achieved this dual testing. Black and Anderson report that the use of aspartame-sweetened water leads to an acute short-term increase in subjective appetite in lean men, but that aspartame-sweetened carbonated soft drinks induce a transient suppression of appetite in similar subjects over a similar time frame.[76] The issue is complicated by the fact that satiety can be transiently conditioned by starch-containing drinks that are paired with a given sensory cue, such as flavor (see Booth[72]). Once conditioned, similar levels of satiation can be transiently induced by the conditioning stimulus alone. Therefore the effects of prior conditioning could influence the outcome of studies using vehicles that mimic the sensory properties of familiar foods.

Dietary restraint may also influence the response of subjects to sweetness, sugar, and artificial sweeteners. Lavine *et al.* (in press) have recently shown sucrose-containing drinks rather than water induce caloric compensation in restrained young women, whereas aspartame-sweetened lemonade produces a counter-compensatory increase in EI on the subsequent day. This effect is unlikely, because of the long time, to have been due to cephalic-phase responses and is more likely to be due to cognitive responses to subtle differences in the taste of the drinks. Thus, they probably recognized the taste of aspartame and cognitively responded to a perceived caloric deficit on the previous day. Again there is a notable lack of longer-term studies that address EB.

In summary, there is little evidence that artificial sweeteners reliably decrease appetite or reduce EI, but they could perhaps prevent any excess EI, which would otherwise occur when calories were provided as drinks. There are conditions where artificially sweetened drinks have been found to stimulate appetite and less often EI, but there is little evidence to suggest that sweeteners reduce intake. Understanding the applicability of these findings to free-living humans is an important area yet to be resolved.

How Robust Is the Fat-Sugar Seesaw, and Does It Mean That Sugar Intakes Are Protective against HF Hyperphagia?

It is now generally accepted that the views of the early 1970s are wrong, that is, that sweetness provided in the form of calories stimulates EI and contributes to increases in obesity. The epidemiological data suggest that consumption of sugars, that is, sweetness with calories, is associated with thinness. Yet the same studies tend to show that as sugar intake increases, so does EI. This suggests that more physically active people select more sugars and therefore does not necessarily imply that increased sugar intake spontaneously promotes thinness. When considering these data, the limitations of epidemiological studies must therefore be taken into account. As already observed in this paper, (1) increasing the energy density of the diet with maltodextrins can lead to excess *ad libitum* EIs, and (2) energy-containing drinks are poorly compensated for. Nevertheless, fat intake under naturalistic conditions does appear to be more of a risk factor for weight gain. This does not, of course, mean that increasing the energy density of the diet with sweet CHOs will never increase EIs. Naismith and Rhodes[77] found that the covert removal of 2.1 MJ/d of sugar from the diet initially decreased EI but was followed by an increased fat intake from 3.57 to 3.97 MJ/d. The authors concluded that "the inverse relationship between dietary sugar and fat poses problems for those seeking to lose weight...." It is difficult to accept this conclusion, inasmuch as subjects were subsequently in an energy deficit of 1.7 MJ on the diet with the higher fat intake. This example highlights the importance of relating dietary and feeding studies to EB or useful proxies thereof. Although there is evidence of some reciprocity in the population between CHO and sugar intake on the one hand and fat intake on the other, this probably reflects the fact that people eat to defend against energy deficits, rather than implying that there is some active process whereby sugar intake promotes dietary fat avoidance. There is little or no evidence that increasing sugar intake promotes a negative EB and weight loss: the critical experiments have not been conducted. The effects on food and nutrient selection of titrating fats and sugars into the diet need to be examined and are currently being initiated at the Rowett Research Institute.

SUMMARY

In the early 1970s carbohydrates (CHOs) were believed to induce overconsumption and excess fat deposition. They are now perceived to protect against these consequences. This paper evaluates the evidence for this change of interpretation by considering (1) the energy content of CHOs, (2) the energetic efficiency with which they are handled by the body, and (3) their effects on appetite, relative to other macronutrients. CHOs are the least energy-dense macronutrients (ΔHc) and exhibit the greatest variability in digestibility. Doubling the usual levels of nonstarch polysaccharides (fiber) may decrease digestibility of a Western diet by 5%. *De novo* lipogenesis from dietary CHO is energetically inefficient but very limited on Western diets, which are relatively high in fat. There appears to be a hierarchy (protein > CHO > fat) in the extent to which the stores of the macronutrients are autoregulated by oxidation. Excess CHO intake tends to promote storage (but not *de novo* synthesis) of fat. The thermogenic effects of CHO are therefore relatively limited on Western diets. Per MJ of energy ingested, macronutrients differentially affect satiety (protein > CHO > fat) under conditions where fat is disproportionately energy dense. Isoenergetically dense loads of fat and CHO exert less pronounced differences on satiety. Under some conditions HC diets promote excess energy intakes. There is little evidence that a CHO-rich diet, or one with intense sweeteners, promotes spontaneous weight loss.

REFERENCES

1. NATIONAL RESEARCH COUNCIL OF THE USA. 1989. Diet and Health: Implications for reducing chronic risk. National Academic Press. Washington DC.
2. ROYAL COLLEGE OF PHYSICIANS. 1993. Obesity report. J. R. Coll. Physicians Lond. **17:** 3-58.
3. SEIDELL, J. 1995. Obesity in Europe: Scaling an epidemic. Int. J. Obesity 19(Suppl. 3): S1-S4.
4. DANFORTH, E. 1985. Diet and obesity. Am. J. Clin. Nutr. **41:** 1132-1145.
5. LIVESEY, G. & M. ELIA. 1988. Estimations of energy expenditure, net carbohydrate utilisation in calorimetry: Evaluation of errors with special reference to the detailed composition of fuels. Am. J. Clin. Nutr. **47:** 608-628.
6. MCCANCE, R. A. & E. M. WIDDOWSON. 1991. The Composition of Foods. 5th ed. B. Holland, A. A. Welch, I. D. Unwin, D. H. Buss, A. A. Paul & D. A. T. Southgate, Eds. Her Majesty's Stationary Office. London.
7. RUBNER, M. 1885. Calorimetrische untersuchungen. Z. Biol. **19:** 535-562.
8. ATWATER, W. O. 1902. On the digestibility and availability of food materials. Agricultural Experiment Station 14th Annual Report. Storrs, Connecticut.
9. ATWATER, W. O. 1910. Principles of Nutrition and Nutritive Value of Foods. Farmer's Bulletin No. 142. US Department of Agriculture. Washington, DC.
10. MCCANCE, R. A. & E. M. WIDDOWSON. 1978. The Composition of Foods. 4th ed. A. A. Paul & D. A. Southgate, Eds. Her Majesty's Stationary Office. London.
11. BURSZTEIN, S. *et al.* 1989. Energy metabolism indirect calorimetry and nutrition. Williams and Wilkins. Baltimore, Maryland.
12. BLAXTER, K. 1989. Energy metabolism in animals and man. Cambridge University Press. Cambridge, UK.
13. LIVESEY, G. 1992. The energy values of dietary fibre and sugar alcohols in man. Nutr. Res. Rev. **5:** 61-84.
14. LIVESEY, G. 1990. Energy values of unavailable carbohydrate and diets: An inquiry and analysis. Am. J. Clin. Nutr. **51:** 617-637.
15. BRITISH NUTRITION FOUNDATION. 1990. Complex Carbohydrates in Foods. The report of the British Nutrition Foundation's Taskforce. Chapman and Hall. London.
16. MUNRO, H. N. 1951. Carbohydrate and fat as factors in protein utilisation. Physiol. Rev. **32:** 449-488.
17. CALLOWAY, D. H. & H. SPECTOR. 1954. Nitrogen balance as related to caloric and protein intake in active young men. Am. J. Clin. Nutr. **2:** 405-412.
18. YOUNG, V. R., Y-M. YU & N. K. FUKAGAWA. 1992. Whole body energy and nitrogen relationships. *In* Energy Metabolism: Tissue Determinants and Cellular Corollaries. J. M. Kinney & H. N. Tucker, Eds.: 138-160. Raven Press Ltd. New York, NY.
19. FAO/WHO/UNU ENERGY AND PROTEIN REQUIREMENTS. 1985. Report of a joint FAO/WHO/UNU consultation, WHO Geneva. Technical Report Series No. 724. World Health Organization. Geneva.
20. JEQUIER, E. 1992. Calorie balance versus nutrient balance. *In* Energy Metabolism: Tissue Determinants and Cellular Corollaries. J. M. Kinney & H. N. Tucker, Eds.: 123-137. Raven Press Ltd. New York, NY.

21. RAVUSSIN, E. et al. 1986. Short-term mixed diet overfeeding man: No evidence for "luxuskonsumption." Am. J. Physiol. **24:** E470-E477.
22. FORBES, G. B. et al. 1986. Deliberate overfeeding in women and men: Energy cost and composition of the weight gain. Br. J. Nutr. **56:** 1-9.
23. NORGAN, N. G. & J. V. G. A. DURNIN. 1980. The effect of weeks of overfeeding on the body weight, body composition and energy metabolism of young men. Am. J. Clin. Nutr. **33:** 978-988.
24. DIAZ, E. et al. 1992. Metabolic response to experimental overfeeding in lean and overweight healthy volunteers. Am. J. Clin. Nutr. **56:** 641-655.
25. FLATT, J. P. 1978. The biochemistry of energy expenditure. *In* Recent Advances in Obesity Research. G. D. Bray, Ed.: Vol. II: 211-228. Newman Publishing. London.
26. ACHESON, K. J. et al. 1988. Glycogen storage capacity and *de novo* lipogenesis during massive carbohydrate overfeeding in man. Am. J. Clin. Nutr. **48:** 240-247.
27. PULLICCINO, E. & M. ELIA. 1991. Intravenous carbohydrate overfeeding: A method for rapid nutritional repletion. Clin. Nutr. Edinb. **10:** 146-154.
28. HELLERSTEIN, M. K., M. CHRISTIANSEN & S. KAEMPFER. 1991. Measurement of *de novo* hepatic lipogenesis in human beings using stable isotopes. J. Clin. Invest. **87:** 1841-1852.
29. ABBOT, W. G. H. 1988. Short-term energy balance: Relationship with protein, carbohydrate and fat balances. Am. J. Physiol. **255:** E332-E337.
30. SUTER, P. M., Y. SCHUTZ & E. JEQUIER. 1992. The effect of ethanol on fat storage in healthy subjects. N. Engl. J. Med. **326:** 983-987.
31. STUBBS, R. J. 1995. Macronutrient effects on appetite. Int. J. Obesity **19**(Suppl. 5): S11-S20.
32. ACHESON, K. J. & E. JEQUIER. 1982. Glycogen synthesis versus lipogenesis after a 500 gram carbohydrate meal in man. Metabolism **31:** 1234-1240.
33. RANDLE, P. J. 1986. Fuel selection in animals. Biochem. Soc. Trans. **14:** 799-804.
34. FLATT, J. P. 1988. Effects of dietary fat on postprandial substrate oxidation and on carbohydrate and fat balances. J. Clin. Invest. **7:** 1019-1024.
35. FRAYN, K. 1995. Physiological regulation of macronutrient balance. Int. J. Obesity **19**(Suppl. 5): S4-S10.
36. STUBBS, R. J. 1993. Carbohydrate balance and day-to-day food intake in man. Am. J. Clin. Nutr. **57:** 897-903.
37. SHETTY, P. S. 1994. Alterations in fuel selection and voluntary food intake in response to iso-energetic manipulation of glycogen stores in man. Am. J. Clin. Nutr. **60:** 534-543.
38. LEIBEL, R. L. et al. 1992. Energy required to maintain body weight is not affected by wide variation in diet composition. Am. J. Clin. Nutr. **55:** 350-355.
39. MCNEILL, G. et al. 1992. The effect of changes in dietary carbohydrate vs. fat intake on 24 h energy expenditure and nutrient oxidation in post-menopausal women. Proc. Nutr. Soc. **51:** 91A.
40. HORTON, T. J. et al. 1995. Fat and carbohydrate overfeeding in humans: Different effects on energy storage. Am. J. Clin. Nutr. **62:** 19-25.
41. JAMES, W. P. T., G. MCNEILL & A. RALPH. 1990. Metabolism and nutritional adaptation to altered intakes of energy substrates. Am. J. Clin. Nutr. **51:** 264-269.
42. WHITEHEAD, J. M. 1994. Effects of diet composition on energy expenditure during energy restriction. MSc Thesis, University of Aberdeen.
43. MAYER, J. 1955. Regulation of energy intake and the body weight: The glucostatic theory and the lipostatic hypothesis. Ann. N.Y. Acad. Sci. **63:** 15-43.
44. RUSSEK, M. 1963. An hypothesis on the participation of hepatic glucoreceptors in the control of food intake. Nature (Lond.) **197:** 79-80.
45. FLATT, J. P. 1987. The difference in the storage capacities for carbohydrate and for fat, and its implications in the regulation of body weight. Ann. N.Y. Acad. Sci. **499:** 104-123.

46. FERNSTROM, J. D. & R. J. WURTMAN. 1972. Brain serotonin content: Physiological regulation by plasma neutral amino acids. Science **178:** 414-416.
47. FERNSTROM, J. D. 1987. Food induced changes in brain serotonin synthesis: Is there a relationship to appetite for specific macronutrients? Appetite **81:** 63-82.
48. BLUNDELL, J. E. 1990. Serotonin and the biology of feeding. Am. J. Clin. Nutr. **55:** 155S-160S.
49. LISSNER, L. & B. L. HEITMANN. 1995. Dietary fat and obesity: Evidence from epidemiology. Eur. J. Clin. Nutr. **49:** 79-90.
50. BLACK, A. E. et al. 1991. Critical evaluation of energy intake data using fundamental principles of energy physiology: 2. Evaluating the results of published surveys. Eur. J. Clin. Nutr. **45:** 583-599.
51. LISSNER, L. et al. 1987. Dietary fat and the regulation of energy intake in human subjects. Am. J. Clin. Nutr. **46:** 886-892.
52. STUBBS, R. J. et al. 1995. Covert manipulation of dietary fat and energy density: Effect on substrate flux and food intake in men feeding *ad libitum*. Am. J. Clin. Nutr. **62:** 316-330.
53. KENDALL, A. et al. 1991. Weight-loss on a low fat diet: Consequence of the impression of the control of food intake in humans. Am. J. Clin. Nutr. **53:** 1124-1129.
54. JOHNSTONE, A. M., C. G. HARBRON & R. J. STUBBS. 1996. Macronutrients, appetite and day-to-day food intake in humans. Eur. J. Clin. Nutr. **50:** 418-430.
55. TREMBLAY, A. et al. 1991. Nutritional determinants of the increase in energy intake associated with a high-fat diet. Am. J. Clin. Nutr. **53:** 1134-1137.
56. VAN STRATUM, P. et al. 1978. The effect of dietary carbohydrate: Fat ratio on energy intake by adult women. Am. J. Clin. Nutr. **31:** 206-212.
57. STUBBS, R. J., C. G. HARBRON & A. M. PRENTICE. 1996. The effect of covertly manipulating the dietary fat to carbohydrate ratio of isoenergetically dense diets on *ad libitum* food intake in free-living humans. Int. J. Obesity **20:** 651-660.
58. CAMPFIELD, L. A. & F. J. SMITH. 1990. Transient declines in blood glucose signal meal initiation. Int. J. Obesity **14**(Suppl 3): 15-33.
59. CAMPFIELD, L. A. et al. 1992. Human hunger: Is there a role for blood glucose dynamics? Appetite **18:** 244 (letter).
60. FRIEDMAN, M. I. & M. G. TORDOFF. 1986. Fatty acid oxidation and glucose utilisation interact to control food intake in rats. Am. J. Physiol. **251:** R840-R845.
61. RABEN, A. 1995. Appetite and carbohydrate metabolism. PhD thesis, Royal Veterinary and Agricultural University. Copenhagen.
62. WALLS, E. K. & H. S. KOOPMANS. 1992. Differential effects of intravenous glucose, amino acids and lipid on daily food intake in rats. Am. J. Physiol. **262:** R225-R234.
63. GIL, K. et al. 1991. Parenteral nutrition and oral intake: Effect of glucose and fat infusion. J. Pen. **15:** 426-432.
64. RITTER, S. & N. Y. CLINGASAN. 1994. Neural substrates for metabolic controls of feeding. *In* Appetite and Body Weight Regulation: Sugar, Fat and Macronutrient Substitutes. J. D. Fernstrom & G. D. Miller, Eds. CRC Press. Boca Raton, Florida.
65. MATTES, R. D. 1996. Dietary compensation by humans for supplemental energy provided as ethanol or carbohydrate in fluids. Physiol. Behav. **59:** 179-187.
66. BLUNDELL, J. E. 1996. Food intake and body weight regulation. *In* Regulation of body weight: Biological and behavioural mechanisms. Dahlem Workshop Reports, Life Sciences Research Report 57. C. Bouchard & G. Bray, Eds. John Wiley and Sons Ltd. Chichester, England.
67. FRYER J. H. 1958. The effects of a late-night caloric supplement upon body weight and food intake in man. Am. J. Clin. Nutr. **6:** 354-364.
68. LEVINE, A. S. & C. J. BILLINGTON. 1994. Dietary fibre: Does it affect food intake and body weight? *In* Appetite and Body Weight Regulation: Sugar, Fat and Macronutrient Substitutes. J. D. Fernstrom & G. D. Miller, Eds. CRC Press. Boca Raton, Florida.

69. BLUNDELL, J. E. & V. J. BURLEY. 1987. Satiation, satiety and the action of fibre on food intake. Int. J. Obesity **11** (Suppl. 1): 9.
70. BURLEY, V. J. & J. E. BLUNDELL. 1990. Action of dietary fibre on the satiety cascade. *In* Dietary Fibre: Chemistry, Physiology and Health Effects. D. Kritchevsky, C. Bonfield & J. W. Anderson, Eds. Plenum Press. New York, NY.
71. STEVENS, J. 1988. Does dietary fibre affect food intake and body weight? J. Am. Diet. Assoc. **88**: 939.
72. BOOTH, D. A., J. RODIN & G. L. BLACKBURN, Eds. 1988. Sweeteners, Appetite and Obesity. Proceedings of the workshop entitled. The Effect of Sweeteners on Food Intake, held by the North American Association for the Study of Obesity. Boston, Massachusetts, 14 October 1987. Appetite **11**(Suppl. 1).
73. CLYDESDALE, F. M. Ed. 1995. Nutritional and health aspects of sugars. Proceedings of a workshop held in Washington DC, May 2-5, 1994. Am. J. Clin. Nutr. **62**(Suppl. 1).
74. PORIKOS, K. P. & T. B. VAN ITALLIE. 1984. Efficacy of low-calorie sweeteners in reducing food intake. *In* Aspartame: Physiology and Biochemistry. L. D. Stegink, Ed. Marcel Dekker Inc. New York, NY.
75. BLUNDELL, J. E. & P. J. ROGERS. 1994. Sweet carbohydrate substitutes (intense sweeteners) and the control of appetite: Scientific issues. *In* Appetite and Body Weight Regulation: Sugar, Fat and Macronutrient Substitutes. J. D. Fernstrom & G. D. Miller, Eds. CRC Press. Boca Raton, Florida.
76. BLACK, R. M. & G. H. ANDERSON. 1994. Sweeteners, food intake and selection. *In* Appetite and Body Weight Regulation: Sugar, Fat and Macronutrient Substitutes. J. D. Fernstrom & G. D. Miller, Eds. CRC Press. Boca Raton, Florida.
77. NAISMITH, D. J. & C. RHODES. 1995. Adjustment in energy intake following the covert removal of sugar from the diet. J. Hum. Nutr. Diet. **8**: 167-175.

Impact of Macronutrient Substitutes on the Composition of the Diet and the U.S. Food Supply

REBECCA MORGAN,[a] MADELEINE SIGMAN-GRANT,[b]
DENISE S. TAYLOR,[a] KRISTIN MORIARTY,[a]
VALERIE FISHELL,[a]
AND PENNY M. KRIS-ETHERTON[a,c]

*Departments of Nutrition[a] and Food Science[b]
The Pennsylvania State University
University Park, Pennsylvania 16802*

INTRODUCTION

Contemporary dietary recommendations target total fat and saturated fat reductions as ways to lower the risk of the major chronic diseases in the United States. Numerous governmental and health organizations recommend that dietary total fat and saturated fat be reduced to ≤ 30% and ≤ 10% of energy, respectively, and that dietary cholesterol be less than 300 mg/day.[1,2] In addition, these dietary recommendations include achieving and maintaining a healthy weight; increasing fruit, vegetable, and fiber intake; reducing sodium in the diet; and consuming alcohol in moderation, if at all.

Dietary recommendations must be translated into food practices that are practical and easy to implement. Recently, several reports used computer simulations and mathematical models to examine the effect of various dietary manipulations, including dietary fat-reduction strategies, on both the nutrient profile and the energy content of the diet.[3-5] These studies were conducted using databases from the Continuing Survey of Food Intake by Individuals (CSFII) prior to 1989, population intake data from the second National Health and Nutrition Examination Survey (NHANES II), as well as use of fat-modified products available at that time. Collectively, these studies showed that a variety of strategies can be used to reduce total and saturated fat and achieve recommended levels of key nutrients. Moreover, these studies suggest that relatively moderate changes in selected food groups (*e.g.*, dairy products; meat, poultry and fish; and fat-modified products) can readily result in achieving contemporary dietary recommendations.

Since the original modeling and simulation studies were conducted, the average American diet appears to have changed. NHANES III data[6] indicate that the intake (as a percent of energy) of total fat and saturated fat has decreased. Presently, total fat comprises approximately 34-35% of energy and saturated fat provides 11-12%

---

[c] Address correspondence to P.M. Kris-Etherton, Department of Nutrition, the Pennsylvania State University, S-126 Henderson Building, University Park, PA 16802. Tel: (814) 863-2923; fax: (814) 863-6103; e-mail: pmk3@psu.edu.

of energy. Other surveys conducted prior to NHANES III reported that total fat was 36–37% of energy and saturated fat was 14% of energy.[7] Thus, the results of NHANES III have provided more recent intake data for total and saturated fat. In addition, the availability of fat-modified products has markedly increased. The introduction of an unprecedented number of fat-modified products include many that were unimaginable a few years ago (*e.g.,* fat-free meat products, snacks, and desserts). Recently, the Nutrition Committee of the American Heart Association released dietary recommendations, including for the first time a lower limit of 15% of calories from fat.[8] Therefore, there is a need to provide a more up-to-date perspective regarding the impact of various fat-reduction strategies on the nutrient profile of the diet. The availability of a large number of fat-modified products makes it plausible that individuals could reduce their fat intake too much. In addition, there is a growing scientific consensus that a diet higher in total fat (~35% of calories), yet low in saturated fat, may be preferable for certain individuals (most notably, persons with diabetes and Syndrome X).[9,10] With this in mind, we used various fat-reduction strategies to reduce both total and saturated fat. In addition, food sources rich in monounsaturated fat were isocalorically added back to the model, allowing modification of fat quality but not fat quantity.

The purpose of this paper was to examine the impact of applying single and multiple fat-reduction strategies on the energy content and macronutrient profile of a typical American diet. The impact of making isocaloric adjustments with food sources high in carbohydrate or monounsaturated fat also was assessed. Any fat-modified diet certainly must be nutritionally adequate. Thus, the nutritional quality of the dietary simulations generated also was evaluated. In addition, because population-based dietary changes clearly will have a significant impact on the food supply, an estimate of how changes in food practices in the United States might affect the food supply has been included.

COMPUTER SIMULATIONS: EFFECTS OF THE APPLICATION OF VARIOUS FAT-REDUCTION STRATEGIES ON THE MACRO- AND MICRONUTRIENT PROFILE OF THE DIET

Methods

Three one-day menus for both men and women were developed using the Nutritionist IV database (N-Squared Computing, First Data Bank Division, San Bruno, CA). Recent NHANES III data indicate that men consume an average of 2600 calories per day and 34% energy from fat, whereas women consume an average of 1800 calories per day and 34% energy from fat.[6] Thus, these were the target goals for both calories and percent energy from fat for the baseline diets for men and women. TABLES 1A and 1B show the baseline diets for men and women, respectively, across a three-day simulation period. These menus include a wide variety of food items in all food groups. For example, different meat products (such as chicken, turkey, ground beef, bacon, and hot dogs) and various fruits, vegetables, grains, and dairy products (including carrots, salads, broccoli, peas, bananas, strawberries, apples, breads, cereals, toaster pastries, cheese, and yogurt) were used. In addition, these diets included

TABLE 1A. Three-day Menus for Men

Breakfast
  Cereal, granola (0.75 c)
  Milk, whole (6 oz)
  Orange juice (8 oz)
Lunch
  Turkey sandwich
    Whole wheat bread
      (2 slices)
    Turkey breast (4 oz)
    Swiss cheese (1 oz)
    Mayonnaise (1 T)
    Lettuce (1 leaf)
    Tomato (2 slices)
  Carrots (2)
  Apple (1 medium)
  Soda (12 oz)
Snack
  Wheat crackers (12)
  Apple juice (12 oz)
Dinner
  Chicken pot pie (1 serving)
  French roll (2)
    Margarine (2 t)
  Green salad (1 serving)
    Ranch dressing (1 T)
  Fruit salad (1 c)
  Milk, whole (6 oz)
  Cookie, chocolate chip (2)
	Breakfast
	  Scrambled eggs (2)
	  Bacon (2 slices)
	  White toast (2 slices)
	    Margarine (2 t)
	  Strawberries, whole
	    (1.5 c)
	  Milk, whole (8 oz)
	  Coffee (12 oz)
	    Sugar, white (2 t)
	    Milk, whole (2 T)
	Lunch
	  Cheese pizza (1 serving)
	  Green salad (1 serving)
	    Italian dressing (1 T)
	  Banana (1 small)
	  Lemonade (12 oz)
	Snack
	  Pretzels (1.5 c)
	  Grape juice drink (8 oz)
	Dinner
	  Beef patty (1 serving)
	  White rice (1 c)
	  Snap beans (2 c)
	  Minestrone soup (1 c)
	  Milk, whole (8 oz)
	  Chocolate cake (1 slice)
		Breakfast
		  Toaster pastry (1)
		  Yogurt (1 serving)
		  Fruit cocktail (1 c)
		  Coffee (12 oz)
		    Sugar, white (2 t)
		    Milk, whole (2 T)
		
		Lunch
		  Cheese sandwich
		    Wheat bread (2 slices)
		    Cheddar cheese (2.5 oz)
		    Margarine (1 T)
		  Potato chips (1 oz)
		  Peas and carrots (8 oz)
		  Soda (12 oz)
		Dinner
		  Hot dog (2)
		    Hot dog roll (2)
		    Ketchup (2 T)
		    Relish (2 T)
		  Baked beans (0.5 c)
		  Green salad (1 serving)
		    Italian dressing (1 T)
		  Fruit punch (6 oz)
		Snack
		  Milk, whole (8 oz)
		  Brownie (2)

common foods that could be modified to incorporate lower-fat versions of milk and meat products, snacks, and desserts.

Food Substitutions

After developing the baseline menus, fat-modified foods were substituted for their higher-fat counterparts, and changes in energy, percent energy from fat and saturated fat, and other nutrients averaged over three days were determined. For men, whole milk was used in the baseline menus. The baseline menus for women contained 2% milk. "Baseline milk" was replaced with 2%, 1%, skim milk, or whole milk (for women). Leaner, and in some cases, nonfat meats were substituted for their higher-fat counterparts. There are many fat-modified products available to consumers. These include both low-fat and nonfat versions of foods classified for the present

TABLE 1B. Three-day Menus for Women

Breakfast
  Cereal, granola (0.5 c)
  Milk, 2% (6 oz)
  Orange juice (6 oz)
 	
Lunch
  Turkey sandwich
    Whole wheat bread
      (2 slices)
    Turkey breast (2 oz)
    Swiss cheese (0.5 oz)
    Mayonnaise (1 T)
    Lettuce (1 leaf)
    Tomato (2 slices)
  Soda (8 oz)
 	
Snack
  Wheat crackers (6)
  Apple (1 medium)
 	
Dinner
  Chicken breast (0.75)
  French roll (1)
    Margarine (2 t)
  Green salad (1 serving)
    Ranch dressing (1 T)
  Broccoli (1.5 c)
  Milk, 2% (6 oz)
  Cookie, chocolate chip (2)
	Breakfast
	  Scrambled egg (1)
	  White toast (2 slices)
	    Margarine (1 T)
	  Strawberries, whole (1 c)
	  Milk, 2% (6 oz)
	  Coffee (12 oz)
	    Sugar, white (2 t)
	    Milk, 2% (2 T)
	
	Lunch
	  Cheese pizza (1 serving)
	  Banana (0.5 small)
	  Soda (12 oz)
	
	Dinner
	  Beef patty (1 serving)
	  White rice (1 c)
	  Snap beans (1 c)
	  Minestrone soup (0.5 c)
	  Milk, 2% (8 oz)
	  Chocolate cake (1 slice)
		Breakfast
		  Toaster pastry (1)
		  Yogurt (0.5 serving)
		  Fruit cocktail (0.5 c)
		  Coffee (12 oz)
		    Sugar, white (2 t)
		    Milk, 2% (2 T)
		
		Lunch
		  Cheese sandwich
		    Wheat bread (1 slice)
		    Cheddar cheese (1.5 oz)
		    Margarine (1 T)
		  Potato chips (0.5 oz)
		  Peas and carrots (8 oz)
		  Tea, unsweetened (12 oz)
		
		Dinner
		  Hot dog (1)
		  Hot dog roll (1)
		  Ketchup (1 T)
		  Relish (1 T)
		  Baked beans (0.75 c)
		  Green salad (1 serving)
		    Italian dressing (1 T)
		  Fruit punch (6 oz)
		
		Snack
		  Milk, 2% (8 oz)
		  Brownie (1)

computer analysis as follows: cheese and yogurt, desserts (cookies, cakes, brownies), eggs and beans, grains (bread, cereals, toaster pastries), other (margarine, mayonnaise, salad dressing), and snacks (chips, crackers, pretzels). In addition to assessing the substitution of either low-fat or nonfat versions of single food categories on the nutrient profile of the diet, exclusive use of all fat-modified products was examined (*e.g.*, the sum of the six categories). Because assessing the impact of carbohydrate substitutes on the diet also was of interest, and because diet soda is the most widely used carbohydrate-modified product, diet soda was substituted for regular soda in the menus, and the impact was assessed.

After performing these single strategies, a combination of strategies, including both moderate and extreme changes, was implemented. For example, for men, changes from whole to 2% milk and from regular to lean meat were considered to be moderate changes, whereas changes from regular to very lean meat, from whole to skim milk, and from regular to nonfat products were classified as extreme. Realizing that a decrease in fat often results in a decrease in calories as well, several simulations were performed for both men and women in which calories were added back as either carbohydrate (in the form of fruits and fruit juices) or monounsaturated fat (as olive oil or peanuts) to make the menus isocaloric. This was done to assess the magnitude of a further decrease in percent energy from fat (when carbohydrate calories were added) and the change in the fat composition of the diets when food sources of monounsaturated fat were added isocalorically.

In addition to these manipulations, the nutrient profile of the diets was evaluated to see if any nutrients were low (*e.g.,* < 2/3 of the RDA). The following micronutrients were examined: vitamin A, vitamin D, vitamin E, vitamin C, vitamin B_6, folate, sodium, iron, calcium, zinc, and magnesium. All micronutrients met at least 67% of the RDA at baseline.

Results

TABLES 2A through 2D present the results of the computer-simulated fat-reduction strategies for total fat, saturated fat, monounsaturated fat, and polyunsaturated fat, as well as for protein, carbohydrate, dietary fiber, and cholesterol. The effects of these strategies on the micronutrient content of the diets for both men and women are shown in TABLES 3A and 3B.

Percent energy from fat decreased for men and women when lower-fat versions of milk were included in the diets (TABLES 2A, 2B). Percent energy from fat decreased from 34% (whole milk) to 33% (2% milk), 32% (1% milk), or 31% (skim milk) for men, and from 34% (2% milk) to 33% (1% milk) or 32% (skim milk) for women. Thus, a gradual decrease was noted in percent energy from fat with the substitution of milk containing progressively less fat for higher-fat counterparts (*e.g.,* either whole milk or 2% milk).

When a variety of lean meats or very lean meats were substituted for their higher-fat counterparts, similar decreases in percent energy from fat were noted (TABLES 2A, 2B). Percent energy from fat for men decreased from 34% (higher-fat versions) to 31% with lean meats and to 30% with very lean meats, whereas, for women, the total percentage from fat decreased from 34% to 32% with both lean meats and very lean meats.

Substitution of some low-fat and nonfat products for their full-fat counterparts (*e.g.,* snacks or desserts, which are consumed in relatively small amounts) revealed that there was little or no effect on total percent energy from fat, whereas other strategies, such as substitutions with the other product category (including foods eaten frequently: margarine, mayonnaise, and salad dressing), showed a greater impact (TABLES 2C, 2D). Dietary fat levels for men were unchanged with the use of low-fat snacks, but decreased to 33% with low-fat desserts and grains, to 32% with low-fat cheese and yogurt, and to 31% with substitutions in the "other" product category. In women, the same trend was observed with the inclusion of these low-fat products. When the sum of these low-fat strategies was applied in women, total fat decreased to 24%, and in men total fat decreased to 26% (TABLES 2A, 2B).

Substitution of nonfat products for their full-fat counterparts in the diets of men and women showed similar, albeit, more extreme trends (TABLES 2A, 2B, 2C, 2D).

TABLE 2A. Use of Fat-modified Products in Men on the Nutrient Profile of the Diet

	Baseline	Milk Substitutions			Meat Substitutions		Fat-modified Products	
		2%	1%	Skim	Lean Meats[a]	Very Lean Meats[b]	Low fat	Nonfat
Energy (kcal)	2719	2673	2643	2617	2630	2606	2417	2245
Fat (g)	104	98	95	91	90	88	69	45
SFA[c] (g)	37	34	32	30	33	32	26	18
MUFA[d] (g)	34	33	32	31	27	27	21	16
PUFA[e] (g)	21	20	20	20	18	18	12	6
Fat (% energy)	34	33	32	31	31	30	26	18
SFA (% energy)	12	11	11	10	11	11	10	7
MUFA (% energy)	11	11	11	10	9	9	8	6
PUFA (% energy)	7	7	7	7	6	6	4	2
Protein (% energy)	13	14	14	14	14	14	15	17
Carbohydrate (% energy)	53	53	54	55	55	56	59	65
Cholesterol (mg)	350	326	313	305	332	302	313	150
Fiber (g)	19	19	19	19	20	20	25	27

[a] Lean meats include lower-fat versions of turkey lunch meat, bacon, ground beef, hot dogs, chicken, and chicken pot pies.
[b] Very lean meats include nonfat turkey lunch meat and hotdogs, as well as lower-fat versions of bacon, ground beef, chicken, and chicken pot pies.
[c] Saturated fat.
[d] Monounsaturated fat.
[e] Polyunsaturated fat.

TABLE 2B. Use of Fat-modified Products in Women on the Nutrient Profile of the Diet

		Milk Substitutions			Meat Substitutions		Fat-modified Products	
	Baseline	2%	1%	Skim	Lean Meats[a]	Very Lean Meats[b]	Low fat	Nonfat
Energy (kcal)	1845	1889	1817	1792	1793	1778	1639	1490
Fat (g)	71	76	68	64	65	63	45	27
SFA (g)	24	28	22	20	22	22	16	11
MUFA (g)	23	25	22	21	20	20	13	9
PUFA (g)	14	15	14	14	13	13	9	3
Fat (% energy)	34	36	33	32	32	32	24	16
SFA (% energy)	12	13	11	10	11	11	9	7
MUFA (% energy)	11	12	11	11	10	10	7	6
PUFA (% energy)	7	7	7	7	7	7	5	2
Protein (% energy)	16	16	17	17	17	17	19	21
Carbohydrate (% energy)	50	48	50	51	51	51	57	63
Cholesterol (mg)	233	256	220	212	225	210	206	123
Fiber (g)	16	16	16	16	16	16	20	21

[a] Lean meats include lower-fat versions of turkey lunch meat, bacon, ground beef, hot dogs, chicken, and chicken pot pies.
[b] Very lean meats include nonfat turkey lunch meat and hot dogs, as well as lower-fat versions of bacon, ground beef, chicken, and chicken pot pies.

TABLE 2C. Use of Individual Fat-modified Products in Men on the Nutrient Profile of the Diet

	Cheese & Yogurt		Desserts[a]		Eggs & Beans	Grains[b]		Other[c]		Snacks[d]	
	Low fat	Nonfat	Low fat	Nonfat	Nonfat	Low fat	Nonfat	Low fat	Nonfat	Low fat	Nonfat
Energy (kcal)	2683	2635	2672	2645	2690	2610	2598	2624	2562	2704	2711
Fat (g)	95	93	98	94	100	97	96	91	84	102	98
SFA (g)	33	30	37	35	36	34	33	35	34	37	36
MUFA (g)	30	31	32	31	33	33	32	30	29	33	31
PUFA (g)	20	20	18	18	20	20	20	16	12	21	19
Fat (% energy)	32	32	33	32	33	33	33	31	30	34	32
SFA (% energy)	11	10	12	12	12	12	12	12	12	12	12
MUFA (% energy)	10	11	11	10	11	11	11	10	10	11	10
PUFA (% energy)	6	7	6	6	7	7	7	5	4	7	6
Protein (% energy)	14	14	13	14	13	14	14	14	14	13	14
Carbohydrate (% energy)	54	54	54	54	54	53	53	55	56	53	54
Cholestrol (mg)	335	313	332	332	209	350	350	346	354	350	350
Fiber (g)	20	19	20	21	18	23	24	19	19	20	21

[a] Desserts include chocolate-chip cookies, chocolate cake, and brownies.
[b] Grains include wheat bread, granola cereal, and toaster pastries.
[c] Other includes mayonnaise, margarine, and salad dressing.
[d] Snacks include wheat crackers, pretzels, and potato chips.

TABLE 2D. Use of Individual Fat-modified Products in Women on the Nutrient Profile of the Diet

	Cheese & Yogurt		Desserts[a]		Eggs & Beans		Grains[b]		Other[c]		Snacks[d]	
	Low fat	Nonfat	Low fat	Nonfat	Low fat	Nonfat	Low fat	Nonfat	Low fat	Nonfat	Low fat	Nonfat
Energy (kcal)	1829	1799	1801	1778		1834	1770	1762	1764	1699	1837	1845
Fat (g)	65	65	66	64		69	66	65	60	53	70	68
SFA (g)	21	20	24	23		24	22	22	23	21	24	24
MUFA (g)	20	21	21	20		22	22	22	19	18	22	22
PUFA (g)	14	14	13	13		14	14	14	11	7	14	14
Fat (% energy)	32	32	33	32		34	33	33	31	28	34	33
SFA (% energy)	11	10	12	11		12	11	11	11	11	12	12
MUFA (% energy)	10	11	11	10		11	11	11	10	9	11	11
PUFA (% energy)	7	7	6	6		7	7	7	6	4	7	7
Protein (% energy)	17	17	17	17		16	17	17	17	18	17	17
Carbohydrate (% energy)	51	51	50	51		50	50	50	52	54	49	50
Cholesterol (mg)	225	212	219	219		163	233	233	229	229	233	233
Fiber (g)	17	16	17	18		15	19	19	16	16	16	17

[a] Desserts include chocolate-chip cookies, chocolate cake, and brownies.
[b] Grains include wheat bread, granola cereal, and toaster pastries.
[c] Other includes mayonnaise, margarine, and salad dressing.
[d] Snacks include wheat crackers, pretzels, and potato chips.

TABLE 3A. Use of Fat-modified Products in Men on the Micronutrient Profile of the Diet

		Milk Substitutions			Meat Substitutions		Fat-modified Products	
	Baseline	2%	1%	Skim	Lean Meats[a]	Very Lean Meats[b]	Low fat	Nonfat
Vitamin A (RE[d])	2908	3008	3016	3024	2989	2989	2848	2960
Vitamin D (μg)	6	6	6	6	6	6	5	4
Vitamin C (mg)	198	198	198	198	190	189	200	200
Vitamin B$_6$ (mg)	1.8	1.8	1.8	1.8	1.7	1.7	1.8	1.5
Folate (μg)	352	353	353	353	342	342	326	275
Sodium (mg)	4201	4204	4206	4210	4040	4177	4275	4064
Iron (mg)	15	15	15	15	15	15	15	16
Calcium (mg)	1290	1299	1304	1307	1311	1310	1268	1292
Magnesium (mg)	339	340	340	331	328	329	281	247
Zinc (mg)	12	12	12	12	11	11	11	9
Vitamin E (mg α-TE)[c]	9	−0%	−0%	−0%	−0%	−0%	−50%	−75%

[a] Lean meats include lower-fat versions of turkey lunch meat, bacon, ground beef, hot dogs, chicken, and chicken pot pies.
[b] Very lean meats include nonfat turkey lunch meat and hot dogs, as well as lower-fat versions of bacon, ground beef, chicken, and chicken pot pies.
[c] Baseline value was obtained from the University of Minnesota Nutrient Data System (NDS) due to missing values in Nutritionist IV. However, percent decreases were calculated based on values reported by Nutritionist IV. α-TE=alpha tocopherol equivalents.
[d] Retinol equivalents.

TABLE 3B. Use of Fat-modified Products in Women on the Micronutrient Profile of the Diet

	Milk Substitutions				Meat Substitutions		Fat-modified Products	
	Baseline	2%	1%	Skim	Lean Meats[a]	Very Lean Meats[b]	Low fat	Nonfat
Vitamin A (RE)	1521	1529	1537	1426	1511	1511	1473	1547
Vitamin D (µg)	5	5	5	5	5	5	4	4
Vitamin C (mg)	152	152	152	152	148	147	154	153
Vitamin B$_6$ (mg)	1.5	1.5	1.5	1.5	1.5	1.5	1.5	1.3
Folate (µg)	302	302	302	301	301	301	283	235
Sodium (mg)	2603	2605	2609	2600	2493	2561	2579	2385
Iron (mg)	11	11	11	11	11	11	10	12
Calcium (mg)	1032	1037	1040	1023	1030	1029	1041	1059
Magnesium (mg)	272	272	264	271	270	270	232	201
Zinc (mg)	10	10	10	10	9	9	9	7
Vitamin E (mg α-TE)[c]	8	–0%	–0%	–0%	–25%	–25%	–75%	–75%

[a] Lean meats include lower-fat versions of turkey lunch meat, bacon, ground beef, hot dogs, chicken, and chicken pot pies.
[b] Very lean means include nonfat turkey lunch meat and hot dogs, as well as lower-fat versions of bacon, ground beef, chicken, and chicken pot pies.
[c] Baseline value was obtained from the University of Minnesota Nutrient Data System (NDS) due to missing values in Nutritionist IV. However, percent decreases were calculated based on values reported by Nutritionist IV.

For men, total fat decreased to 33% with nonfat eggs and beans and grains, to 32% with nonfat snacks, desserts, and cheese and yogurt, and to 30% with the "other" product category (nonfat margarine, mayonnaise, and salad dressing). The sum of these categorized substitutions decreased total fat to 18%. Nonfat eggs and beans did not impact the diets of women (possibly due to smaller portion sizes), but nonfat snacks and grains decreased total fat to 33%, whereas nonfat desserts, and cheese and yogurt decreased total fat to 32%. Substitution of the "other" category resulted in 28% energy from total fat, whereas use of all nonfat products resulted in 16% energy from fat in the diets of women.

Reductions in saturated fat were also observed with the implementation of various strategies (TABLES 2A, 2B). Percent energy from saturated fat decreased from 12% to 11%, 11%, or 10% with the use of 2%, 1%, or skim milk, respectively, in men. Also, implementation of 1% or skim milk in women decreased percent energy from saturated fat from 12% to 11% or 10%, respectively. Use of lean and very lean meats showed reductions in percent energy from saturated fat, with the implementation of either lower-fat version decreasing saturated fat to 11% in both men and women. Use of nonfat cheese and yogurt as a single fat-reduction strategy was able to meet the saturated fat goal of ≤10% of energy from saturated fat (TABLES 2C, 2D). Implementation of other single fat-modified strategies did not achieve the dietary goal for saturated fat. Obviously, the large decreases in saturated fat observed with the use of lower-fat versions of milk and meat products reflects the greater amount of saturated fat present in these food sources. However, dramatic decreases in total fat can likewise result in marked decreases in saturated fat (TABLES 2A, 2B). Exclusive use of nonfat products resulted in a reduction of saturated fat to 7% of energy in both men and women. Thus, reasonable reductions in saturated fat may be achieved by decreasing dietary fat intake from specific food groups (*e.g.,* meat and dairy products) or by significantly reducing total fat intake in general.

Dietary recommendations might be better met with the implementation of multiple fat-reduction strategies. We defined moderate strategies as the use of either 2% milk, lean meat, or low-fat products; whereas, skim milk, very lean meats, and nonfat products were considered extreme. The effects of these multiple strategies are shown in FIGURE 1. Percent energy from fat was reduced to 29% in men and to 31% in women with the implementation of two moderate strategies (*e.g.,* 2% milk and lean meats). Combination of a moderate and extreme strategy (*e.g.,* 2% milk and nonfat products) decreased percent energy from fat even further—to 16% in men and 15% in women. It is possible to markedly decrease dietary fat by using all three extreme strategies (skim milk, very lean meats, and nonfat products). When all of these very low and nonfat versions were substituted for their higher-fat counterparts, the percent energy from total fat decreased to 7% in men and to 8% in women, respectively. Thus, various multiple fat-reduction strategies can be applied, and, depending upon the strategies implemented, small or nominal, to very marked, effects on dietary fat can be achieved.

A decrease in the total energy content of the diets resulting from the implementation of different fat-reduction strategies was also observed (TABLES 4 and 5). In men, a change from whole to 2% milk led to an average daily reduction of 46 kcals, a change to 1% milk of 76 kcals, and a change to skim milk of 102 kcals per day. Similarly, in women a change from 2% to 1% milk reduced energy content by 28

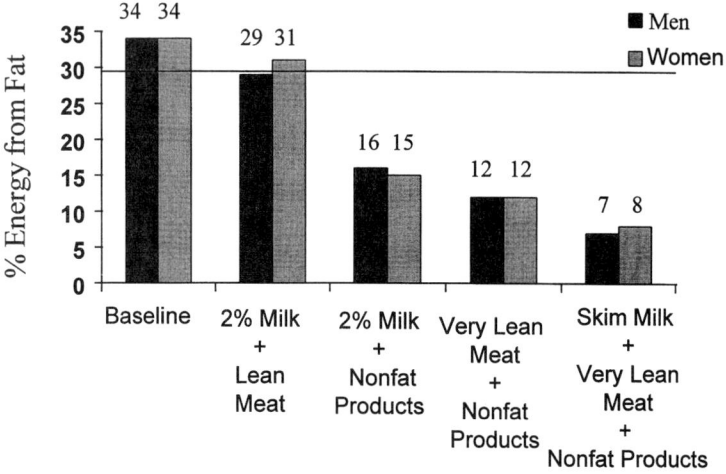

FIGURE 1. Percent energy from fat in the diets of men and women at baseline and compared to four combination strategies. Combination strategies include two moderate strategies (2% milk and lean meat), a moderate and extreme strategy (2% milk and nonfat products), two extreme strategies (very lean meat and nonfat products), and three extreme strategies (skim milk, very lean meat, and nonfat products).

TABLE 4. Reduction in Average Daily Energy with Milk and Meat Strategies (kcals)

Baseline	Men 2719	Women 1845
Strategy		
Whole ⇒ 2% milk	46	—
Whole or 2% ⇒ 1% milk	76	28
Whole or 2% ⇒ skim milk	102	53
Higher fat ⇒ lean meat	89	52
Higher fat ⇒ very lean meat	113	67

kcals, and use of skim milk led to a reduction of 53 kcals per day. Replacement with lean or very lean meat for their higher-fat counterparts led to a reduction of 89 or 113 kcals, respectively, in men. Likewise, these same fat-reduction strategies resulted in a reduction of 52 and 67 kcals in women.

Fat-modified strategies (low-fat and nonfat) had moderate to extreme effects on the total energy content of the diet (TABLE 5). Nonfat snacks had the most modest effect on energy, leading to an 8 kcal reduction in men and no decrease in energy in women. The "other" category (margarine, mayonnaise, and salad dressing) had the greatest impact on the energy content of the diet. Use of low-fat products in this

TABLE 5. Reduction in Energy with Fat-modified Products (kcals)

Fat-modified Product	Men		Women	
	Low fat	Nonfat	Low fat	Nonfat
Snacks	15	8	8	0
Eggs & beans	–	29	–	11
Cheese & yogurt	36	84	16	46
Desserts	47	74	44	67
Grains	109	121	75	83
Other	95	157	81	146
Total	**302**	**473**	**224**	**353**

TABLE 6. Percent Energy from Fat with Isocaloric Substitution of Carbohydrates

	Men	Women
Skim milk		
Hypocaloric	31%	32%
Isocaloric	30% (+102 kcal)	31% (+39 kcal)
Very lean meat		
Hypocaloric	30%	32%
Isocaloric	29% (+113 kcal)	31% (+67 kcal)
Nonfat products		
Hypocaloric	18%	16%
Isocaloric	15% (+474 kcal)	13% (+355 kcal)

category led to a 95 kcal reduction per day in men and a decrease of 81 kcals in women. Nonfat products in this same category almost doubled the decrease in energy in both men and women, leading to a reduction of 157 kcals in men and 146 kcals in women. Marked decreases in energy content were observed if the sum of these low-fat and nonfat strategies were applied. Use of all nonfat products resulted in a 473 kcal reduction in men and a decrease of 353 kcals in women.

It is interesting to note that when the menus were made isocaloric by adding back energy as carbohydrate, percent energy from fat was decreased even further (TABLE 6). With skim milk and very lean meats, isocaloric substitutions decreased percent energy from fat by an additional 1% in both men and women. For nonfat products, isocaloric substitutions led to a 3% further decrease in men and women.

Amounts of specific oils (olive or canola) and nuts (peanuts or mixed nuts), products high in monounsaturated fat, that could be added to the diets of men and women after implementation of various fat-reduction strategies to make them isocaloric are shown in TABLES 7 and 8. Effects of isocaloric substitutions of either peanuts or olive oil on the fat composition of the diets of men and women appear in TABLES

TABLE 7. Amounts of Different Foods High in Monounsaturated Fat Required for Isocaloric Substitution of Fat-modified Menus for Men

	Olive or Canola Oil (tsp)	Peanuts or Mixed Nuts (# of nuts)
Milk		
Whole ⇒ 2%	~1	11
Whole ⇒ 1%	~2	18.5
Whole ⇒ skim	~2.5	25
Meat		
Higher fat ⇒ lean	~2	22
Higher fat ⇒ very lean	~2.75	27.5

TABLE 8. Amounts of Different Foods High in Monounsaturated Fat Required for Isocaloric Substitution of Fat-modified Menus for Men

	Olive or Canola Oil (tsp)	Peanuts or Mixed Nuts (# of nuts)
Cheese and yogurt		
Regular ⇒ low fat	~1	9
Regular ⇒ nonfat	~2.5	24
Desserts		
Regular ⇒ low fat	~2	11.5
Regular ⇒ nonfat	~2	18
Grains		
Regular ⇒ low fat	~2.75	26.5
Regular ⇒ nonfat	~3.75	37.5
Other		
Regular ⇒ low fat	~2.5	23
Regular ⇒ nonfat	~3.75	38.5
Snacks		
Regular ⇒ low fat	~1/12	0.75
Regular ⇒ nonfat	~1/10	2
Eggs and beans		
Regular ⇒ nonfat	~1	10.5

9A and 9B. Although both peanuts and olive oil are rich sources of monounsaturated fat, peanuts are a source of protein as well, and, as a result, isocaloric substitutions of these two products have slightly different impacts on the fat content of the diets. When peanuts were isocalorically added back to the diets containing skim milk or lean meats, total fat decreased from baseline in men (*e.g.*, from 34% to 33% energy from fat). In addition, a greater decrease in percent energy from fat was observed in the menus containing all low-fat products (31%) and all nonfat products (28%) with the isocaloric substitution of peanuts in men. A similar trend was observed for

TABLE 9A. Isocaloric Substitutions in Men

Isocaloric substitutions with peanuts

	Total Fat (g)	Total Fat (%)	SFA (g)	SFA (%)	MUFA (g)	MUFA (%)	PUFA (g)	PUFA (%)
Baseline	104	34	37	12	34	11	21	7
Skim milk	100	33	31	10	35	12	23	7
Lean meats	98	33	34	11	31	10	20	6
Low-fat substitutions	95	31	30	10	34	11	20	7
Nonfat substitutions	85	28	24	8	36	12	19	6

Isocaloric substitutions with olive oil

	Total Fat (g)	Total Fat (%)	SFA (g)	SFA (%)	MUFA (g)	MUFA (%)	PUFA (g)	PUFA (%)
Baseline	104	34	37	12	34	11	21	7
Skim milk	103	34	31	10	39	13	21	7
Lean meats	100	33	34	11	35	11	19	6
Low-fat substitutions	103	34	30	10	46	15	15	5
Nonfat substitutions	99	33	26	9	55	18	11	4

TABLE 9B. Isocaloric Substitutions in Women

	Total Fat (g)	Total Fat (%)	SFA (g)	SFA (%)	MUFA (g)	MUFA (%)	PUFA (g)	PUFA (%)
Isocaloric substitutions with peanuts								
Baseline	71	34	24	12	23	11	14	7
Skim milk	69	34	21	10	24	11	16	8
Lean meats	69	34	23	11	22	11	15	7
Low-fat substitutions	62	30	19	9	21	11	14	7
Nonfat substitutions	57	28	15	8	24	12	13	6
Isocaloric substitutions with olive oil								
Baseline	71	34	24	12	23	11	14	7
Skim milk	70	34	21	10	26	13	15	7
Lean meats	71	34	23	11	25	12	14	7
Low-fat substitutions	68	33	19	9	30	15	11	5
Nonfat substitutions	67	33	17	8	39	19	6	3

TABLE 10. Selected Nutrients That Decrease in Response to Fat-reduction Strategies in Women

	Vitamin E (mg α-tocopherol equivalents)[a]	Zinc (mg)
Baseline	8	10
Skim milk	−0%	10
Very lean meat	−25%	9
Nonfat products	−75%	7

[a] Baseline value was obtained from the University of Minnesota Nutrient Data System (NDS) due to missing values in Nutrionist IV. However, percent decreases were calculated based on values reported by Nutritionist IV.

women. This reflects the fact that a greater addition of peanuts (as a result of a greater reduction in calories with more extreme strategies) alters both the fat and protein content of these diets. As expected, percent energy from fat was not notably altered with isocaloric additions of olive oil in any fat-modified strategy. Monounsaturated fat became the greatest contributor of percent energy from fat in the diets containing skim milk, low-fat products, and nonfat products with the isocaloric additions of either peanuts or olive oil. It is important to note that when olive oil was isocalorically substituted in the diet containing all nonfat products, percent energy from monounsaturated fat was approximately twice as high as percent energy from saturated fat in the diets of both men and women. Thus, the greater the amount of fat that can be isocalorically added back to a diet containing fat-modified products, the greater the decrease in saturated fat and the greater the increase in monounsaturated fat.

Implementation of various fat-reduction strategies (milk, meats, and fat-modified products) did not significantly alter the nutrient quality of the diets. With the exception of two nutrients (vitamin E and zinc), micronutrient content continued to be ≥2/3 the RDA when averaged over three days (TABLE 10).

NUTRIENT ADEQUACY OF FAT-MODIFIED DIETS

A key question that a number of investigators have addressed is how the nutrient quality of the diet changes in response to decreasing total fat. Although computer simulations are useful, they do not provide information about actual nutrient changes that accompany dietary modifications to lower total fat. It is important to note that investigators report the nutrient quality of fat-modified diets on the basis of the nutrient:energy ratio of the diet,[11–13] or alternatively, as a percent of the RDA.[14] A limitation of looking solely at the nutrient:energy ratio of the diet is that it is still possible for the target nutrient not to meet the RDA. The data shown in TABLES 11, 12, and 13 reveal nutrients that are low, as well as those that increase in free-living subjects following Step-One and Step-Two diets.[15–18] These data are reported on the basis of the percent of the RDA achieved, the percent of the subjects consuming less

TABLE 11. Percentage of Subjects on Step-One Diets Who Report Consuming less than Two-Thirds of the RDA of Selected Nutrients

Micronutrient	Study	
	Bae et al. [15,a]	RLRC[b] Bassett/PSU
Vitamin A	21	41
Vitamin D	21	42
Vitamin E	21	37
Vitamin C	9	6
Vitamin B_6	26	1
Folic Acid	9	8
Calcium	21	38
Copper	26	—
Magnesium	16	26
Zinc	37	50

[a] Subjects were on a Step-One diet for 18 weeks.
[b] Subjects were on a Step-One diet for 3 months. RLRC = Rural Lipid Resource Center.

TABLE 12. Nutrients That Increase in Subjects following a Step-One Diet

Micronutrient	Study[a]		
	McCarron et al.[17,b]		Retzlaff et al.[18,c]
	Female	Male	Male
Vitamin A	197 (55%)	187 (52%)	180 (29%)
Vitamin D	99 (4%)	146 (18%)	NC[d]
Vitamin C	223 (27%)	298 (45%)	210 (17%)
Vitmain B_6	113 (9%)	133 (17%)	110 (7%)
Folate	170 (21%)	207 (24%)	140 (14%)
Riboflavin	144 (4%)	165 (5%)	110 (3%)
Thiamin	—	—	115 (10%)
Calcium	100 (10%)	132 (11%)	NC

[a] Values are percent of RDA (values are percent increase).
[b] Subjects self-selected a Step-One diet for 10 weeks.
[c] Subjects were on a Step-One/Step-Two diet for 2 years.
[d] No change.

than two-thirds of the RDA for key nutrients, as well as the percent increase in certain nutrients in the fat-modified diets.

The nutrients of greatest concern in subjects following a Step-One diet are vitamin E, copper, and zinc (TABLE 13). In addition, other nutrients of concern include vitamins A, D, B_6, and folic acid, and the minerals, calcium and magnesium (TABLE 11). By contrast, some investigators have reported increased intakes of certain nutrients in individuals on fat-modified diets (TABLE 12). It is important to note that for certain nutrients (*e.g.*, vitamins A, D, C, B_6, folic acid, and calcium) some individuals increase, whereas others decrease their intake of these nutrients. Furthermore, in some instances these changes are substantial, whereas other changes are of smaller magnitude.

IMPACT OF FAT-MODIFIED PRODUCTS ON THE U.S. FOOD SUPPLY

Low-fat and nonfat products are now the fastest growing food items in supermarkets in the U.S. The most popular reduced-fat product is 2% or skim milk, with 66% of the U.S. population using a lower-fat milk.[19] It is of interest to look at the effect of these proposed dietary changes on recent estimated milk consumption. Based on data from the 1996 Food Consumption, Prices, and Expenditures Report,[20] consumption of whole milk has declined appreciably, whereas consumption of 2% and skim milk has increased (TABLE 14).

Based on the data in TABLE 14, consider the following scenario: one-third of all men consuming whole milk in 1994 switch to 2% milk, and one-third of all women consuming 2% milk in 1994 switch to skim milk. What effect would this dietary change have on U.S. milk consumption? Whole milk consumption would decrease to 25%, 2% milk would decrease to 45%, and skim milk would increase to 30% of milk consumed in the United States.

Meat and pork products, such as hotdogs, luncheon meats, and bacon represent another food category in which consumption of low-fat products is on the rise. TABLE 15 depicts a recent estimate of consumption of regular and low-fat versions of such products in the United States. Based on data from this table, 15% of all hot dogs, 24% of all luncheon meats, and 7% of all bacon consumed in 1995 were low fat. These figures illustrate recent trends toward consumption of lower-fat meat and pork products. As food companies work to develop better tasting products at lower prices, we can expect a continual increase in the consumption of low-fat versions of meat and pork products.

The effect of population-based dietary recommendations on consumption data of meat and pork products could prove significant, as was shown with the U.S. milk consumption data. For example, suppose one-third of consumers of regular (not low-fat) hot dogs, luncheon meat, and bacon switched to the respective low-fat versions of these products. As a result, 42% of all hot dogs, 38% of all luncheon meats, and 33% of all bacon consumed would be low fat.

These examples demonstrate the significant impact that substitutions with reduced-fat products can have on overall consumption data of various foods. Similar effects can be shown with consumption data of salad dressings, mayonnaise, and snack foods, for example, which have regular, low-fat, and some nonfat versions.

TABLE 13. Selected Intake of Nutrients Providing less than 100% of the RDA for Subjects following a Step-One/Step-Two Diet

	Study[a]		
	McCarron et al.[17,b]		Retzlaff et al.[18,c]
Micronutrient	Female	Male	Male
Vitamin E	77	82	~90
Copper	56	75	—
Zinc	75	86	~75

[a] Values are percent of RDA.
[b] Subjects self-selected a Step-One diet for 10 weeks.
[c] Subjects were on a Step-One/Step-Two diet for 2 years.

TABLE 14. Milk Consumption Trends

	1970	1994
Whole milk	82%	37%
2% Milk	14%	49%
Skim milk	4%	14%

TABLE 15. 1995 Annual Pounds Purchased per Household[a]

	Regular	Low fat
Hotdogs	7.7	1.2
Luncheon meats	17.5	4.2
Bacon	7.4	0.5

[a] Data obtained from National Pork Producers Council/National Cattlemen's Beef Association.

EFFECTS OF IMPLEMENTATION OF FAT-REDUCTION STRATEGIES ON MACRONUTRIENT AND MICRONUTRIENT INTAKE OF FREE-LIVING INDIVIDUALS

Computer-modeling studies provide important insights about strategies that can be used to decrease total fat and, in turn, the impact that these strategies have on the nutrient profile of the diet. Although this is a useful exercise, it nonetheless is important that the effect of these various fat-reduction strategies on the nutrient profile of the diet be assessed in free-living subjects on self-selected diets. Thus, to determine the actual impact of specific fat-reduction strategies on macro- and micronutrient intakes of American males and females, an analysis of the CSFII data from 1989 through 1991 was performed. Fat-reduction strategies included the exclusive use of skim milk when consuming milk, lean meats when consuming meats, and/or fat-modified versions of cheese, salad dressing, cake, pudding, and yogurt in place of their higher-fat counterparts. A unique procedure was developed to sort food codes from the combined three-year database for those respondents who supplied records for three days (n = 11,912).[21] A comparison of energy and nutrient intake between groups was made using ANOVA. Relatively few Americans used only the fat-modified counterpart of a full-fat product over the three-day diet assessment period studied (n = 991 for skim milk only, n = 350 for lean meats only, n = 228 for fat-modified products only). For those who did, this favorably impacted their nutrient intake. Dietary fat, saturated fat, cholesterol, and energy intakes[22] were lower, whereas intake of most vitamins and minerals was higher with use of any strategy. Of importance was that the single fat-reduction strategy that decreased total and saturated fat most while favorably affecting micronutrient content of the diet was exclusive use of skim milk. Adults (n = 117) who used two or three fat-reduction strategies achieved the National Cholesterol Education Program goals for total fat (≤30% energy from fat), saturated fat (≤10% energy), and cholesterol (< 300 mg), and reduced their total energy intake while maintaining adequate micronutrient intakes. The results of this study demonstrate that individuals are using both single and multiple fat-reduction strategies to modify their diet. In addition, these results suggest that a simple way for individuals and families to reduce their intake of fat, saturated fat, and cholesterol would be to use skim milk in place of higher-fat milk as their initial fat-reduction strategy. Multiple fat-reduction strategies can also be applied to facilitate meeting contemporary dietary recommendations.

IMPLICATIONS

The application of different fat-reduction strategies results in variable decreases in total and saturated fat in the diet. Some fat-reduction strategies applied to typical American diets for men and women result in small to modest decreases in total and saturated fat, whereas others have a much greater impact. It is of interest to note that substitution of skim milk for higher-fat milks decreases total fat 2 to 3 percentage points, and use of very lean meats instead of higher-fat meats decreases total fat 2 to 4 percentage points. In men, these modifications had a slightly greater impact (by 1 to 2 percentage points) because men consume larger quantities of milk and meat than do women. In fact, in men, use of very lean meats achieved the total fat goal of 30% energy from fat, although not the saturated fat goal of ≤10% of calories. In women, use of skim milk achieved the saturated fat goal, whereas the total fat goal was not met. Use of lean meats and very lean meats had comparable effects on total fat and saturated fat. The computer simulations (which represent the theoretical application of different fat-reduction strategies) showed that the substitution of either skim milk or very lean meats did not achieve contemporary dietary recommendations for total fat or saturated fat. Each had a small impact on lowering dietary total fat and saturated fat. Additional dietary modifications would be required to achieve current dietary recommendations if skim milk and lean meats were used as single fat-reduction strategies.

Substitution of all low-fat products for their higher-fat counterparts achieved the total fat and saturated fat targets. As would be expected, therefore, substitution of nonfat products for all of the higher-fat versions resulted in a very substantial reduction in total and saturated fat. In fact, inclusion of all nonfat products decreased total and saturated fat by almost one-half. Interestingly, however, exclusive use of any one of the fat-modified foods included in the low-fat and nonfat groupings resulted in a small decrease in total fat (by as little as 0 to 2 percentage points) with the exception of exclusive use of products in the "other" category (*e.g.,* salad dressing, margarine, and mayonnaise). Because of their widespread usage, greater reductions, especially in total fat, resulted when all low-fat (*e.g.,* 8 to 10 percentage points) or all nonfat (*e.g.,* 16 to 18 percentage points) products were used. In addition, depending on the specific fat-modified food item substituted, there can be little impact on saturated fat. The effect reflects the type of fat (*e.g.,* unsaturated) that is used or is present in the different foods in this category. As would be expected, the greater the use of foods grouped in these two categories (*e.g.,* low-fat and nonfat modified products), the greater the impact on total fat (as well as saturated fat) content of the diet.

Application of multiple strategies affects dietary total and saturated fat differently, depending on the specific fat-reduction strategies used. Implementation of two moderate strategies (*e.g.,* 2% milk and lean meats) has a modest effect on the amount of total fat in the diet, decreasing it by 3 to 5 percentage points. When the most extreme single strategy (exclusive use of nonfat products) was used together with moderate strategies (*e.g.,* low-fat milk and lean meats), the impact was appreciable, achieving the lower limit for dietary fat that presently is recommended (*e.g.,* 15% of calories). However, when all fat-reduction strategies are applied maximally, dietary fat is reduced to very low, possibly dangerously low, levels of 7 to 8% of energy. These levels of total fat are approximately 50% lower than the lower limits currently recommended by the American Heart Association (15% energy from fat).

The reduction of total fat in the diet is associated with decreased energy, obviously with greater decreases accompanying larger reductions in total fat. Thus, implementation of dietary fat-reduction strategies could potentially be an effective approach to weight loss. For individuals who do not need or want to lose weight, diets can be made isocaloric by adding either carbohydrate calories or unsaturated fat calories. The addition of carbohydrate calories would further decrease the percent energy from fat. Replacing calories with monounsaturated fat results in a decrease in percent energy from saturated fat despite total fat being high (>30% of calories). This latter approach is gaining greater recognition among scientists as a possible blood cholesterol lowering diet for certain persons (*e.g.,* those with diabetes, insulin resistance, Syndrome X, hypertriglyceridemia).[10] In this latter situation, fat-reduction strategies are used mainly to decrease dietary saturated fat. Because some strategies have a greater impact than others, it will be necessary to use multiple strategies to achieve ≤10% of calories from saturated fat.

In recent years the availability of many fat-modified foods has increased. Consumers have countless choices with respect to using low-fat, nonfat and even full-fat foods to plan healthy diets that meet current dietary recommendations. In fact, 88% of adult Americans use reduced-fat foods and beverages at least once every two weeks.[19] The computer-modeling simulations employed herein have shown that different approaches can be used to achieve present dietary recommendations. It is clear, however, that the various fat-reduction strategies consumers can employ have different effects on dietary total and saturated fat, with only some of them enabling dietary recommendations to be achieved. With application of several fat-reduction strategies, however, it is possible to achieve dietary recommendations that also include consuming a nutritionally adequate diet. However, widespread application of fat-reduction strategies could be problematic with respect to meeting both nutrient and energy requirements. For example, nutrients of potential concern in fat-modified diets include vitamin E and zinc, especially with widespread application of fat-reduction strategies. In extremely low-fat diets (*e.g.*, ≤10% of calories from fat), vitamin E is negligible and, as is apparent, could lead to a deficiency. Thus, nutrition education efforts are needed to teach consumers appropriate application of fat-reduction strategies. For some well-intentioned individuals, in particular, it will be important to educate them on the possible adverse consequences of long-term consumption of extremely low-fat diets that provide inadequate calories and nutrients. For others, they will require information about how to effectively apply multiple (and even more moderate) fat-reduction strategies to achieve contemporary dietary recommendations. Furthermore, for individuals who would benefit from a diet high in monounsaturated fat and low in saturated fat, nutrition education efforts are required to effectively teach implementation of this fat-modified diet.

Although the results of the computer simulations presented here are informative in suggesting the potential impact of different fat-reduction strategies, there are limitations to this type of approach. First of all, menus were developed to include many foods that could be modified with lower-fat versions. Although these foods appeared to be common to the American diet, possible food combinations are endless, and thus the results could be highly variable depending on the specific foods used in the baseline diets. In fact, many people may not include these exact foods in their diets and are not likely to employ exclusive use of one particular fat-reduction strategy. More likely, consumers may purchase certain fat-modified products that do not fit into the specific categories outlined in this paper. Nevertheless, these types of simulations are useful in predicting changes that could occur in the diets of Americans if certain fat-reduction strategies were employed.

The availability of so many different fat-modified products in the marketplace offers numerous choices to consumers to facilitate decreasing dietary total and saturated fat. In theory, seemingly simple dietary modifications are all that are required to decrease total and saturated fat to recommended levels. Consumer education is necessary to assure that various fat-reduction strategies are applied appropriately. In addition, it will be important to evaluate how consumers are applying various fat-reduction strategies and how it affects the quality of their diet. Perhaps more importantly, it will be of greater significance to evaluate the effects of all fat-modified products on the food consumption practices of individuals who use them, as well as their overall impact (*e.g.*, on energy and nutrients) on the U.S. diet.

REFERENCES

1. NUTRITION AND YOUR HEALTH: DIETARY GUIDELINES FOR AMERICANS. 1995. 4th edition. USDA, USDHHS; Home and Garden Bulletin no. 232.

2. EXPERT PANEL ON DETECTION, EVALUATION, AND TREATMENT OF HIGH BLOOD CHOLESTEROL IN ADULTS. 1993. Summary of the Second Report of the National Cholesterol Education Program (NCEP) Expert Panel on Detection, Evaluation, and Treatment of High Blood Cholesterol in Adults (Adult Treatment Panel II). J. Am. Med. Assoc. **269**(23): 3015-3023.
3. CLEVELAND, L. E., A. J. ESCOBAR & S. M. LUTZ. 1993. Method for identifying differences between existing food intake patterns and patterns that meet nutrition recommendations. J. Am. Diet. Assoc. **93:** 556-563.
4. LYLE, B. J., K. E. MCMAHON & P. A. KREUTLER. 1991. Assessing the potential dietary impact of replacing dietary fat with other macronutrients. J. Nutr. **122:** 211-216.
5. SMITH-SCHNEIDER, L. M., M. J. SIGMAN-GRANT & P. M. KRIS-ETHERTON. 1992. Dietary fat reduction strategies. J. Am. Diet. Assoc. **92:** 34-38.
6. MCDOWELL, M. A., R. R. BRIEFEL, K. ALAIMO, A. M. BISCHOF, C. R. CAUGHMAN, M. D. CARROLL, C. M. LORIA & C. L. JOHNSON. 1994. Energy and macronutrient intakes of persons ages 2 months and over in the United States: Third National Health and Nutrition Examination Survey, Phase 1, 1988-91. Advance data from vital and health statistics; No. 255. National Center for Health Statistics. Hyattsville, MD.
7. ERVIN, B. & D. REED, Eds. 1993. Nutrition Monitoring in the United States. Chartbook I: Selected Findings from the National Nutrition Monitoring and Related Research Program. Public Health Service, 41. Hyattsville, MD.
8. KRAUSS, R. M., R. J. DECKELBAUM, N. ERNST, E. FISHER, B. V. HOWARD, R. H. KNOPP, T. KOTCHEN, A. H. LICHTENSTEIN, H. C. MCGILL, T. A. PEARSON, T. E. PREWITT, N. J. STONE, L. VAN HORN & R. WEINBERG. 1996. Dietary guidelines for healthy American adults: A statement for health professionals from the nutrition committee, American Heart Association. Circulation **94:** 1795-1800.
9. Anonymous. 1992. Dietary recommendations for people with diabetes: An update for the 1990s. Diabetic Med. **9**(2): 189-202.
10. REAVEN, G. M. 1995. Pathophysiology of insulin resistance in human disease. Physiol. Rev. **75**(3): 473-486.
11. BUZZARD, I. M., E. H. ASP, R. T. CHLEBOWSKI, A. P. BOYAR, R. W. JEFFERY, D. W. NIXON, G. L. BLACKBURN, P. R. JOCHIMSEN, E. F. SCANLON, W. INSULL, R. M. ELASHOFF, R. BUTRUM & E. L. WYNDER. 1990. Diet intervention methods to reduce fat intake: Nutrient and food group composition of self-selected low-fat diets. J. Am. Diet. Assoc. **90:** 42-50, 53.
12. GORBACH, S. L., A. MORRILL-LABRODE, M. N. WOODS, J. T. DWYER, W. D. SELLES, M. HENDERSON, W. INSULL, S. GOLDMAN, D. THOMPSON, C. CLIFFORD & L. SHEPPARD. 1990. Changes in food patterns during a low-fat dietary intervention in women. J. Am. Diet. Assoc. **90:** 802-809.
13. PEITINEN, P., R. DOUGHERTY, M. MUTANEN, U. LEINO, S. MOISIO, J. IACONO & P. PUSKA. 1984. Dietary intervention study among 30 free-living families in Finland. J. Am. Diet. Assoc. **84:** 313-318.
14. BURROWS, E. R., H. J. HENRY, D. J. BOWEN & M. M. HENDERSON. 1993. Nutritional application of a clinical low fat dietary intervention to public health change. J. Nutr. Ed. **25:** 167-175.
15. BAE, C-Y., J. M. KEENAN, P. FONTAINE, J. WENZ, C. M. RIPSIN & D. J. MCCAFFREY. 1993. Plasma lipid response and nutritional adequacy in hypercholesterolemic subjects on the American Heart Association Step-One Diet. Arch. Fam. Med. **2:** 765-772.
16. NAGLAK, M. C. 1996. Evaluation of the diet cost, diet patterns and food choices of hypercholesterolemic adults participating in the rural lipid resource center: A physician assist model. PhD Dissertation, The Pennsylvania State University, University Park, PA.
17. MCCARRON, D. A., S. OPARIL, A. CHAIT, R. B. HAYNES, P. KRIS-ETHERTON, J. S. STERN, L. M. RESNICK, S. CLARK, C. D. MORRIS, D. C. HATTON, J. A. METZ, M. MCMAHON, S. HOLCOMB, G. W. SNYDER & F. X. PI-SUNYER. 1997. Nutritional management of cardiovascular risk factors: A randomized clinical trial. Arch. Int. Med. **157:** 169-177.

18. RETZLAFF, B. M., A. A. DOWDY, C. E. WALDEN, B. S. MCCANN, G. GEY, M. COOPER & R. H. KNOPP. 1991. Changes in vitamin and mineral intakes and serum concentrations among free-living men on cholesterol-lowering diets: The dietary alternatives study. Am. J. Clin. Nutr. **53**: 890–898.
19. CALORIE CONTROL COUNCIL. 1996. Fat replacers: Food ingredients for healthy eating. Calorie Control Commentary **18**(1): 4–5.
20. PUTNAM, J. J. & J. E. ALLSHOUSE. 1996. Food consumption, prices, and expenditures: Annual data, 1970–1994. Food and Consumer Economics Division, Economic Research Service, U.S. Department of Agriculture. Statistical Bulletin No. 928.
21. PETERSON, S., M. SIGMAN-GRANT & C. ACHTERBERG. Development of a food code level sorting procedure using the 1989–91 CSFII data base. Fam. Econ. Nutr. Rev. In press.
22. PETERSON, S. L. 1996. Adoption of lower-fat food choices by American men, women, and children: Impact on macro- and micronutrient intake. PhD Dissertation, The Pennsylvania State University, University Park, PA.

Impact of Macronutrient-substituted Foods on Food Choice and Dietary Intake[a]

DAVID J. MELA [b]

Consumer Sciences Department
Institute of Food Research
Earley Gate, Whiteknights Road
Reading RG6 6BZ, United Kingdom

Public concern with body weight control and other perceived health implications of high fat and sugar consumption have prompted massive industrial efforts toward the development and marketing of novel formulations of traditional foods, nutritionally modified by the replacement or removal of macronutrients, primarily fats and sugars. Scientific evaluations of the potential influences of fat or sugar replacement on energy intake or weight control have been largely derived from animal research and from numerous laboratory-based human feeding studies that have focused on appetite and eating behavior under controlled and generally short-term conditions. This latter body of work is reviewed elsewhere in this volume and in other sources.[1-4]

Although laboratory-based studies have provided a wealth of information relating to the psychobiological determinants and correlates of hunger, satiety, and regulation of energy balance, it is not clear how closely the results of such experiments relate to "real-life" consumer behaviors. Indeed, there are many reasons why the results of these types of experiments should not be used as the principal basis for predicting actual dietary implications of macronutrient-substituted food product use by consumers in natural situations.[5] In most of this work, studies have been conducted (or at least meals consumed) in a controlled research setting, a restricted range of foods has been provided free of cost by investigators, and subjects have not had access to normal packaging or nutrition information. Appropriate consumer research requires more realistic food acquisition and eating environments and allows for broader external influences on food choice, including cognitive behavioral responses. This review will focus on the potential implications for food choice and dietary intake of purchase and consumption of macronutrient-substituted foods by normal consumers in the domestic environment, primarily relying on data from population-based studies and prospective trials.

A broad range of existing and proposed intense sweeteners, bulk replacers, and ingredients and technologies for fat reduction are discussed at length in the food technology literature and other sources.[6] Fat and sugar replacement will be considered here as generic categories, although acknowledging that the use, acceptance, or dietary

---

[a] This paper and most of the author's research described herein have been made possible by Competitive Strategic Grants from the UK Biotechnology and Biological Sciences Research Council.

[b] Tel: +44 118 935 7000; fax: +44 118 926 7917; e-mail: david.mela@bbsrc.ac.uk.

implications of certain materials can be important. In particular, approval of new fat or bulk replacers and applications could markedly expand the range and degree of macronutrient substitution in the food supply, potentially augmenting opportunities for dietary impact or raising other specific nutritional issues.[7] Similarly, considerable differences in the biological and epidemiological links of fat versus sugar in the development of overeating and obesity are discussed elsewhere.[5,8-10]

POPULATION STUDIES

Predictive Models

Given the high-level academic, public health, commercial interest, and occasionally heated scientific debates on the effects of macronutrient substitution, there are surprisingly few analyses or predictive models based on large population dietary intake data sets, although this is a growing area of research. Beaton *et al.*[11] computed the possible impacts of use of fat and carbohydrate (CHO, primarily sugars) substitutes, using models that assume casual use and compensatory energy intake by consumption of a mixed diet. This work suggests that use of intense sweeteners might be predicted to result in lower CHO and greater fat intakes, whereas fat replacement would have the opposite effect. There now appears to be a limited amount of empirical support for this predictive analysis from other such analyses and from prospective trials (discussed below). The majority of this work has focused on fat rather than sugar replacement.

Lyle *et al.*[12] used a combination of marketing/sales data and nutritional analyses to show that marked reductions in fat intake could be achieved through use of a limited number of reduced-fat (RF) alternative products, at least among individuals who would usually have eaten such items with high frequency. Using a roughly analogous computer-modeling approach, Smith-Schneider *et al.*[13] showed that use of fat-modified foods could be helpful in achieving reduction in fat intakes, although many different dietary approaches could be taken to reach the same effect. More recently, Patterson *et al.*[14] carried out a simulation based around estimated energy and fat intakes from a food-frequency questionnaire that included options for respondents to specify their use of a range of fat-reduction practices, including consumption of RF alternatives. Although the study does not make a direct comparison between groups of subjects based on their use of these specific fat-reduction behaviors or food choices, the investigators computed the impact of recoding these options to their high-fat alternatives. This approach suggests that such practices could markedly influence estimates of fat and energy intakes, and the report provides an indication of the relative impacts that would be attributed to specific behaviors or food exchanges in their study population based on these substitutions.

A drawback of such predictive and modeling studies is that they typically make a number of fixed assumptions. In general, simulations are based around the use of macronutrient-substituted foods as a direct replacement for the traditionally formulated alternatives, although market and research data suggest that this is not always how such products are incorporated into the diet. Assumptions must also be made about degree and food sources of caloric compensation occurring when replacements have a lower energy content. Also, the models generally assume no major shifts in other food-selection patterns occurring as a result of the use or nonuse of specific macronutrient-substituted foods. Both laboratory studies and the consumer trials discussed below have generally not observed evidence of macronutrient-specific caloric compensation; however, information or beliefs relating to the energy or macronutrient composition of foods have been shown to influence eating behavior in experimental studies.[15-17] Furthermore, not all subgroups within the population may respond the same way, or have the same motivations or intent to achieve particular dietary outcomes.

Dietary Intake Studies

There are few full publications of analyses relating energy and macronutrient intakes and body weight status to consumption of macronutrient-substituted foods. Such studies have the tremendous advantage of assessing what is occurring in practice among large numbers of consumers; however, they necessarily rely upon self-report data of questionable quality, and they can identify only associations, not causality. As a result, assignment of cause and effect in any identified relationships is always disputable.

Stellman and Garfinkel[18] analyzed data on self-reported body weights and intense sweetener use from a survey of subjects entering a prospective cancer trial. The authors concluded that their results did not constitute evidence that use of intense sweeteners ". . . either helps weight loss or prevents weight gain." However, there was widespread reporting of parts of their results indicating that consumption of intense sweeteners was positively related to body weight and that users were more likely to report weight gains over the preceding 12 months. The weaknesses in the collection and interpretation of these data are clearly acknowledged in the original paper and noted by most subsequent papers citing it. However, the outcomes were sufficiently provocative that the producers of one intense sweetener collaborated in an aggressive critique of the work eight years later[19]—not, unfortunately, supported by any additional analyses of large-scale dietary surveys or epidemiological studies that might afford direct comparison.

A much smaller cross-sectional study[20] found no clear evidence that use of intense sweeteners was associated with lower sugar intakes. Although the extent of data presented and statistical analyses in that study are limited, computations based on available data indicate no consistent association between intense sweetener use and relative macronutrient composition of the diet, including sugars. The results, therefore, suggest that intense sweeteners were added to the diet, rather than directly substituting for or otherwise causing a reduction in the consumption of dietary sugar sources. However, there is no information on specific food selections that might give an indication of the manner in which intensely sweetened products were incorporated into the diet, replaced certain foods, or perhaps generated increases in the consumption of others.

At this writing, there are also few cross-sectional studies relating specifically to the use of RF foods, and there is clearly a general need for additional and more extensive comparative studies evaluating food choice patterns and macro- and micronutrient intakes of users and nonusers of different macronutrient-substituted foods. Existing databases from individual dietary intake studies, national surveys, and dietary intervention trials should be suitable for this purpose and typically generate a range of data on food and nutrient intakes, and anthropometric, demographic, and biochemical measures. It should be possible to use these to characterize individuals practicing particular dietary patterns, for example, levels of use of macronutrient-substituted foods. Indeed, the same national databases have been extensively used to assess population exposure to specific macronutrient substitute materials and to examine dietary trends and relationships between nutrient intakes and measures of health status. However, there are difficulties in doing this in practice. In particular, the limited specificity of the nutritional data and the constantly changing composition of modified foods are significant problems, and the interpretation of the results (cause and effect) is problematic. Prospective trials provide an alternative approach, with different advantages and drawbacks.

PROSPECTIVE CONSUMER TRIALS

Prospective trials to assess the benefits of macronutrient substitutes are also notable for their absence from the literature. Until recently, relevant data were derived from a few studies on weight loss or examining a range of strategies undertaken to achieve specific dietary changes. Kanders *et al.*[21] reported results of a "pilot" study indicating that obese women, but not men, had slightly greater weight loss on a diet that included intense sweeteners. The study is often cited as evidence of the weight-control benefits of reduced-sugar (RS) food use,[19,22] although the actual results provide little direct evidence for such an interpretation. Use of fat-substituted foods has been reported to be easily adopted and highly acceptable, although not necessarily the most effective of several approaches used to achieve reductions in fat intakes by subjects given extensive dietary and behavioral counseling.[23] However, that study used a highly motivated population, and did not specifically quantify the impact of use of RF food per se. Reports of trials focusing on the changes in macronutrient or energy intakes occurring as a result of casual consumption of macronutrient-substituted foods by nonobese or nondieting consumers have only just begun to appear.

We have now completed two prospective dietary trials in which free-living consumers purchased their own foods in retail supermarkets and consumed them *ad libitum* at home over periods of 6 weeks[24] or, more recently, 10 weeks.[25] A third study was also carried out in conjunction with other strategies for promoting reduced fat consumption.[26] The first study[24] examined the use of RF foods, whereas the second[25] included two intervention groups, one using RF and another using RS foods. Subjects for these studies were not initially users of such products. In both trials, following a baseline period, a control group continued with their usual diet, whereas intervention subjects were instructed to incorporate RF (or RS) product alternatives into their diets. Subjects were allowed to select the specific modified products they wished to use, and also to use the full-fat or full-sugar versions of these or other foods, if they wished. Like normal consumers, therefore, they were not fixed into a strict diet or food-selection regimen and had the opportunity to simultaneously purchase and consume modified and traditional items of any composition, and hence

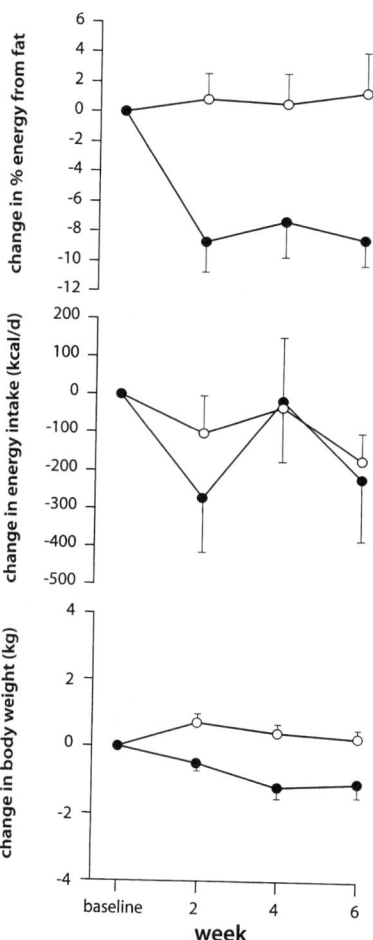

FIGURE 1. Mean (± SEM) changes from baseline in percent energy from fat (top), total energy intakes (middle), and body weights (bottom) occurring during use for 6 weeks of reduced-fat products (●), compared to a normal diet control group (○). (Adapted from Gatenby et al.[24] With permission from Academic Press.)

the potential to achieve any final level of relative macronutrient intake. This contrasts with studies where subjects have been placed on regimens of relatively fixed composition (such as Kendall et al.[27]) or had very clear dietary targets (e.g., for fat intake).[23,28–30] Diet records were collected and body weights recorded at periodic intervals over the course of the studies.

In the first trial,[24] subjects using RF foods immediately and consistently achieved a substantial reduction in percent energy from fat throughout the six-week intervention period (FIG. 1, top). Carbohydrate and protein intakes spontaneously increased, such

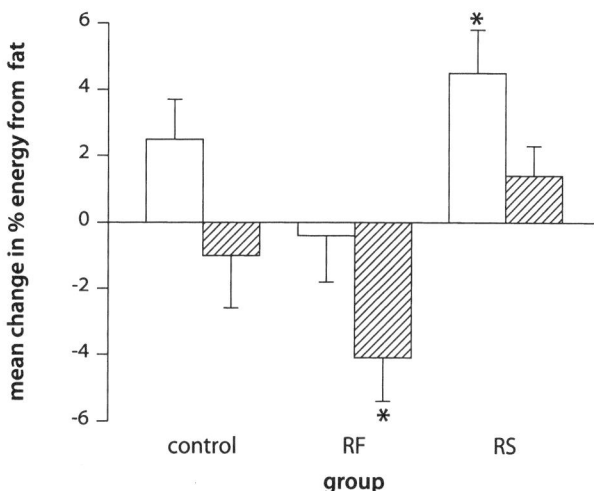

FIGURE 2. Mean (± SEM) of changes from baseline over 10 weeks (mean of 4 time points) in percent energy from fat, in relation to initial fat intakes, by reduced-fat (RF) and reduced-sugar (RS) intervention groups, and a normal diet control group. * indicates difference from 0 at p ≤ 0.01. Initial fat intake: ☐, ≤ 35% energy; ▨, ≥ 35% energy.

that overall energy intakes did not differ significantly from those of controls (FIG. 1, middle). However, as can be seen in FIGURE 1 (bottom), subjects experienced a modest weight loss over the first four weeks of the trial. This may have occurred due to an initial period of undereating (although changes in energy intakes did not reach statistical significance vs. controls at any time point) or may perhaps represent an effect of the substantially lowered fat intakes per se.[31] This small but significant weight loss is completely consistent with the results of other recent studies in which nonobese subjects have been placed on low-fat diet regimens.[27-30,32,33]

In a more recent trial,[25] users of RF foods also achieved a significant reduction in fat intakes; however, the magnitude of change was about half that seen in Gatenby et al.[24] Users of RS foods showed a significant reduction in sucrose intakes, though not total sugars. Energy intakes of both intervention groups closely paralleled those of controls, and there were no differential treatment effects on body weights over the 10-week intervention period.

Further (unpublished) analyses of these data have revealed important differences in the responses of subjects with differing initial diets. In particular, it is apparent that the reductions in fat intake of the RF group are almost entirely attributable to those subjects with a starting fat intake above 35% of energy, with little change occurring among subjects with moderate or low initial fat intakes (FIG. 2). A similar result was also observed in the Multicentre Study on Fat Reduction (MSFAT) trial,[34,35] described below (FIG. 3).

More intriguing results appear when one considers the effect of changes in fat and sucrose consumption on intakes of each other. A fat-sugar "seesaw" is commonly

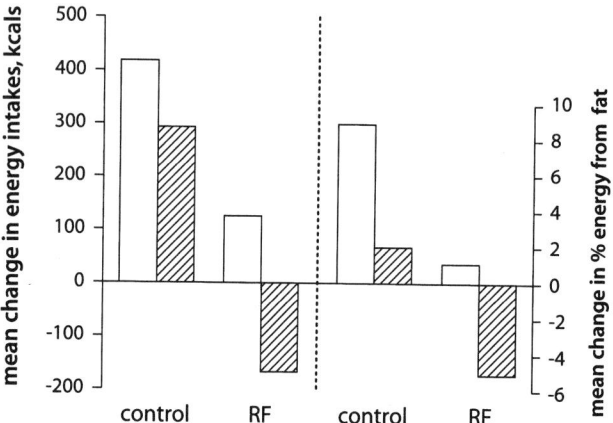

FIGURE 3. Mean change from baseline over 6 months (mean of 3 time points) in total energy intake and percent energy from fat, in relation to initial fat intakes, by reduced-fat (RF) and full-fat control groups. MSFAT study data from de Graaf et al.[34] Initial fat intake: ☐, ≤ 35% energy; ▨ ≥ 35% energy.

seen in dietary intake data, such that diets lower in sugars are invariably found to be higher in fat,[36-40] and this issue has been emphasized in recent work examining dietary outcomes of covert replacement of sugar with intense sweeteners.[41] We found that RF food use and associated reductions in fat intakes were not related to any consistent directional changes in sucrose intakes in any subgroup examined thus far. However, for subjects starting from an initial low-fat intake, use of RS foods prompted a marked increase in percent energy from fat (FIG. 2). A further result was that when subjects were classified by initial sucrose intake, high-sucrose consumers changing to the use of RS foods were found to increase their fat intake (not shown). These outcomes raise questions regarding the uptake of RS food use by individuals for whom reductions in fat intake is an important dietary goal.[41] However, the presence and magnitude of this effect is clearly dependent upon the type and macronutrient composition of the modified foods, the foods (if any) that are replaced in the initial diet, and the overall macronutrient profile of the initial diet. Analyses based on our subjects' initial diets have revealed no statistically significant differences in changes in total energy intakes or body weights.

Results from the MSFAT trial, a large, multicenter study of RF food use, have recently begun to appear in publication.[34,35,42,43] In this trial, nonobese subjects were assigned to groups consuming full-fat and equivalent RF products for six-month intervention periods, during which they were allowed access at no cost to a high number of commercial food products through shops set up at the research centers. A number of procedures ensured that RF subjects incorporated a certain minimum amount of RF products into their diets. In addition to dietary intakes and anthropometric data,[34,35] extensive biochemical and physiological measurements were made, to more fully identify possible effects of the use of these commercial products of differing composition.[42,43]

The main dietary outcomes of the MSFAT trial were that, in agreement with our studies,[24,25] subjects adopting the use of RF foods reduced their intakes of fat, but not of energy,[34] and showed no changes in body weights over the study period.[35] The design gave controls free access to a wide range of full-fat items, and these subjects significantly increased their fat energy intakes, and gained weight.[34,35] Hence, changes in energy intakes and body weight significantly differed between the RF and control groups. Extensive analyses by de Graaf *et al.*[34] have examined the extent to which energy compensation in the RF users was derived from increased consumption of the RF items versus the rest of the diet. As with our 10-week study[25] (FIG. 2), it is apparent that a major effect of the interventions was to reduce the fat intakes of RF subjects initially having high fat intakes, but also a marked rise in the fat intakes of MSFAT control subjects whose fat intakes were initially low[34,35] (FIG. 3).

CONSUMER BEHAVIOR ISSUES

Do consumers respond to the use of macronutrient-substituted foods by consciously or unconsciously increasing their selection of macronutrients from other sources? There are still far too few data that can be used to reliably predict the influences that existing or future macronutrient substitutes might have on overall food selection patterns, and the issue warrants investigation as nutritionally modified foods proliferate on supermarket shelves. The prospective studies above, and a large number of studies using covert manipulations, suggest that energy compensation for macronutrient substitution is not macronutrient specific.[1,44] However, these experimental data do not eliminate the possibility of cognitive behavioral responses, such as those observed by Caputo and Mattes,[15] who found that subjects exhibited increases in self-selected fat intakes during periods in which they had been given what they believed to be lower-fat meals. This issue clearly warrants further consideration, and it should be possible to extract evidence relating to this type of behavior from analyses of large cross-sectional dietary intake data sets. Such information, which may be crucial in determining overall dietary implications of macronutrient substitutes, will require combinations of survey and dietary intake and should be a focus of future research.

Concern has also been expressed that increased interest might be directed towards certain foods (*e.g.*, those traditionally high in fat or sugar) that some consumers presently avoid on nutritional grounds, and consumption of these products might therefore increase at the expense of other, more nutrient-dense items.[45,46] This scenario remains speculative, as there are few if any relevant data addressing the issue. Particular attention may need to be paid toward groups with special needs (*e.g.*, children, very elderly people, and clinical populations), those who might be expected to incorporate macronutrient-substituted foods into their diets at relatively high levels, or those who may be predisposed to developing eating disorders.

Use of macronutrient-substituted foods could have other effects on food choices. Data from our laboratory suggest that many consumers may have unrealistic views regarding the extent to which they have already reduced their fat consumption, for example, and grossly miscategorizing their own personal fat intakes.[47] Not surprisingly, this can be linked to reduced likelihood of adopting further dietary changes.[26]

Several other studies have also found that consumers commonly judge both their relative fat intake and their risk of diet-related diseases as optimistically low.[48-50] The extent to which casual use of macronutrient-substituted foods might contribute to such misperceptions, and perhaps resistance to other dietary changes, is not known.

Lastly, there are consumer issues relating to the potential cost associated with use of macronutrient-substituted and reduced-energy versions of foods. If these specialized products cost as much or more than their traditional counterparts, and their use is accompanied by at least partial (and more likely, complete) caloric compensation, it follows that the total volume or number of food products consumed, and hence cost to the consumer, must increase to sustain this level of caloric intake. Although this could provide economic benefits to sectors of the food industry, it may create a hidden burden for individuals with limited financial resources, with possible consequences for overall food purchasing and dietary intake patterns.

CONCLUSIONS

What are the dietary implications for ordinary consumers purchasing macronutrient-substituted foods in the shops and using them *ad libitum?* Do consumers compensate for the macronutrient substitutes, and in what way? To what extent do product promotions and information, and consumer beliefs and knowledge, influence this compensatory behavior? Research to date has largely focused on appetite regulation but not on the actual behavior or overall diets of consumers in more natural situations.

The data presented here are largely consistent with the view that, unless part of a willful effort to reduce intakes or strictly control diet composition, consumers are likely to compensate for most or all of the energy reduction of macronutrient-substituted foods, probably by consumption of a mixed diet. Nevertheless, marked reductions in fat intakes or energy density seem to prompt modest spontaneous weight loss. Casual use of RF foods appears likely to produce significant reductions in fat intake, at least for individuals starting from a high-fat intake. However, there is rather less clear evidence for the overall dietary impact of RS food use, and recent data highlight concerns regarding possible adverse influences on fat intakes. Counterproductive, cognitive behavioral responses to macronutrient-substituted foods also remain possible, perhaps likely for some groups. There is a lack of relevant population and prospective data with which to assess the extent of such responses in natural settings.

Overall, it is clear that the dietary implications of macronutrient-substituted foods will reflect the manner in which they are incorporated into the diet, the overall behavioral response of consumers, the nutritional profile of the initial diet, and the resultant shifts in food choice. Future research should particularly focus on analyses of cross-sectional and longitudinal population data, and prospective dietary intervention trials conducted under extended, realistic-use conditions, to assess the actual patterns of nutrient and energy intakes that result from informed use in normal eating.

REFERENCES

1. BELLISLE, F. & C. PEREZ. 1994. Low-energy substitutes for sugars and fats in the human diet: Impact on nutritional regulation. Neurosci. Biobehav. Rev. **18:** 197–205.

2. BLUNDELL, J. E. & P. J. ROGERS. 1994. Sweet carbohydrate substitutes (intense sweeteners) and the control of appetite: Scientific issues. *In* Appetite and Body Weight Regulation. J. D. Fernstrom & G. D. Miller, Eds.: 113–124. CRC Press. Boca Raton, FL.
3. ROLLS, B. J. 1991. Effects of intense sweeteners on hunger, food intake and body weight: A review. Am. J. Clin. Nutr. **53:** 872–878.
4. ROLLS, B. J. 1991. The impact of low-fat foods on energy and nutrient intakes. Trends Food Sci. Technol. **2:** 325–328.
5. MELA, D. J. 1996. Assessing the potential dietary implications of macronutrient substitutes. *In* Progress in Obesity Research: 7. A. Angel, H. Anderson, C. Bouchard, D. Lau, L. Leiter & R. Mendelson, Eds.: 423–430. John Libbey & Co. London.
6. KHAN, R., Ed. 1993. Low-Calorie Foods and Food Ingredients. Blackie. London.
7. MELA, D. J. 1996. Implications of fat replacement for nutrition and food intake. Fett/Lipid **98:** 50–55.
8. WESTRATE, J. A. 1995. Fat and obesity. Int. J. Obesity **19**(Suppl. 5): S38–S43.
9. ASTRUP, A. & A. RABEN. 1995. Carbohydrate and obesity. Int. J. Obesity **19**(Suppl. 5): S27–S37.
10. PRENTICE, A. M. 1995. Are all calories equal? *In* Weight Control. The Current Perspective. R. Cottrell, Ed.:8–33. Chapman & Hall. London.
11. BEATON, G. H., V. TARUSAK & G. H. ANDERSON. 1992. Estimation of possible impact of non-caloric fat and carbohydrate substitutes on macronutrient intake in the human. Appetite **19:** 87–103.
12. LYLE, B. J., K. E. MCMAHON & P. A. KREUTLER. 1991. Assessing the potential dietary impact of replacing dietary fat with other macronutrients. J. Nutr. **122:** 211–216.
13. SMITH-SCHNEIDER, L. M., M. J. SIGMAN-GRANT & P. M. KRIS-ETHERTON. 1992. Dietary fat reduction strategies. J. Am. Diet. Assoc. **92:** 34–38.
14. PATTERSON, R. E., A. R. KRISTAL, R. J. COATES, F. A. TYLAVSKY, C. RITENBAUGH, L. VAN HORN, A. W. CAGGIULA & L. SNETSELAAR. 1996. Low-fat diet practices of older women: Prevalence and implications for dietary assessment. J. Am. Diet. Assoc. **96:** 670–676, 679.
15. CAPUTO, F. A. & R. D. MATTES. 1993. Human dietary responses to perceived manipulation of fat content in a mid-day meal. Int. J. Obesity **17:** 241–244.
16. WOOLEY, O. W., S. C. WOOLEY & R. B. DUNHAM. 1972. Can calories be perceived and do they affect hunger in obese and nonobese humans? J. Comp. Physiol. Psychol. **80:** 250–258.
17. SHIDE, D. J. & B. J. ROLLS. 1995. Information about the fat content of preloads influences energy intake in healthy women J. Am. Diet. Assoc. **95:** 993–998.
18. STELLMAN, S. D. & L. GARFINKEL. 1986. Artificial sweetener use and one-year weight change among women. Prev. Med. **15:** 195–202.
19. LAVIN, P. T., P. G. SANDERS, M. A. MACKEY & F. N. KOTSONIS. 1994. Intense sweeteners use and weight change among women: A critique of the Stellman and Garfinkel study. J. Am. Coll. Nutr. **13:** 102–105.
20. CHEN, L.-N. A. & E. S. PARHAM. 1991. College students' use of high-intensity sweeteners is not consistently associated with sugar consumption. J. Am. Diet. Assoc. **91:** 686–690.
21. KANDERS, B. S., P. T. LAVIN, M. B. KOWALCHUCK, I. GREENBERG & G. L. BLACKBURN. 1988. An evaluation of the effect of aspartame on weight loss. Appetite **11**(suppl): 73–84.
22. RENWICK, A. G. 1994. Intense sweeteners, food intake, and the weight of a body of evidence. Physiol. & Behav. **55:** 139–143.
23. KRISTAL, A. R., E. WHITE, A. L. SHATTUCK, S. CURRY, G. L. ANDERSON, A. FOWLER & N. URBAN. 1992. Long-term maintenance of a low-fat diet: Durability of fat-related dietary habits in the Women's Health Trial. J. Am. Diet. Assoc. **92:** 553–559.
24. GATENBY, S. J., J. I. AARON, G. MORTON & D. J. MELA. 1995. Nutritional implications of reduced-fat food use by free-living consumers. Appetite **25:** 241–252.

25. GATENBY, S. J., J. I. AARON, V. M. JACK & D. J. MELA. Extended use of foods modified in fat and sugar content: Nutritional implications in a free-living female population. Am. J. Clin. Nutr. In press.
26. PAISLEY, C. M. 1994. Barriers to the adoption and maintenance of reduced-fat diets. Ph.D. thesis, University of Reading, UK.
27. KENDALL, A., D. A. LEVITSKY, B. J. STRUPP & L. LISSNER. 1991. Weight loss on a low-fat diet: Consequence of the imprecision of the control of food intake in humans. Am. J. Nutr. **53**: 1124–1129.
28. RABEN, A., N. DUE JENSEN, P. MARCKMANN, B. SANDSTRÖM & A. ASTRUP. 1995. Spontaneous weight loss during 11 weeks' ad libitum intake of a low fat/high fiber diet in young, normal weight subjects. Int. J. Obesity **19**: 916–923.
29. SCHAEFER, E. J., A. H. LICHTENSTEIN, S. LAMON-FAVA, J. R. MCNAMARA, M. M. SCHAEFER, H. RASMUSSEN & J. M. ORDOVAS. 1995. Body weight and low-density lipoprotein cholesterol changes after consumption of a low-fat ad libitum diet. J. Am. Med. Assoc. **274**: 1450–1455.
30. SIGGAARD, R., A. RABEN & A. ASTRUP. 1996. Weight loss during 12 weeks' ad libitum carbohydrate-rich diet in overweight subjects at a Danish work site. Obesity Res. **4**: 347–356.
31. PREWITT, T. E., D. SCHMEISSER, P. E. BOWEN, P. AYE, T. A. DOLECEK, P. LANGENBERG, T. COLE & L. BRACE. 1991. Changes in body weight, body composition, and energy intake in women fed high- and low-fat diets. Am. J. Clin. Nutr. **54**: 304–310.
32. SHEPPARD, L., A. R. KRISTAL & L. H. KUSHI. 1991. Weight loss in women participating in a randomized trial of low-fat diets. Am. J. Clin Nutr. **54**: 821–828.
33. CHLEBOWSKI, R. T., G. L. BLACKBURN, I. M. BUZZARD, D. P. ROSE, S. MARTINO, J. D. KHANDEKAR, R. M. YORK, R. W. JEFFERY, R. M. ELASHOFF & E. L. WYNDER. 1993. Adherence to a dietary fat intake reduction program in postmenopausal women receiving therapy for early breast cancer. J. Clin. Oncol. **11**: 2072–2080.
34. DE GRAAF, C., J. J. M. M. DRIJVERS, J. H. ZIMMERMANNS, K. H. VAN HET HOF, J. A. WESTRATE, H. VAN DEN BERG, E. J. M. VELTHUIS-TE WIERIK, K. R. WESTERTERP, M. S. WESTERTERP-PLANTENGA & W. P. H. G. VERBOEKET-VAN DE VENNE. Energy and fat compensation during long-term consumption of reduced-fat products. Appetite. In press.
35. ZIMMERMANNS, N. & K. VAN HET HOF. MSFAT-Study: The effect of light products on food intake and indicators of health [undated pamphlet]. Unilever Research Laboratorium. Vlaardingen, The Netherlands.
36. LEWIS, C. J., Y. K. PARK, P. B. DEXTER & E. A. YETLEY. 1992. Nutrient intakes and body weights of persons consuming high and moderate levels of sugars. J. Am. Diet. Assoc. **92**: 708–713.
37. GIBSON, S. A. 1993. Consumption and sources of sugars in the diets of British schoolchildren: Are high-sugar diets nutritionally inferior? J. Hum. Nutr. Diet. **6**: 355–371.
38. GIBSON, S. A. 1996. Are diets high in non-milk extrinsic sugars conducive to obesity? An analysis from the Dietary and Nutritional Survey of British Adults. J. Hum. Nutr. Diet. **9**: 283–292.
39. GIBNEY, M. J. 1980. Dietary guidelines: A critical appraisal. J. Hum. Nutr. Diet. **3**: 245–254.
40. BAGHURST, K. I., P. A. BAGHURST & S. J. RECORD. 1994. Demographic and dietary profiles of high and low fat consumers in Australia. J. Epidemiol. Community Health **48**: 26–32.
41. NAISMITH, D. J. & C. RHODES. 1995. Adjustment in energy intake following the covert removal of sugar from the diet. J. Hum. Nutr. Diet. **8**: 167–175.
42. VERBOEKET-VAN DE VENNE, W. P. H. G., K. R. WESTERTERP, T. J. F. M. B. HERMANS-LIMPENS, C. DE GRAAF, K. VAN HET HOF & J. A. WESTRATE. 1996. Long term consumption of full-fat or reduced-fat products in healthy non-obese volunteers: Assessment of energy expenditure and substrate oxidation. Metabolism **45**: 1004–1010.

43. Velthuis-te Wierik, E. J. M., H. van den Berg, J. A. Westrate, K. H. van het Hof & C. de Graaf. 1996. Consumption of reduced-fat products: Effects on parameters of anti-oxidative capacity. Eur. J. Clin. Nutr. **50:** 214-219.
44. Westerterp-Plantenga, M. S., W. J. Pasman, M. J. W. Yedema & N. E. G. Wijckmans-Duijsens. 1996. Energy intake adaptation of food intake to extreme energy densities of food by obese and non-obese women. Eur. J. Clin. Nutr. **50:** 401-407.
45. Munro, I. C. 1990. Issues to be considered in the safety evaluation of fat substitutes. Food Chem. Toxicol. **28:** 751-753.
46. Owen, A. L. 1990. The impact of future foods on nutrition and health. J. Am. Diet. Assoc. **90:** 1217-1222.
47. Lloyd, H. M., C. M. Paisley & D. J. Mela. 1993. Changing to a low fat diet: Attitudes and beliefs of UK consumers. Eur. J. Clin. Nutr. **47:** 361-373.
48. Raats, M. M. & P. Sparks. 1995. Unrealistic optimism about diet-related risks: Implications for interventions. Proc. Nutr. Soc. **54:** 737-745.
49. Sparks, P., R. Shepherd, N. Weiringa & N. Zimmermanns. 1995. Perceived behavioural control, unrealistic optimism and dietary change: An exploratory study. Appetite **24:** 243-255.
50. Sparks, P. & R. Shepherd R. 1994. Public perceptions of the potential hazards associated with food production and food consumption: An empirical study. Risk Analysis **14:** 799-806.

Impact of the Use of Reduced-fat Foods on Nutrient Adequacy

JAMES T. HEIMBACH,[a] BROOKE E. VAN DER RIET, AND S. KATHLEEN EGAN

TAS, Inc.
1000 Potomac Street, NW
Washington, D.C. 20007

INTRODUCTION

The U.S. government and a variety of medical and public health associations and authorities have advised the American public to limit average fat intake to 30% of calories to decrease health risks, and to restrict energy intake to the level needed to achieve or maintain desirable body weight. These recommendations apply to healthy Americans two years of age and older, of all ethnic groups, male and female. The advice to limit fat and energy intake are found in the Dietary Guidelines for Americans,[1] which form the basis for all Federal nutrition policy and consequently are reflected in the National School Lunch Program, the WIC Program, the National Cholesterol Education Program's Step 1 Diet, and other nutrition programs.

However, available data indicate that the average consumer is far from reaching the goal limiting fat intake to 30% of calories. Two years ago, in a paper on this same topic presented at the American Chemical Society's Annual Meeting and recently published as a chapter in *Hypernutritious Foods,*[2] we reported on results of the 1989-90 and 1990-91 Continuing Surveys of Food Intakes by Individuals (CSFII). At that time, fat intake accounted for 35% of the calories in the diets of survey respondents, averaging 69 g/person/day for the average American.

The number of reduced fat foods for which significant consumption was reported in the 1989-90 and 1990-91 CSFII was quite small and was almost exclusively composed of low-fat and skim milk, low-fat cheeses, low-fat table spreads, and low-fat or fat-free salad dressings. Although there were other types of reduced fat products available, little consumption was reported for them.

We learned a number of things at that time, including the following: reduced fat foods were generally consumed in similar portion sizes to the higher fat foods they replaced, and thus fat intakes from these foods were indeed reduced; these fat reductions were not obviated by increased consumption of fat elsewhere in the diet, and so users of these products had lower total intakes of fat than did users of the higher-fat counterparts; users of reduced-fat foods had, quite consistently, higher intakes of vitamin A than did users of the higher-fat alternatives; and users of reduced-fat foods tended to have lower intakes of vitamin E than did users of the regular products.

---

[a] Tel: (202) 337-2625; fax: (202) 337-1744; e-mail: jth@tasinc.com.

Since this research was completed, the food industry has not been idle: many new reduced-fat foods have become available to consumers in a wide range of food categories. Consequently, it is of interest to examine the trends in the use of reduced-fat foods as well as to determine the nutritional impact of use of these products.

METHODS

All food and nutrient consumption data are derived from surveys conducted by the U.S. Department of Agriculture. The five surveys used in this research are the 1987-88 Nationwide Food Consumption Survey (NFCS), Individual Intake Component;[3] the 1989-90 CSFII;[4] the 1990-91 CSFII;[5] the 1991-92 CSFII;[6] and the 1994 CSFII.[7]

All of these surveys were based on stratified area probability samples of individuals residing in households. The 1994 CSFII included the entire country, whereas the previous surveys included only the conterminous states. Interviewing for the 1987-88 NFCS took place between April 1987 and August 1988. The first three CSFIIs were in the field from April through March of the following year; the 1994 CSFII was executed during the 1994 calendar year.

All surveys prior to 1994 measured dietary intake of all individuals in sampled households for a three-day period. The day-1 individual intake was collected using a 24-hour recall of foods consumed the previous day, whereas day-2 and day-3 intakes were based on records maintained by the respondent. In the 1994 CSFII, dietary intake of individuals in sampled households was measured for two nonconsecutive days, both using 24-hour recalls. The second day was randomly chosen from 3 to 10 days after the first, omitting seven days.

In all surveys, individuals were surveyed in all four seasons and on all days of the week. In addition to information on food consumption, the survey collected physiological and demographic data, such as sex, age, self-reported height and weight, ethnic group, pregnancy and lactation status, and household income. This information permitted assessment of food consumption by specific population groups of interest.

Quantities of foods and beverages consumed were recorded in household measures, weights, dimensions, or common units (*e.g.,* slice, piece). All quantities were converted to grams by the USDA.

The 1994 CSFII included 5,589 respondents, representing an 80% response rate.[7] Sample sizes and response rates for the other USDA surveys have been reported elsewhere.[3-6]

Foods regarded as "reduced fat" for the purpose of analysis were those identified in the USDA food description as "reduced fat," "low fat," "nonfat," "fat free," or the like. Categories of such foods were skim milk, low-fat milk, diet frozen dairy desserts, reduced-fat cheese, low-fat luncheon meats, diet frozen meals, egg substitutes, reduced-fat sweet baked goods, reduced-fat salty snacks, low-calorie and low-fat salad dressings, and reduced-fat nonsweet crackers. Foods were not regarded as "reduced fat" unless they had higher fat counterparts; thus, for example, low-fat yogurt was not included because full-fat yogurt no longer has a significant market share.

Because the 1994 CSFII collected only two days of data, whereas the previous surveys collected three, it was not appropriate to compare intakes across the entire survey period. Consequently, all analyses were based on person-days. In this approach, each day's consumption of an individual is regarded as a separate record. Consequently, a finding that a product was consumed on x% of person-days does not mean that only x% of the population ever uses it.

We examined several population subgroups defined by age/sex and by racial/ethnic identification in addition to the total U.S. population: males and females, age 1-6; males and females, age 7-12; males, age 13-19; females, age 13-19; males, age 20-39; females, age 20-39; males, age 40-59; females, age 40-59; males, age 60+; females, age 60+; whites; blacks; and Asian-Americans.

RESULTS

A number of reduced fat foods were reported for the first time in the 1994 survey. The category with the greatest number of new products was sweet baked goods (especially cookies), with 15 new foods reported in addition to the 28 that were reported in previous surveys. As a percentage, the largest growth was in nonsweet crackers, which had only a single food reported prior to 1994, but 7 reported in the 1994 CSFII.

Between 1987-88 and 1994, there was a 41% increase in the proportion of person-days in the U.S. population on which consumption of at least one of these foods was reported, from 30.5% in 1987-88 to 42.9% in 1994. However, for the total population, nearly all of this increase was between 1987-88 and 1989-90. Blacks showed the largest percentage increase in reported use, from 7.8% in 1987-88 to 15.7% in 1994, but they still remained far below the white population (49.0%) in reported use of reduced-fat foods on a given day.

In all surveys, low-fat milk (1% and 2%) accounted for over half of reported use of reduced-fat foods. In 1987-88, low-fat milk was reported on 22.7% of person-days; that figure climbed to 26.4% in 1994. However, its share is declining: in 1987-88, about 74% of all reduced-fat foods reported consumed was low-fat milk, whereas in 1994 low-fat milk accounted for only about 62% of reported use of reduced-fat foods. Skim milk was the second most frequently reported reduced-fat food, and its use nearly doubled from 5.4% in 1987-88 to 9.5% in 1994. This substantial increase in reported consumption of skim milk was found in all population subgroups examined with one exception: among blacks, use of skim milk increased only from 1.7% in 1987-88 to 1.8% in 1994.

Other than low-fat and skim milk, no other reduced-fat food was reported by more than about 5% of respondents on a given day.

In terms of percentage increase in consumption, the leading categories were salty snacks and nonsweet crackers, which had no reported consumption of reduced-fat versions in 1987-88 and were reported by 1.4% and 0.7% of respondents in 1994.

On days when use of a reduced-fat food was reported, only a single food was reported about 70% of the time, although that food may have been consumed on multiple occasions. ("Single food" refers to a given food code, not a given category of foods. Thus, consumption of two different kinds of reduced-fat cookies was counted as two different foods.) Obviously, this single reduced-fat food is usually low-fat milk. This tendency to use only a single reduced-fat food was particularly pronounced among blacks: 83% of blacks who consumed reduced-fat foods reported only a single food on a given day compared with 68% of whites. Generally, women who used reduced-fat foods were more likely than were men to report consumption of more than a single food. An exception was teenagers: 26% of males but only 22% of females who used reduced-fat foods reported more than one food.

It was rare for an individual to report consuming more than two different reduced-fat foods on a single day. Overall, only about 8% of person-days included reports of three or more different reduced-fat foods. Among blacks, only 2% reported consumption of more than two different such foods. The group with the highest frequency of reported consumption of three or more reduced-fat foods was women age 60 or older, with 15%. No participant in the 1994 CSFII reported use of more than five different reduced-fat foods on a given day.

When reduced-fat foods were consumed, they were usually consumed in the same or smaller amounts than their full-fat counterparts. For example, the mean amount of reduced-fat sweet baked goods consumed on a single eating occasion by users of these products was about 61 g (2.2 oz), whereas the mean amount consumed of regular sweet baked goods was about 84 g (3.0 oz). This difference was due to a complete shifting of the intake distribution and not to some extreme intakes of regular products raising the mean. Over 70% of users of the reduced-fat versions consumed 2 oz or less versus only 54% of users of the full-fat alternatives. On the other hand, amounts of reduced-fat sweet baked goods in excess of 5 oz were consumed on less than 3% of days, whereas their regular counterparts were consumed at this level on nearly 12% of days. This same pattern was found across age/sex and racial/ethnic groups.

Turning to the impact of consumption of reduced-fat foods on nutrient intake, there was a pronounced change in the sources of calories in the diet. Whereas those who did not report consumption of any reduced-fat foods derived 35% of their calories from fat, those who consumed one or two reduced-fat foods lowered this to 32%, whereas those consuming three or more such foods reduced their calories from fat to only 26%. Somewhat surprisingly, there was little difference in protein consumption between those who did or did not consume reduced-fat foods. There was, then, an increase in the proportion of calories from carbohydrates for those using reduced-fat foods, from 49% among nonusers to 59% among those who reported using three or more reduced-fat foods on a given day.

For the total population, the ratio between intakes of polyunsaturated and saturated fatty acids (the P/S ratio) did not differ much between users and nonusers of low-fat foods; that is, there was a reduction in intake of saturated fatty acids that paralleled the reduction in total fat. Nonusers of reduced-fat foods derived 12% of their calories from saturated fatty acids, whereas those who reported using three or more reduced-fat products derived only 8 percent.

These same patterns, to a greater or lesser degree, were found for all population groups examined: in all subpopulations, users of three or more reduced-fat foods showed substantially lower intakes of total fat and of saturated fatty acids than did nonusers of these foods. However, these were not always to the same degree, and so the P/S ratio increased with increasing use of reduced-fat foods for some population groups and decreased for others.

As a matter of some interest, the only subpopulation that reached the target of 30% of calories from fat even among nonusers of reduced-fat foods was Asian-Americans. Those Asian-Americans who did use three or more such foods reached a level of only 13% of calories from fat and only 4% of calories from saturated fatty acids.

At the other end of the spectrum, males age 20 to 39 failed to reach the target of 30% of calories from fat or that of 10% of calories from saturated fatty acids, even among those using three or more reduced-fat products on a given day. This was the only subpopulation examined in which heavy users of reduced-fat products failed to reach the recommended intake levels for either total fat or saturated fatty acids.

In most—but not all—population groups examined, those who used three or more reduced-fat foods had higher total caloric intake than did those who consumed none. For the total population, this difference was quite small (1805 kcal for nonusers, 1860 kcal for users of one or two reduced-fat foods, and 1837 kcal for users of three or more such foods). The difference was greater for teenage males (users of three or more reduced-fat foods consumed 3772 kcal vs. only 2549 kcal for nonusers), whereas it was in the opposite direction for teenage females (1610 kcal for users of three or more reduced-fat foods vs. 1804 kcal for nonusers).

Intake of vitamin A was substantially higher among those who consumed three or more reduced-fat foods on a given day than among those who did not report using these foods; for the total population, high users of reduced-fat foods had a mean vitamin A intake of 10,000 IU (1540 RE) versus 4900 IU (790 RE) among nonusers. This finding was invariable across all population groups examined.

On the other hand, in the total population, vitamin E intake was about the same among users and nonusers of reduced-fat foods. Although nonusers had a mean daily intake of 7.3 mg of vitamin E, users of three or more reduced-fat foods averaged 7.5 mg/day. However, this varied considerably across subpopulations. For example, among teenage males, heavy users of reduced-fat foods had a mean intake of 14.1 mg of vitamin E versus only 9.0 mg for nonusers; for teenage females the situation was reversed, with users of three or more products averaging only 4.6 mg of vitamin E versus 6.9 mg for nonusers. In fact, intakes of vitamin E across groups closely paralleled calorie intakes rather than use of reduced-fat foods.

Intake of iron was higher for those reporting consumption of three or more reduced-fat foods (17.7 mg/day in the total population) than for nonusers (12.8 mg). This difference was found across the various subpopulations examined. Like iron, zinc showed higher levels of intake for users of reduced-fat products; in the total population, the mean daily zinc intake was 9.6 mg for nonusers of these foods, 10.7 mg for users of one or two different reduced-fat foods, and 11.5 mg for users of three or more. However, this trend was not found for all population groups. Teenage males, for example, showed a strong increase in zinc intake with increasing use of reduced-fat foods, whereas teenage females who were heavy users of reduced-fat products had lowered intake of zinc.

DISCUSSION

It is clear that consumption of reduced-fat foods increased substantially between 1987–88 and 1994, both in the variety of products consumed and in the proportion of the population who consumed them. However, this has not been a monotonic function over the period. For most population groups, the largest change in the proportion of people using these products took place between 1987-88 and 1989-90; since that time, many subpopulations have shown little further change, while some have actually shown regression.

The increase in the variety of products used reflects market availability. Although recent rapid growth is seen in some food categories, the picture is still dominated by low-fat milk and skim milk. No other reduced-fat food is reported by more than about 5% of respondents on a given day.

Several findings of the current research confirmed those found previously. Although it has been suggested that consumers of reduced-fat products may obviate their advantages by increasing the amount consumed, in fact this does not happen. Indeed, in many cases the average amount consumed is less for the reduced-fat product that for its full-fat counterpart.

As was found previously, consumption of reduced-fat foods does indeed result in lower fat consumption overall; that is, fat "savings" from use of reduced-fat products are not "compensated for" by increased intake of fat from other sources during the day. For nearly all population groups studied, users of three or more reduced-fat foods per day achieved fat intakes of less than 30% of calories and saturated fatty acid intakes of less than 10% of calories. However, energy reductions were not seen from use of reduced-fat foods for the majority of the population groups. This suggests that heavy users of reduced-fat foods are eating more foods from other groups.

Again confirming earlier findings, vitamin A intake is actually considerably higher among heavy users of reduced-fat products than among nonusers, as are, in most cases, iron and zinc. Although additional research on the overall food intake patterns of these groups is required, this result appears to reflect a dietary pattern containing a variety of sources of vitamins and essential minerals.

The impact on intake of vitamin E of the use of reduced-fat foods is less clear. For the total population, vitamin E intake does not appear to be related to use of reduced-fat products. However, some population groups showed substantial differences, but in opposite directions. The results demonstrate that many consumers are able to choose a diet low in fat, based on extensive use of reduced-fat foods, and still obtain the same level of vitamin E as others obtain from a diet higher in fat.

Clearly, more in-depth examination of the data is required to fully understand the nutritional impact of use of reduced-fat foods and, by implication, of products using fat substitutes. There do appear to be different dynamics at work for different individuals. For example, there is the finding that teenage males who use many reduced-fat products have higher intakes of energy, vitamin A, vitamin E, iron, and zinc than do nonusers of these foods, whereas for teenage females the pattern is reversed: those using three or more reduced-fat products have lower intakes of energy and several nutrients. This suggests that perhaps teenage males tend to consume these products as part of an expanded diet, whereas teenage females may be using these products in a restricted diet.

One finding is exceptionally clear, and that is that blacks are not using reduced-fat foods. The proportion reporting use of even a single such food is less than a third of that for whites. Further, among those who do use at least one reduced-fat food, only about half as many blacks as whites use more than a single food. This represents a clear challenge to nutrition educators.

Overall, the results of this research demonstrate that use of reduced-fat foods can play a valuable part in helping consumers achieve dietary goals pertaining to consumption of fat and saturated fat while still obtaining adequate intakes of vitamins and minerals.

REFERENCES

1. U.S. DEPARTMENT OF AGRICULTURE AND U.S. DEPARTMENT OF HEALTH AND HUMAN SERVICES. 1995. Nutrition and your health: Dietary Guidelines for Americans. Fourth Edition. Home and Garden Bulletin. No. 232.
2. DOUGLASS, J. S., J. T. HEIMBACH, D. K. WAYLETT, B. E. SEVER & B. J. PETERSEN. 1996. Dietary Impact of Fat-Free Food Products. *In* Hypernutritious Foods. J. W. Finley, D. J. Armstrong, S. Nagy & S. F. Robinson, Eds. Agscience. Auburndale, FL.
3. HUMAN NUTRITION INFORMATION SERVICE, USDA. 1990. Nationwide Food Consumption Survey 1987-88 (Individual Intake Component). Dataset.
4. HUMAN NUTRITION INFORMATION SERVICE, USDA. 1992. Nationwide Food Consumption Survey: Continuing Survey of Food Intakes by Individuals 1989-90. Dataset.
5. HUMAN NUTRITION INFORMATION SERVICE, USDA. 1993. Nationwide Food Consumption Survey: Continuing Survey of Food Intakes by Individuals 1990-91. Dataset.
6. AGRICULTURAL RESEARCH SERVICE, USDA. 1994. Nationwide Food Consumption Survey: Continuing Survey of Food Intakes by Individuals 1991-92. Dataset.
7. AGRICULTURAL RESEARCH SERVICE, USDA. 1996. Nationwide Food Consumption Survey: Continuing Survey of Food Intakes by Individuals 1994. Dataset.

Consumer Attitudes and Practices

LYN O'BRIEN NABORS [a]

Calorie Control Council
5775 Peachtree-Dunwoody Road
Suite 500-G
Atlanta, Georgia 30342

Reduced-fat foods and beverage products are extremely important to the consumer and, consequently, to the food industry as well. Fat continues to be consumers' number one nutritional concern. According to the Food Marketing Institute, 60% of consumers state that the fat in their food is their greatest area of concern. This figure has quadrupled since 1987, when only 16% of consumers rated fat as their most important concern.[1]

Indeed, it is difficult to pick up a magazine or newspaper these days without finding some mention of the need to reduce dietary fat intake to 30% or less of calories. Numerous health and government authorities, including the surgeon general, the National Academy of Sciences, the American Heart Association, and the American Dietetic Association, advocate this reduction in fat intake. Even the percent daily value of fat now appearing on food labels is based on 30% of calories.

As a result of this increasing emphasis, there has been an increase in new product introductions and percentage of market share for fat-modified products. According to *New Product News,* 1995 was another banner year for product introductions bearing reduced-fat claims. A total of 1,914 new products bearing reduced- and low-fat claims were introduced in 1995. This is the highest it has ever been, and up from 1,439 new products introduced in 1994.[2]

The U.S. Department of Health and Human Services considered the availability of reduced-fat foods and beverages so important that it included this as a goal of its "Healthy People 2000" program. The program, which began in 1986, set a goal of having at least 5,000 such products available to consumers by the year 2000.[3] And the food and beverage industry has responded. In a 1995 update on the program, HHS said that more than 5,600 low- and reduced-fat products were on the shelves, exceeding the goal set by HHS and doing so five years early. This is one of only two nutritional goals of the program already met.[4]

A couple of specific examples further illustrate the point. The market share for fat-modified cookies increased from zero in 1991 to 15% in 1995, and fat-modified cheese sales more than doubled from 4 to 10%. During the same period, the number of fat-modified cheeses available tripled.[5]

Since 1978 the Calorie Control Council has conducted surveys to gauge public opinion on low-calorie foods and beverages. Reduced fat products were introduced into council surveys in 1991. More than simply tracking consumer usage of reduced-fat foods and beverages, the council's data provide insights into consumer attitudes

[a] Tel: (404) 252-3663; fax: (404) 252-0774; e-mail: naborly@assnhq.com.

toward the products, and into what areas may have growth potential in the next few years. These data will be the primary focus of this discussion.

Qualified respondents for the 1996 survey were males and females age 18 or older. For the survey, a total of 1,500 telephone interviews were completed in February, using a national random probability sample. The data were weighted by sex, age, and region to produce a sample that would be projectable to the entire U.S. population. The sample reliability is +/-2.5 percent. The survey was conducted by Booth Research Services of Atlanta, Georgia, for the Calorie Control Council.

According to the 1996 survey, reduced-fat products are consumed regularly by over 172 million American adults—88% of the adult population.[6] That number has increased by almost 50 million since 1991, when 124 million men and women used these products.[7]

Women are, and have consistently been, more likely to be users than men, but the differences are narrowing. In 1991, 61% of males and 72% of females used these products. In 1996 the numbers increased to 87% of males and 90% of females.

REASONS FOR USING REDUCED-FAT PRODUCTS

The top five reasons for use of reduced-fat products are to stay in better health, to reduce fat, to eat or drink healthier foods and beverages, to reduce cholesterol, and to reduce calories. "To stay in better overall health" (at 79%) is clearly the top reason for consuming low-fat/reduced-fat/fat-free foods and beverages, and has been historically in council surveys.[6]

Important reasons for using reduced-fat products vary between men and women, and by age. Women are more likely to cite the following reasons: to reduce fat, to reduce calories, to lose weight, and because they taste good. Men, significantly more than women, do not cite any specific reason for using reduced-fat products.

Those 50 and older are more likely to view reducing cholesterol, reducing calories, and helping with a medical condition as important, whereas younger respondents (18 to 49) are more likely to say that maintaining an attractive physical appearance or the product's good taste are reasons for using reduced-fat products.

The council's 1996 survey also provides other indicators of American consumers' continued commitment to good health and healthful eating. This survey found that more than three-fourths (78%) of American adults say they are eating a healthier diet today than three years ago. Additionally, the vast majority of consumers of light foods (also 78%) consume light foods and beverages because these products allow them to eat a healthy diet without sacrificing all the foods they like to eat.

Consumers are also reading labels for nutrition information. Sixty-eight percent of adults say they always try to check the nutrition label of the foods and beverages they buy for fat content. Sixty-one percent check for calories.

MOST POPULAR REDUCED-FAT PRODUCTS

A great deal of data presented here clearly indicate that reduced-fat foods and beverages are more popular than ever. It might, therefore, be easy to interpret from this that the reduced-fat phenomenon has "peaked." Indeed, some have tried to argue this very point, and there have been statements to that effect in various trade publications.

The first response to that charge would be simply to point out that the abundance of data, much of which is summarized above, strongly indicate that reduced-fat products continue their popularity unabated, whereas those who have made claims to the contrary have also acknowledged that they have no real data to back their claims. Further to the point, however, the following data demonstrate that, even with the tremendously high level of enjoyment and acceptance of reduced-fat products, opportunities for successful new product introductions exist, and they exist within specific product categories.

The council survey provides data on which products are the most popular and, through comparison with previous surveys, which ones have shown the most promise. First, the most popular reduced-fat products: low-fat or skim milk is consumed by 66% of adults; reduced-fat salad dressings/sauces/mayonnaise are next, with 60%; reduced-fat cheese/dairy products are used by 53%; and reduced-fat margarine is enjoyed by 50 percent.[6]

As for the product categories that show the greatest growth between 1993 and 1996, there are a number: low-fat or skim milk has shown strong growth, up from 48% to 66% usage among consumers today. With regard to percentage growth, though, reduced-fat candy has done best, up 53% since 1993. Reduced-fat chips/snack foods are up 51%, from 29% usage in 1993 to 43 percent, and the reduced-fat cakes/baked goods category has grown 22 percent.[8] With the increasing availability of ingredients and technology to improve baked goods, chips, and candy, these three categories are excellent future growth prospects as well. Tremendous opportunities also abound within many other light-product categories.

DAILY USAGE

One of the council survey's most compelling findings has to do with daily usage of reduced-fat products. It also is a key area of opportunity for such products in the years ahead. The number of people who use reduced-fat products has grown by 22% since 1993.

The segment of those consumers who use the products daily also has grown, but not as much—up 9% among reduced-fat users. Among the total population, however, daily usage of reduced-fat products has soared, up 32% since 1993.

What has happened is that the overall category of reduced-fat food and beverage users has expanded. As it has, and as new consumers have been added, they have entered at a "lower usage level." That is, they are just starting out in their use of reduced-fat products, and they're using them with lower frequency right now. The overall growth in the number of people who use reduced-fat products could be masking what seems like only modest growth in daily usage, but is, in fact, dramatic growth.

More than half (51%) of reduced-fat product consumers enjoy these products on a daily basis. Another 25% use them several times a week. Those who use them daily consume them, on average, 3.3 times per day. Here again, some noteworthy age differences emerge from the data. Those aged 18 to 34 are less likely to be daily users than those 35 and older, but the younger reduced-fat consumers who *do* use the products daily are likely to use more total reduced-fat products per day than older consumers. Daily reduced-fat consumers aged 18 to 34 consume an average of 3.6 products a day, whereas those 35 and older consume 3.1 on average.[6]

DESIRE FOR ADDITIONAL PRODUCTS

Today, 41% of reduced-fat consumers would like to see additional reduced-fat products available, down from 60% in 1993 and 67% in 1991. This finding is not surprising, however. It attests to the improved quality of products reduced in fat. Products garnering the most interest were meat products, named by 17% of those who would like to see more reduced-fat products available, and snacks/chips, which were named by 16 percent. The interest in additional reduced-fat snacks/chips is significantly higher than in 1993—up from 10 percent. This is interesting because reduced-fat snacks and chips have been one of the fastest-growing categories in America, and yet interest in having additional products has grown right along with it.

DIETING

Because consumer attitudes toward dieting and weight loss often affect attitudes toward fat and fat reduction, the 1996 survey's data on dieting also are of interest. Today, 24% of adults are on a diet—a level that has remained relatively constant, ranging between 24% and 27%, since 1989, when the council's survey was the first to identify a significant decline in dieting.[9] In the 1986 survey, 37% of respondents said they were dieting.[10] By 1989, that number dropped to 26%, and it has hovered in that range ever since.

The methods for dieting are largely unchanged. That is good news for the reduced-fat food and beverage industry, because using foods and beverages reduced in fat is the second most popular method of dieting. This method is used by 93% of those who are on a diet. Cutting down on foods high in sugar, starch, or fat is the top method, used by 95 percent. Exercise is third at 88%, and use of low-calorie, sugar-free foods and beverages is a close fourth, at 84 percent.[6]

The data seem to show that dieters understand how to diet sensibly, the majority of them say they are cutting back on fat and calories, and exercising.

PREFERRED LABEL DESCRIPTORS

Additionally, the council's 1996 survey provides insight into what attracts consumers with regard to food label descriptors, which can have significant implications for future product introductions.

Reduced-fat consumers were asked in the survey to choose between a number of descriptors having to do with fat reduction. The term "fat-free" was the most preferred descriptor, named by 29% of reduced-fat consumers. The other descriptors scored as follows, as a favorite among reduced-fat product consumers: low fat at 20%, no fat at 18%, light at 15%, and reduced fat at 11 percent.[6] These levels are generally the same as they were 1993.

In addition, 84% of reduced-fat users reported that it is important for them to know the actual percent that a product is reduced in fat. Among reduced-fat consumers who are also dieting, an overwhelming number (93%) rated the actual percent reduction in fat as important.[6]

CALORIES STILL COUNT

Clearly, light and reduced-fat products are more popular than ever. There is little doubt that Americans are concerned about the fat content of their diet and are taking steps to decrease it. U.S. Department of Agriculture food consumption surveys bear this out, indicating that Americans got 33% of their calories from fat in 1994, down from 40 percent in 1977-78.[11]

So why aren't Americans thinner than ever? The answer is not a simple one. Experts believe a number of factors contribute to the increasing incidence of overweight in this country—currently about 33%, according to National Center for Health Statistics.[12] The continuing level of physical inactivity of Americans has been cited by numerous researchers as a major factor. Only 15% of Americans exercise strenuously three times a week, according to the recently released Surgeon General's Report on Physical Activity and Health.[13]

In America today, there is, we hope, an increasing and converging scientific and public awareness of the need to reduce both obesity and intake of fat and calories in food, and the concomitant need to increase levels of physical activity. This point was emphasized in a February 1996 study released by The National Academy of Sciences. The study concluded that, in terms of cancer causation, far greater than any risk from chemicals in food is the risk associated with fat and excess calories in foods. The researchers stated that, "... the contribution of calories and fat outweighs that of all other individual food chemicals, both the naturally occurring and synthetic" and "Americans would benefit most from eating fewer calories and fats."[14]

CONCLUSION

To a large degree, the food and beverage industry is succeeding in introducing a wide variety of reduced-fat and fat-free products that closely mimic the taste, texture, and mouthfeel of their higher-fat counterparts. The prospects for increasing the array of light foods and beverages has never been better, particularly when the wide range of reduced-fat ingredients currently available is considered, as well as many that lie just over the horizon.

Consumer education, however, about the proper role of these products as part of a healthy lifestyle and in weight control, including exercise, is necessary. We hope that the E of NLEA (the Nutrition Labeling and Education Act) will become a reality and that consumers will increasingly understand that calories still count.

As the council's study has shown, there are still many positive indicators for overall reduced-fat market growth. Of course, the final determination on whether or not a particular light product will succeed is simple: Does the product taste good? This is what has always separated the winners from the losers, and it will continue to be the challenge for light food and beverage processors. Among the relatively few people who do not consume light products (only 12%), the number one reason, according to the council's survey, is taste.[6] Where once consumers demanded low-calorie and reduced-fat products that they hoped tasted good, now they demand good taste as well. The burden for food processors has shifted: now they must satisfy the public's desire for better health *and* indulgence.

REFERENCES

1. FOOD MARKETING INSTITUTE. 1996. Trends in the United States: Consumer Attitudes and the Supermarket. Washington, D.C.
2. PREPARED FOODS. 1996. New Products Watch. April, p. 37.
3. U.S. DEPARTMENT OF HEALTH AND HUMAN SERVICES. 1990. Healthy People 2000. National Health Promotion and Disease Prevention Objectives. DHHS Publication No. (PHS) 91-50212. U.S. Government Printing Office, Washington, D.C.
4. U.S. DEPARTMENT OF HEALTH AND HUMAN SERVICES. 1995. Healthy People 2000 Midcourse Review and 1995 Revisions.
5. FOOD LABELING & NUTRITION NEWS. 1996. NLEA Affecting Consumer Nutrition Label Usage, Market Trends: FDA Survey, June 13, p. 10.
6. CALORIE CONTROL COUNCIL. 1996. Light Products Survey, Booth Research Services, Inc., Atlanta, GA. (unpublished)
7. CALORIE CONTROL COUNCIL. 1991. Dieting and Low-Calorie/Reduced-Fat Products Survey, Booth Research Services, Inc., Atlanta, GA. (unpublished)
8. CALORIE CONTROL COUNCIL. 1993. Dieting and Low-Calorie/Reduced-Fat Products Survey, Booth Research Services, Inc. (unpublished)
9. CALORIE CONTROL COUNCIL. 1989. Low-Calorie Products Survey, Booth Research Services, Inc., Atlanta, GA. (unpublished)
10. CALORIE CONTROL COUNCIL. 1986. Dieting and Low-Calorie Products Survey, Booth Research Services, Inc., Atlanta, GA. (unpublished)
11. PUTNAM, J. J. & L. A. DUEWER. 1995. FoodReview, May-August. p. 10.
12. KUCZMARSKI, A. J. *et al.* 1994. J. Am. Med. Assoc. **272** (3):205.
13. MANLEY, A. F. 1996. Physical Activity and Health: A Report of the Surgeon General. U.S. Government Printing Office, Pittsburgh, PA.
14. NATIONAL RESEARCH COUNCIL. 1996. Carcinogens and Anticarcinogens in the Human Diet; National Academy Press. Chapter 5, p. 308.

Social Determinants of Food Intake

LOUIS E. GRIVETTI [a]

Department of Nutrition
University of California
Davis, California 95616

INTRODUCTION

Interest and study of food patterns of individuals and societies stems from antiquity. Ancient Egyptian scribes documented rations of soldiers and servants; Greek and Roman naturalists and physicians described characteristic foods of ancient Mediterranean societies; ancient Indian and Chinese texts have provided details of everyday and festival foods; and medieval and early modern travel and exploration accounts reported aspects of food production, food storage, cooking, and dietary practice throughout most regions of the world.[1–7]

Systematic investigations of the social determinants of food intake, however, stem from the 20th century. Such studies initially were associated with resupply efforts directed toward war-torn populations after World War I.[8] Although basic principles of effective food relief were developed at the end of World War I, there has been an unevenness of subsequent food relief efforts, especially at the conclusion of World War II, and during subsequent decades. Nutritional and medical problems associated with food relief following widespread social unrest, civil war, and environmentally produced disasters reveal that the principles were not easily learned and applied.[9]

The basic principles that determine how and why people accept or reject food were reexamined and published in two important documents produced by the Committee on Food Habits of the National Research Council during World War II.[10,11] In subsequent years the number of nutritional anthropologists and others interested in food patterns and the social determinants of food intake behavior has increased sharply. These professionals have produced a wide range of bibliographies[12,13] and manuals.[14,15] Contemporary social scientists interested in food and diet have drawn extensively from this rich twentieth century literature, but, collectively, we owe our methods and research paradigms to the numerous pioneers who laid the methodological foundations for our investigations.

FOOD-SELECTION PRINCIPLES

Availability

Four principles influence and determine food patterns in individuals, families, or societies. The principal of availability can be stated as a truism: humans cannot eat

---

[a] Tel: (916) 752-2078; fax: (916) 752-8966; e-mail: legrivetti@ucdavis.edu.

what is not available. Specific foods, however, may be constant or available throughout the calendar year due to natural characteristics of the food, or available because of advances in food technology, improved storage, expanded world trade networks, and improved food distribution systems. Food availability, on the other hand, may be seasonal or irregular due to environmental constraints or because of limited access to advanced preservation, storage, and distribution technology. Food availability also is driven by economic concepts, specifically supply and demand: foods may be geographically available, but may be too expensive for purchase and consumption.[16]

Familiarity

The principal of familiarity holds that although potential foods may be available, if humans do not perceive items as edible and fit for consumption, such potential foods will go unrecognized. Individuals and societies within all environmental settings establish norms that identify a broad range of specific items as edible and suitable for consumption. Familiarity, however, does not correlate with nutritional quality, whether high or low caloric, or vitamin or mineral content. Each culture and society throughout history has determined what is suitable and fit, and conversely unsuitable and forbidden.[17] In many instances these decisions are codified in formal religious codes and tenants expressed in Buddhism, Christianity, Hinduism, Islam, Judaism, or in animistic and natural spirit faiths throughout the world.[18-21]

The concept of familiarity is driven initially by availability, then by nonnutritional food-related functions, that is, how foods and consumables are used culturally, economically, and politically within society. Because an item is perceived familiar and deemed suitable or fit for consumption does not imply that the food has high nutritional value or is safe to eat. Foods familiar and widely consumed in one society may go unrecognized in other social groups and may not be perceived as edible. Beef, chicken, eggs, fish, and pork, for example, are widely eaten in many world societies, but these same foods are viewed with revulsion and disgust by others. Further, edible insects, cats and dogs, carrion, and various barks, flowers, fungi, leaves, resins, roots, stems, and tubers are highly suitable in many world societies, but not to most Americans in 1996. The principle of familiarity, therefore, has led to the old classic saw: "one man's meat is another's poison."[22]

The principle of familiarity, furthermore, may be extended to a singular, logical conclusion: humans starve in the midst of food plenty. With few exceptions humans starve because hungry people are not familiar with, and hence do not recognize, the countless edible items available to them as potential foods. People starve because of cultural–social dictates that identify and "carve-out" a specific spectrum of available, potential items identified as familiar and culturally suitable.[1] It follows, furthermore, that what humans do not recognize as potential food resources cannot be articulated and cannot be passed on as knowledge to future generations. This leads to a rapid decline of food knowledge and awareness that specific available items can serve as human food during time of environmental catastrophe, social–political unrest, or warfare. Ample food resources existed in the Sahel and Kalahari deserts of Africa during recent droughts. In the Sahel these food items went unrecognized; in the Kalahari they were used: in the Sahel there was massive starvation, but in the Kalahari malnutrition and famine were limited.[23]

Selectivity

Potential foods available and recognized as fit for humans to eat present a broad spectrum in any environmental niche and cultural setting. Not all potential items identified fit for consumption are selected or chosen by individuals. Human food selection is primarily based upon individual likes and dislikes based upon sensory evaluation of past experience with the food. If foods are tasted and liked, consumption is likely to be repeated; if foods are tasted and disliked other principles come into play and rejected items may or may not be consumed again.[24] Two corollaries logically follow from the principle of selectivity: (1) individuals or societies do not maximize dietary use of potential foods available and within any environmental niche; and (2) because foods have quite different nutrient composition, diets chosen can be sound, marginal, or deficient.

Despite publications to the contrary,[25,26] research suggests there are no innate mechanisms that "trigger" human food selection for specific nutrients.[27] Although specific mechanisms regulate energy balance and food intake, there are no "felt needs" for specific nutrients. Although sodium intake and thirst regulatory mechanisms are interlinked, zinc-deficient individuals do not recognize they are deficient. Regarding energy, one senses hunger and the need to eat, which leads to behavior regulated by mechanisms associated with appetite and satiety. Although several publications during the 1970s suggested that humans turned to cannibalism because of a "lack of available protein foods," there is no felt need for protein.[28,29] In essence, people throughout the world select dietary components because food items and combinations are available, because foods are familiar and culturally correct, and because specific items taste good. Furthermore, most humans do not select foods for their nutritional value. Those who do primarily are community nutritionists, home economists, dietitians, nutrition scientists, and their professional clients.

Food selection also is driven by historical considerations, economic issues, and by 19th and 20th century marketing decisions. Exploration and contact between the Old and New Worlds after 1492 led to an expansion of available foods, the so-called "Colombian exchange." Between 1492 and 1612, British, French, and Spanish explorers, priests, and military men conquered and occupied portions of the New World. Paralleling the military conquest and settlement was a corresponding "clash of cuisine," as New World foods found acceptance into the national cuisines of Africa, Asia, and Europe. The following foods were not available and known in the Old World before 1492: amaranth, artichoke, avocado, kidney bean, lima bean, blackberry, blueberry, cacao (chocolate), cassava, black cherry, cranberry, concord grape, guava, huckleberry, maize, papaya, peanut, pecan, chili pepper, pineapple, popcorn, potato, pumpkin, quinoa, raspberry, wild rice, sassafras, sunflower, tomato, and turkey. Conversely, a host of Old World foods were imported and spread throughout North, Central, and South America: almond, apple, apricot, asparagus, barley, cabbage, cattle (beef, milk, and dairy products), cucumber, eggplant, garlic, goat (meat, milk, and dairy products), grapes (subsequent European wines), lemon, lettuce, lime, oats (and oatmeal), olive, onion, orange, pig (pork and lard), rice, rye, sheep (lamb, milk, and dairy products), sugar cane, turnip, and wheat.[31]

In the years following 1492, the Colombian exchange led to improved food diversity and diet; in other instances, however, the exchange led to economic and medical-nutritional disasters. Some recently introduced foods were adopted and became new dietary staples. Use of other foods, once dietary staples, declined, became minor food elements, and were nearly forgotten. Former dietary staples or foods once prominent in the New World diet included agouti, añus, calabash, caiman, chuñu, coraçon, duck potato, golden club, guanaco, iguana, jicama, manatee, muskrat, oca, pemmican, pitahaya, sacqwuenummener berry, tapir, or zapote. Who recognizes or eats these items today?[30]

In Europe, Old World wheat gave way to New World potatoes in several geographical regions. With the appearance of potato blight, famine and economic catastrophe occurred in places like Ireland and central Switzerland.[31] The conventional view holds that New World maize brought to Europe by Columbus subsequently dispersed throughout Europe, then into Africa and Asia. Maize consumed alone, without its culturally protective mix of legumes, led to pellagra, which was initially described as a medical problem in Mediterranean Europe. There is no evidence that pellagra existed before 1492. Thus, the combined principles of availability, familiarity, and selectivity were central to the cultural decisions to consume maize in Europe, and pellagra resulted.[32]

Anticipation–Expectation

Individuals anticipate and expect specific sensory properties to be associated with specific foods because of past, learned experience. Consumer anticipation-expectation follows from four categories of information: taste (four dimensions of sweet, sour, salt, and bitter); color (two dimensions of hue and intensity); texture (a subjective continuum anchored by ''smooth'' and ''coarse''); and odor (a second subjective continuum anchored by ''delightful'' and ''terrible'').[33]

Deviation from anticipated, expected sensory properties serves as a warning to consumers that the item may be unsafe. Greenish-blue, iridescent potatoes would not likely be consumed, but how far from the expected ''white'' are consumers willing to accept? In this instance acceptability also may be a function of marketing, inasmuch as potato biodiversity provides a range of cultivars with distinctive nonwhite colors, and blue potatoes have found limited commercial success after being served at upscale restaurants where the menu highlights *nouveau cuisine*.

The principal of anticipation-expectation, further, is related more to the principle of familiarity, than to factors associated with food-related safety. Deviation from expected taste, color, texture, and odor may lead consumers to reject items that are safe for human consumption, an issue that lies more with aesthetics and anticipated taste, color, odor, and texture than with food safety.[34]

FOOD-REJECTION PRINCIPLES

Humans do not have an innate sense of what is edible and inedible. Humans learn to make these distinctions during infancy. Human protection during infancy is the cultural training ground for food acceptance and food avoidance behavior, without which most infants would die. In a classic paper on the origins of human dietary practices, Leopold and Ardry observed that most plants in any ecological niche were toxic to humans. They argued that the ability to make and maintain fire, approximately 500,000 years ago, led to cooking, which allowed a broad range of plant compounds toxic to human consumers to be neutralized. They noted, furthermore, that bitterness generally correlated with toxicity and served as a warning to potential consumers that specific plants could be dangerous.[35] But bitterness, in and of itself, does not automatically serve as a warning to consumers. Human infants, when presented with a bitter beverage challenge, produce an expected facial grimace, but then the infant reaches out for a second taste of the bitter product: they taste the bitter solution, produce further facial grimaces, and continue to reach out for more. This unexpected finding works against the intuitive logic that bitter and potentially toxic items would be rejected as human food. The work of Leopold and Ardry revealed the paramount need for human supervision of food-related behavior of infants and young children. It logically follows from their research that if human infants were left unprotected to forage for food without adult supervision, they would be poisoned and die after consuming toxic plants. Bitterness, therefore, does not necessarily lead to food rejection. How, then, do humans distinguish edible from inedible, safe from toxic, and ultimately select diets that are nutritionally sound? Food avoidance and rejection is determined by a range of factors.

Gatekeepers

Researchers in human food behavior commonly use an analytical concept of the "gatekeeper," initially identified by Kurt Lewin in the 1930s.[25] Lewin coined the term "gatekeeper" to identify persons or economic, political, and social institutions that facilitate or hinder access to food. He perceived human diet and food patterns as the result of the flow of food down "channels," a concept where foods ultimately were produced, processed, transported to markets, purchased, and flowed to households where they were prepared, served, and consumed. Lewin's channels reflected food-related contributions from hunting-gathering, agriculture-horticulture, animal husbandry, as well as from barter, gift, and cash exchanges. His gatekeepers were perceived as factors that facilitated or restricted the flow of food down the channels, from field, to distribution points, to markets, to household pantries.

A Lewin-style analysis of food and energy flow in society reveals the power of gatekeepers and their influence in both food acceptance and food avoidance or rejection. Teamster truckers represent an example of a gatekeeper. Most food in the United States is distributed by truck; if the Teamster's Union goes on strike, for example, one immediately sees their influence on the flow and distribution of food, and ultimately on the availability of foods within the effected geographical area.

Food-rejection Principles

Individual likes and dislikes, however, influence which foods are purchased and ultimately reach the household and human palate. A variety of factors determine why foods are rejected. Some foods are consumed initially, then rejected because of specific individual decisions caused by physical characteristics of the food, whether color, odor, taste, texture. The pattern is basic: eat, evaluate, repeat consumption, or reject. Yet, other foods are rejected before they are consumed because of appearance and unmet consumer expectations. Examples would be blue peas, green carrots, slimy fish, items that probably would be rejected before being tasted. Many Americans, if offered plates of stingless bees, caterpillars, snake eggs, or monkey brains, would immediately reject such fare, whereas others would be willing to taste, evaluate, and eat these foods.

Paul Rozin, the noted food psychologist, coined two words to describe food acceptance and rejection behavior. He used the word *neophobia,* or fear of the new, to describe consumer unwillingness to experiment with different, culturally incorrect cuisines. The opposite condition he called *neophilia,* or love of the new, that represented others who were adventurous, willing to take food-related risks, who regularly sought out unusual, different food resources. Rozin was the first to observe this basic human food-related dichotomy, a pattern that certainly dates to the dawn of human existence. What is intriguing, however, is that twentieth century individuals may pride themselves on being neophiles and exhibit a willingness to experiment with new, unusual foods. When Rozin's concept is placed within an evolutionary context, however, it has been the neophiles who experimented with wild, undomesticated plants and became poisoned, whereas it was the conservative neophobes who stuck with familiar, old favorite items that passed their genes to the next generation.[36,37]

Food rejection is due to learned behaviors. Infants are not born with culturally determined attitudes towards food. Infants do not learn through trial and error, but through the acceptance-rejection patterns of their parents, other caregivers, and the social dictates of the society into which each child is born. Culturally determined visual cues, linked with concepts of expectation-anticipation play significant rolls in understanding food rejection.

Aversive Foods

Some potential foods originally tasted and then rejected by consumers fit a separate category. Paul Rozin and his colleagues also were the first to identify these so-called aversive foods. This category of foods includes items initially perceived as distasteful and nearly always rejected, but because of specific social-cultural circumstances, consumers are regularly exposed to the foods. After repeated consumption the aversive food, once rejected, becomes liked, desired, and craved. Examples include alcoholic beverages (especially beer), chili peppers, and prepared horseradish.[38]

Avoidance Behavior

Psychologists interested in food patterns, especially aversions or avoidance behavior, suggest that cultural transmission of food information is so powerful that humans classify many items as inedible that never have been consumed. Psychologists suggest that individuals recognize foods that are culturally correct or incorrect early in childhood, probably by the age of ten. One result of social-cultural identification of so-called "proper" and "improper" foods is biologically maladaptive: foods are rejected by young children, and the rejection pattern is transmitted through adolescence into adult years and then retransmitted to children born of these parents. As a result many thousands of nutritious foods are not consumed because they are perceived as improper, or are not recognized at all as a potential food.

Cultural Suitability

Another important result of cultural transmission of food-related information and deciding what is "good" and "not good" to eat is seen with the difficulty of introducing new foods into different parts of the world. Food researchers working in the international arena regularly have heard responsible scientists and administrators claim that food habits or food patterns are not important during famine because starving people will eat anything. This is incorrect: many will elect to starve during famine rather than eat food that is culturally or religiously incorrect. Furthermore, it is callous merely to send food that donors, themselves, like to eat. At the very least donor countries should recognize the basic food patterns and attempt to match donated food with needs of the society requesting international food assistance.

Food-rejection Principles

At the most basic level, there are three reasons for rejecting food, sometimes identified as the "3 Ds": danger, rejected because of the anticipated postingestion consequences, whether allergic reaction, indigestion, or vomiting; disgust, rejected because of the origin or nature of the food; and distaste, rejected because of the smell and taste.[39]

Religious issues also are important and determine a broad range of acceptable and forbidden foods. A meal of roast beef and wine, for example, could never be followed by coffee and cream in Orthodox Jewish homes; wine could serve as a central meal beverage in both Jewish and Christian homes, but never in Muslim families; creamed tuna on toast would never be served to Muslims in Egypt, but the same combination is acceptable to both Jews and Christians. In Medieval Europe breads or cookies in human form were never prepared by Christians, and during the Spanish Inquisition, Muslims and Jews who rejected pork were executed.[40]

Food rejection also takes another form, whereby items liked individually are rejected and considered inappropriate or repulsive if served in combination. Examples that could be repugnant in American society might include braised salmon topped with ice cream; asparagus-flavored chocolate; fried potatoes in wine; and spaghetti served with a festive caramel pudding sauce.[41]

Individual foods and combinations considered appropriate at a specific meal setting may be inappropriate at others. An individual may like pepperoni pizza, but consider this food inappropriate at breakfast. Conversely, others would not prepare orange juice and waffles for an evening meal. Following this line, educators who conduct research on food choice regularly are challenged by students in who regularly consume Jell-O and pizza for breakfast, potato chips at dinner, and who think nothing of combining ice cream with garden salad.

Social Status and Prestige

Food selection and rejection also are associated with social status and prestige. Each society determines a set of so-called status foods, items that possess well-defined characteristics. Status foods, for example, tend to be expensive (caviar; vintage wines), time consuming or difficult to prepare (stuffed grape leaves; homemade pasta), complex in recipe with numerous ingredients (moussaka; seven-bean salad), usually animal protein (steak), or have a specific cultural identity (rice in Asia; bread in Greece; homemade apple pie in America).[42] It follows that if certain foods fit a status category, then other foods must be "everyday" or low-status items with opposite characteristics: inexpensive; quick or easy to prepare; simple recipe with few ingredient; and lesser cuts of meat.

Low status or everyday items tend to be served to family members on a regular basis and are not offered to guests when entertaining. Everyday or low-status foods, however, may shift upward in status if the food is fussed-over (grilled hamburgers with special spices), prepared in an unusual manner (barbecued with a secret sauce), shaped differently (carrot curls; tomato stars), or given an unusual name (Sam's special Saturday spaghetti).[43]

Famine Foods

Food selection and rejection considerations also lead to the concept of famine food. These items are defined as foods recognized by individuals or societies, but normally rejected so long as there are abundant other food resources.[44] Hence, individuals turn to famine foods during periods of limited food availability; consumers then return to a regular diet, omitting the famine foods, after the return of food-related security. Famine foods are critical in certain geographical areas of the world because they maintain general energy needs during drought, social unrest, or war.[45] Although famine foods have been the research focus of a wide variety of scholars, most investigations, including nutritional composition, have been conducted during a particular famine or drought.[46-48]

CONCLUSIONS

Although descriptive work on diet and food patterns stems from antiquity, research on the social determinants of food intake is associated with investigations conducted by the League of Nations when both social and environmental aspects of food patterns were undertaken to improve consumer acceptance of food-relief items. Subsequent research by anthropologists, economists, and psychologists were instrumental in improving dietary patterns in America and abroad during and after World War II. Methods and approaches used by recent investigators attracted to food intake patterns and the nutritional consequences of food-related behavior were developed more than 50 years ago and have been refined during recent decades.

REFERENCES

1. GRIVETTI, L. E. 1981. Cultural nutrition. Anthropological and geographical themes. Annu. Rev. Nutr. **1:** 47-68.
2. DARBY, W. J., P. GHALIOUNGUI & L. E. GRIVETTI. 1977. Food, The Gift of Osiris. 2 Vols. Academic Press. London, England.
3. ATHENAEUS. 1927-1941. The Deipnosophists. 7 Vols. Translated by C. B. Gulick. Putnam, New York, NY.
4. PLINY. 1938-1956. Natural History. Translated by H. Rackham and W. H. S. Jones. 8 Vols. William Heinemann, London, England.
5. CARAKA-SAMHITA. 1981. Agnivesa's Treatise, Refined and Annotated by Caraka, and Redacted by Drdhabala. Vol. 1. Sutrasthana to Indriyasthana. Edited by P. Sharma. Chaukambha Orientalia, Delhi, India.
6. SIMOONS, F. J. 1991. Food in China. A Cultural and Historical Inquiry. CRC Press. Boca Raton, Florida.
7. BERNAL DÍAZ [DEL CASTILLO]. 1956. The Discovery and Conquest of Mexico, 1517-1521. Edited from the only exact copy of the original manuscript (and published in Mexico) by Genaro Garcia. Translated by A. P. Maudslay. Farrar, Straus, and Cudahy, New York, NY.
8. BIGWOOD, E. J. 1939. Guiding Principles for Studies on the Nutrition of Populations. League of Nations, Health Organization, Technical Committee on Nutrition. Vol. 3, Number 1. Geneva, Switzerland. League of Nations.
9. AALL, C. 1970. Relief, nutrition, and health problems in the Nigerian/Biafran War. J. Trop. Pediatr. **16:** 70-80.
10. COMMITTEE ON FOOD HABITS. 1943. The Problem of Changing Food Habits. National Research Council Bulletin 108. National Research Council, National Academy of Sciences. Washington, D.C.
11. COMMITTEE ON FOOD HABITS. 1945. Manual for the Study of Food Habits. National Research Council Bulletin 111. National Research Council, National Academy of Sciences. Washington, D.C.
12. FREEDMAN, R. L. 1981. Human Food Uses. A Cross-Cultural, Comprehensive Annotated Bibliography. Greenwood. London, England.
13. WILSON, C. S. 1979. Food—Custom and Nurture. An annotated bibliography on sociocultural and biocultural aspects of nutrition. J. Nutr. Ed. Supplement to Volume 11.
14. DE GARINE, I. 1972. The Socio-cultural aspects of nutrition. Ecol. Food Nutr. **1:** 143-163.
15. QUANDT, S. A. & C. RITENBAUGH. 1986. Training Manual in Nutritional Anthropology. American Anthropological Association. Washington, D.C.
16. GRIVETTI, L. E. 1978. Culture, diet, and nutrition. Selected themes and topics. Bioscience **28:** 171-177.
17. GRIVETTI, L. E. 1997. Food Prejudices and Taboos. *In* Cambridge History and Culture of Human Nutrition. Cambridge University Press. New York, NY. In press.
18. GRIVETTI, L. E. & R. M. PANGBORN. 1974. Origin of selected Old Testament dietary prohibitions. J. Am. Diet. Assoc. **65:** 634-638.
19. JELLIFFE, D. B. & E. F. P. JELLIFFE. 1978. Food habits and taboos: How have they protected man in his evolution? Prog. Hum. Nutr. **2:** 67-76.
20. KILARA, A. & K. K. IYA. 1992. Food and dietary habits of the Hindu. Food Technol. **46**(10): 94-104.
21. REGENSTEIN, J. M. & C. E. REGENSTEIN. 1988. The kosher dietary laws and their implementation in the food industry. Food Technol. **42**(6): 86, 88-94.
22. GRIVETTI, L. E. 1978. Culture, diet, and nutrition. Selected themes and topics. Bioscience **28**(3): 171-177.
23. GRIVETTI, L. E. Nutritional success in a semi-arid land. Examination of Tswana agropastoralists of the Eastern Kalahari, Botswana. Am. J. Clin. Nutr. **31:** 1204-1220.

24. LEWIN, K. 1943. Forces behind food habits and methods of change. *In* The problem of changing food habits. Committee on Food Habits, National Research Council Bulletin, Number 108. pp. 35-65. National Academy of Sciences, Washington, D.C.
25. DAVIS, C. M. 1928. Self-selection of diet by newly weaned infants. Am. J. Dis. Child. **36:** 651-679.
26. DAVIS, C. M. 1939. Results of the self-selection of diets by young children. Can. Med. Assoc. J. **41:** 257-679.
27. STORY, M. & J. E. BROWN. 1987. Do young children instinctively know what to eat? N. Engl. J. Med. **316:** 103-106.
28. HARNER, M. 1977. The enigma of Aztec sacrifice. Natural History **136:** 47-51.
29. ORTIZ DE MONTELLANO, B. 1978. Aztec cannibalism. An ecological necessity? Science **200:** 611-617.
30. GRIVETTI, L. E. 1992. Clash of cuisines. Notes on Christoforo Colombo 1492-1503. Nutr. Today **26**(2): 13-15.
31. UHLE, A. F. & L. E. GRIVETTI. 1993. Alpine and Brazilian Swiss food patterns after a century of isolation. Ecol. Food Nutr. **29:** 119-138.
32. PATWARDEN, V. N. & W. J. DARBY. 1972. The State of Nutrition in the Arab Middle East. pp. 34-56. Vanderbilt University Press. Nashville, Tennessee.
33. AMERINE, M. A., R. M. PANGBORN & B. ROESSLER, 1965. Principles of Sensory Evaluation of Food. Academic Press. New York, NY.
34. KARE, M. R. & O. MALLER. 1967. The Chemical Senses and Nutrition. With a Bibliography on the Sense of Taste, prepared by R. M. Pangborn and I. M. Trabue. Johns Hopkins Press. Baltimore, Maryland.
35. LEOPOLD, A. C. & R. ARDREY. 1972. Toxic substances in plants and the food habits of early man. Science **176:** 512-514.
36. ROZIN, P. & A. E. FALLON. 1980. The psychological categorization of foods and non-foods: A preliminary taxonomy of food rejections. Appetite **1:** 193-201.
37. ROZIN, P. & A. E. FALLON. 1981. The acquisition of likes and dislikes for foods. *In* Criteria of Food Acceptance. How Man Chooses What He Eats. J. Solms & R. L. Hall, Eds.: 35-48. Forster. Zurich, Switzerland.
38. FALLON, A. E. & P. ROZIN. 1983. The psychological bases of food rejections by humans. Ecol. Food Nutr. **13:** 15-26.
39. ROZIN, P. & T. A. VOLLMECKE. 1986. Food likes and dislikes. Annu. Rev. Nutr. **6:** 433-456.
40. GRIVETTI, L. E., S. J. LAMPRECHT, H. J. ROCKE & A. WATERMAN. 1987. Threads of cultural nutrition. Arts and humanities. Progr. Food Nutr. Sci. **11:** 249-306.
41. GRIVETTI, L. E. 1975. Flavor and culture. The importance of flavors in the Middle East. Food Technol. **29**(6): 38-40.
42. JELLIFFE, D. B. 1967. Parallel food classification in developing and industrialized countries. Am. J. Clin. Nutr. **20:** 279-281.
43. GRIVETTI, L. E., S. J. LAMPRECHT, H. J. ROCKE & A. WATERMAN. 1987. Threads of cultural nutrition. Arts and humanities. Progr. Food & Nutr. Sci. **11:** 249-306.
44. SMITH, G. C., M. S. CLEGG, C. L. KEEN & L. E. GRIVETTI. 1995. Mineral values of selected plant foods common to Southern Burkina Faso and to Niamey, Niger, West Africa. Int. J. Food Sci. Nutr. **47:** 41-53.
45. GRIVETTI, L. E., C. J. FRENTZEL, K. E. GINSBERG, K. L. HOWELL & B. M. OGLE. 1987. Bush foods and edible weeds of agriculture. Perspectives on dietary use of wild plants in Africa, their role in maintaining human nutritional status, and implications for agricultural development. *In* Health and Disease in Tropical Africa. Geographical and Medical Viewpoints. R. Akhtar, Ed.: 51-81. Harwood. London.

46. OGLE B. M. & L. E. GRIVETTI. 1985d. Legacy of the chameleon. Edible wild plants in the kingdom of Swaziland, Southern Africa. A cultural, ecological, nutritional study. Part 4. Nutritional Analysis and Conclusions. Ecol. Food Nutr. **17:** 41-64.
47. HUMPHRY, C., M. S. CLEGG, C. L. KEEN & L. E. GRIVETTI. 1993. Food diversity and drought survival. The Hausa example. Int. J. Food Sci. Nutr. **44:** 1-16.
48. SMITH, G. C., S. R. DUEKER, A. J. CLIFFORD & L. E. GRIVETTI. 1996. Carotenoid values of selected plant foods common to Southern Burkina Faso, West Africa. Ecol. Food Nutr. **35:** 43-58.

Macronutrient Substitutes and Weight-reduction Practices of Obese, Dieting, and Eating-disordered Women

ADAM DREWNOWSKI [a]

Human Nutrition Program
University of Michigan School of Public Health
Ann Arbor, Michigan 48109-2029

One in three adult Americans is reported to be obese. Data from the 1989-91 National Health and Nutrition Examination Survey (NHANES III) place the prevalence of obesity at 33%.[1] This represents a sharp increase from the 1976-80 NHANES II survey, which found that 24.4% of men and 26.7% of women were obese.[2] Obesity was defined by the 85th percentile cutpoint of BMI values (BMI = wt/ht^2) for a reference population in the third decade of life.[2] According to some reports, the prevalence of obesity has increased most rapidly among children, teenagers, minorities, and newly immigrant ethnic groups.[3,4] Adolescent women, in particular, showed the greatest increase in both energy intakes and body weights[5] and appear to be the population at most risk.

Dieting to lose weight is a relatively common behavior, particularly among women. Most women, regardless of their body weight, wish to be thinner than they are.[6] However, the precise nature of weight management practices can be difficult to establish, partly because of differing definitions of the word "diet." Survey studies that define dieting as restricting calories for the purpose of losing weight suggest that two out of five adult women are dieting at any one time.[6] Lifetime prevalence of dieting to lose weight is, of course, much higher, and it is estimated that 80 or 90% of the female population have dieted at some point in their lives.[7,8] Psychologists and social scientists have noted that dieting to lose weight has become a normative behavior among young women, even among those women who are not overweight or obese.[9]

The management of body weight is a major societal preoccupation and a multibillion dollar industry. Studies of weight management practices of overweight men and women suggest that reducing the amount of sugar and fat in the diet is the most common option by far.[7,10] Most dieters, whether male or female, have at some point used foods containing macronutrient substitutes for weight control. Such foods are likely to contain intense sweeteners, fat replacement products, or both. Though not intended as appetite suppressants, foods containing macronutrient substitutes help to

---

[a] Address correspondence to Adam Drewnowski, Human Nutrition Program, School of Public Health M-5170, 1420 Washington Heights, Ann Arbor, MI 48109-2029. Tel: (313) 647-0208; fax: (313) 764-5233; e-mail: adamdrew@umich.edu.

maintain the variety and the diversity of energy-restricted diets.[10] The effectiveness of foods containing macronutrient substitutes in the management of body weight is a topic of both clinical and public health interest.

WEIGHT MANAGEMENT PRACTICES

Not all attempts at weight control are benign. Dieting behaviors are distributed along a continuum that ranges from complete lack of concern with body weight to pathological dieting and eating disorders.[11] Among scales and measures designed to assess the degree of concern with dieting and the type of efforts at weight control are the restraint scale,[9] the eating pathology scale,[11] the dieting severity scale,[12] and numerous questionnaires that deal with binge eating and other symptoms of eating disorders.[13,14] Clinically significant eating disorders, anorexia and bulimia nervosa, are generally regarded as the pathological extreme of a broader continuum of dieting behaviors.[11] Epidemiological studies have estimated the prevalence of anorexia nervosa among teenage women at approximately 1%.[15] Bulimia nervosa, a disorder characterized by binge eating and vomiting, is reported to affect between 1 and 3% of college-age women.[16] The recently defined binge-eating disorder (BED), a proposed DSM IV diagnostic category, is characterized by compulsive binge eating that is not followed by purging.[17] BED is reported to affect up to one-third of all obese women, especially those with early onset obesity and a high proportion of obese parents and siblings. Early age at onset and high familial risk are the best current indices of genetic obesity.[18] It is worth noting that the literature on obesity, binge eating, and eating disorders contains numerous references to food "cravings" or food "addictions," generally involving those foods that are either sweet or rich in fat.[19,20]

Human obesities are currently viewed as the outcome of an interaction between genetic predisposition and exposure to environmental variables, including diet. Much of recent research, conducted with animal models, has emphasized the genetic nature of obesity in both humans and rats. The search for the "obese" genotype has led to remarkable discoveries in molecular genetics.[21] However, the heritable component may not be body weight *per se,* but a predisposition to the obese state, and it is well-known that gene expression is modified by nutrients. Linking candidate genes with excess body fat, the common physiological end point for obesity, tells us nothing about the intervening mechanisms that may have led to gene expression in the first place. The search for an obese phenotype, that is, the outcome of the interaction between genetics and the environment, is likely to provide better clues regarding the development of obesity in humans. However, few studies have explored the potential impact of genetic factors on food selection, or examined the interaction between genetic predisposition to obesity and the dietary environment. Given recent evidence that the appetite for fats may carry an inherited component,[22] one strategy for identifying behavioral manifestations of the obese phenotype might be to study human preferences for high-fat foods.

The contribution of sugar and fat intakes to the development of human obesity is a topic of immense theoretical and practical interest. The typical American diet is largely composed of these two ingredients, deriving 22% of energy from simple sugars, both natural and added, and 34–37% of energy from fats.[23,24] It has long been a common belief that obesity was chiefly caused by lack of willpower and overconsumption of good tasting foods.[25] Recent advances in medical research now show that human obesities represent a more complex physiological and metabolic disorder of multiple origin.[21,22] Genetic predisposition, lifestyle factors, and individual food choices contribute in varying degrees to the expression of the obese state. The development of obesity is influenced by familial risk and can be delayed or modified by changes in energy intakes, physical activity, and energy expenditure. The degree of overweight is modified further by dietary factors, such as the energy density or the fat content of the habitual diet.[26]

SWEET TOOTH VERSUS FAT TOOTH

Both obesity and the BED have now been linked to an increased pleasure response to dietary sugars and fats. Taste-related behaviors of obese and dieting women have recently become a focus of renewed research attention. Generally, the pleasure or hedonic response function to sweet stimuli follows an inverted-U shape.[27] Preference ratings for sucrose solutions in water increase up to a certain concentration of sucrose (usually 8-10% wt/v) and then decline as the solution is perceived as sweet and therefore less pleasant. Only children show no hedonic "breakpoint" for sweet, selecting intensely sweet stimuli that often prove unpleasant to adults.[27]

Early research on obesity and taste preferences was largely limited to studies of sugar solutions in water.[27] Following some disagreements as to whether obese women liked or disliked sweet stimuli, most researchers came to the conclusion that there was no single "obese" response to sweet taste.[27] Individual differences in hedonic response profiles were so great as to outweigh any obese/normal differences.[28,29] No obese response profile to sweetness was ever obeserved, and no direct connection was found between taste preferences for sweetness and body weight. Large-scale consumer survey studies showed no link between body weight and reported preferences for sucrose in canned peaches, lemonade, or ice cream.[30]

Later studies focused on the role of dietary fat in determining food acceptance. The earliest studies, conducted with normal-weight students, both male and female, employed 20 sweetened mixtures of milk, cream, and sugar as the sensory stimuli of choice.[31] The stimuli provided a wide range of fat (0-52% wt/wt) and sugar levels (0-20% wt/wt), presented in an orthogonal design. Mixtures of cream (20% fat) and sugar (10% wt/wt) were the most highly preferred. Higher ratings were obtained for stimuli containing 20% fat and 8-10% sugar than for unsweetened dairy products, or for intensely sweet solutions of sucrose in skim milk.[31] This synergistic effect of sugar and fat mixtures was soon confirmed in other studies conducted with other types of sugar/fat mixtures.[31-39] In most cases, the sensory pleasure response was highly interactive and was linked to the proportions of sugar and fat in the stimulus sample. Stimuli used in these studies included sweetened milk and cream, milk shakes, cream cheese, cake frostings, and ice cream.[32-39] The studies focused almost exclusively on sweetened dairy products, inasmuch as ice cream, milk shakes, pastries, and cakes are often mentioned in the context of food cravings and eating binges in women.[19] Studies on sensory preferences for sugar and fat in nonclinical samples of children, adolescents, and adults are summarized in TABLE 1.

TABLE 1. Sensory Preferences for Sugar and Fat Mixtures: Children, Adolescents, and Adults

Subjects	Number	Age (yr)	Stimuli[a]	Percent sugar	Percent fat	Results	Ref.
Children	34 m; 40 f	10–13	20 fromage blanc or heavy cream	0, 5, 10, 20, 40	0, 3, 7, 30	Boys liked sweeter stimuli than girls; preferences for sweet declined with age.	36
Adolescents	30 m; 20 f	13–15					
Adolescents	26 m; 16 f	16–19					
Adults	30 m; 31 f	>19					
Children	10 white	9–15	16 milk or cream	0, 5, 10, 20	0, 3, 11, 36	Black children liked sweeter stimuli.	37
	10 black						
Normal wt adults	5 m; 11 f	18–24	20 milk or cream	0, 5, 10, 20	0, 3, 10, 37, 52	Best liked stimuli: 8% sugar; 20% fat.	31
Normal wt adults	12 m; 13 f	18–24	20 milk or cream	0, 5, 10, 20	0, 3, 12, 37, 52	Best liked: 20% fat in liquids; 35% fat in solids.	33
			20 sandwiches	0, 5, 10, 20	0, 3, 12, 37, 52		
Normal wt adults	50 f	18–24	15 cake frostings	20, 30, 40, 50, 60, 70, 77	15, 25, 35	Best liked: 60% sugar; 35% fat.	34
Normal wt adults	12 m; 25 f	18–21	16 milk or cream	0, 5, 10, 20	0, 3, 11, 36	Taste preferences vary with menstrual cycle.	41
Dancers	23 f	18	15 fromage blanc	1, 5, 10, 20, 40	0, 3, 7, 30	Dancers disliked sweet and high-fat stimuli.	40
Controls	14 f	26					
Swimmers	17 f	17–21	16 milk or cream	0, 5, 10, 20	0, 3, 10, 37	Swimmers disliked sweet and high-fat stimuli.	39
Controls	28 f	17–20					
Young	20	22	16 milk or cream	0, 5, 10, 20	0, 3, 11, 36	Elderly insensitive to fat.	38
Elderly	20	82					

[a] Numbers refer to number of stimuli presented to subjects.

Reported preferences for sugar and fat were influenced by menstrual cycle and by dietary restraint. Dieting and weight-conscious women sometimes disliked all energy-dense foods and gave low ratings to stimuli containing either sugar or fat. As shown in TABLE 1, female varsity swimmers[39] and ballet dancers[40] disliked intensely sweet and fat-rich foods. One question is whether their responses were affected by concerns with weight and dieting and so were subject to cognitive bias.

Clinical studies on the acceptability of sugar/fat mixtures[33,42-45] conducted with obese, dieting, and eating-disordered patients showed that dieting was generally associated with lower-reported preferences for sugar, fat, or both. Studies conducted with massively obese and formerly obese women showed that obese patients selected those stimuli that were relatively low in sugar but were rich in fat. Formerly obese subjects showed elevated preferences for intensely sweet and fat-rich foods.[33] By contrast, women patients with a diagnosis of anorexia or bulimia nervosa sometimes liked sweet taste, when presented in a noningestive context but were invariably averse to the oral sensation of dietary fat.[42-45] These studies are summarized in TABLE 2.

These studies demonstrated an inverse relationship between sensory preferences for fat and body weight. Generally, overweight and obese subjects selected high-fat stimuli, whereas lean subjects did not.[33,42] Even so, the observed relationship between fat preferences and BMI was weak, accounting for no more than 4% of the variance.[33,42] Significantly, obese individuals characterized by massive obesity and weight fluctuations gave higher ratings to fat-rich foods than equally obese individuals whose weights were more stable.[36,45] Massive obesity and weight fluctuations are sometimes taken to be indices of a genetic predisposition to obesity, suggesting again that a selective appetite for fats in foods may be an expression of the obese phenotype.

FOOD CHOICES IN OBESITY AND EATING DISORDERS

In sensory studies, overweight and obese women showed elevated preferences for energy-dense foods, including some foods that were rich in fat. However, linking sensory studies with food intake data continues to challenge most investigators. Taste preference profiles have sometimes been linked with self-reported food preference data, most often obtained using questionnaires or checklists. By contrast, very few studies have managed to link sensory preferences with patterns of food intake. Though we often assume that sensory preferences influence dietary intakes, laboratory evidence on this point is often less firm than might be supposed.

One study[46] examined preferences for different levels of fat in such foods as mashed potatoes, scrambled eggs, pudding, or tuna fish salad. There was no statistically significant link between liking for fat in foods and the amount of fat consumed. On the other hand, the researchers revealed a direct link between fat preferences and the subjects' own body fat. Consistent with previous results,[33,42] preferences for dietary fats appeared to be linked to the degree of overweight.

A more recent study conducted with 3 to 5-year-old children suggests that preferences for fat in foods may carry an additional inherited component. In that study,[47] preferences for fat-containing foods in a group of 18 children were successfully linked to the amount of fat consumed under laboratory conditions. Both measures were significantly linked to a measure of parental overweight, as determined by the

TABLE 2. Sensory Preferences for Sugar and Fat Mixtures: Obesity and Eating Disorders

Subjects	Number	Age (yr)	Stimuli	Percent sugar	Percent fat	Results	Ref.
Obese	12 f	20–60	20 milk or cream	0, 5, 10, 20	0, 3, 10, 36, 52	Best liked: 4% sugar; 32% fat (obese); 8% sugar, 20% fat (normal wt).	32
Ex obese	1 m; 7 f						
Normal wt	15 f						
Obese	32 m; 29 f	20–45	9 frostings	20, 40, 60, 70	15, 25, 35	Higher preferences among the obese.	35
Normal wt	15 m; 16 f						
Obese—High flux	20 f	12–50	9 ice cream	12, 15, 18	10, 15, 20	High-flux group liked ice cream more.	45
Obese—Low flux	17 f		5 sucrose soln	2, 8, 16, 32			
Obese	12 f	21–42	15 fromage blanc	1, 5, 10, 20, 40	0, 3, 7	Best liked: 5% sugar; 7% fat.	56, 59
Normal wt	12 f						
Normal wt	12 m						
Bulimic women	16 f	18–26	15 fromage blanc	1, 5, 10, 20, 40	0, 3, 7	Women with bulimia liked sweet but disliked fat.	43
Controls	16 f						
ED[a]	32 f	14–25	20 milk or cream	0, 5, 10, 20	0, 3, 10, 36, 52	ED patients liked sweet but disliked fat.	42
Controls	16 f						
Diabetic	19 m; 12 f	40–65	juice milk cheese	0, 3, 6, 9, 12	0, 1, 2, 4 20, 40	Sweet and fatty foods liked less after diet therapy.	58
Anorectic women	12 f	26.8	fromage blanc	1, 5, 10, 20, 40	0, 3, 7, 30	AN[b] disliked both sweet and fat.	44
Controls	14 f						
BED women	20 f	18–40	20 milk or cream	2, 4, 8, 16, 32	3, 10, 20, 36	Naloxone suppressed preferences for sweet and fat in both groups.	57
Controls	21 f						

[a] Eating disordered.
[b] Anorexia nervosa patients.

BMI (BMI = kg/m^2). Although none of the parents in that study were overweight, studying fat preferences of lean children of obese parents would be a research project of exceptional interest. Fat preferences and fat consumption may represent a potential behavioral mechanism for the expression of familial obesity.

Other studies have examined food preference profiles as a function of sex and body weight. In a large study of U.S. Army personnel, Meiselman et al.[48] showed that overweight people selected red meat dishes rather than desserts. A study of several hundred obese patients[49] confirmed that self-reported food preferences of obese males typically included steaks and roasts, hamburgers, french fries, pizza, and ice cream. By contrast, obese women tended to list bread, cake, cookies, ice cream, chocolate, pies, and other desserts. In other words, obese men tended to prefer protein/fat mixtures (*i.e.,* meats), whereas obese women listed carbohydrate/fat mixtures, notably those that were sweet. Although food preferences of obese women have been characterized as "carbohydrate cravings," preferences for fat, sugar, or both often seem closer to the mark.

Linking food preferences with food intake data poses a challenge to the investigator. Although dietary intake assessments have often failed to link obesity with excess energy intakes, the main problem may have been underreporting and bias. Studies using the doubly labeled water technique to measure energy expenditure showed conclusively that obese subjects had elevated resting energy expenditure values and probably consumed more calories than did lean controls.[50] Both clinical and epidemiological studies have also linked obesity with excessive consumption of dietary fat. In some studies, percent body fat was linked to percentage of fat calories in the habitual diet or with sensory preferences for fat in foods.[46] In other studies, obesity was linked to an elevated proportion of fat in the diet and lower values of the carbohydrate-to-fat ratio.[26]

MACRONUTRIENT SUBSTITUTES

Has the availability of low-energy foods diminished the prevalence of obesity in the U.S. or had a measurable impact on public health? Despite diverse dietary recommendations and guidelines, the prevalence of obesity in the U.S. continues to rise. Dietary guidelines intended for the general public have long addressed reducing the consumption of sugars and fat. The 1988 Surgeon General's Report on Nutrition and Health[51] recommended replacing foods high in fat, saturated fat, and cholesterol with vegetables, fruits, and whole grain foods. The 1989 Diet and Health Report of the National Academy of Sciences,[52] neutral with respect to sugars, recommended increasing intake of carbohydrates to 55% of total daily calories by doubling the intake of vegetables and fruits.

One problem with high carbohydrate diets is that many people enjoy the taste of fat-rich foods and are reluctant to give them up.[53] Fats endow foods with their characteristic texture and flavor and play a major role in determining the palatability of the diet.[53] By contrast, diets composed solely of grains, legumes, pulses, vegetables, and fruit tend to be viewed as bland, monotonous, and unsatisfying. After two decades of high-carbohydrate diets, signs of consumer backlash are already in place, inasmuch as the best-selling diet books of 1996 recommend weight-loss diets that are relatively low in carbohydrate but high in protein and high in fat.[54]

The development of new low-fat foods by the food industry has become a public health issue. Among the aims of the Healthy People 2000 Report[55] was to increase the number of processed foods that were reduced in fat and saturated fat to at least 5,000 brand items. It was specifically noted that such foods should be made available to schools and to low-income families. Because fat is calorically more dense than sugar (9 kcal/g as opposed to 4 kcal/g), replacing fat in foods offers potentially greater caloric savings to the consumer. Low-energy foods containing macronutrient substitutes offer a way of maintaining a palatable and varied diet, a valuable adjunct to dietary compliance and weight control.

ACKNOWLEDGMENTS

The author wishes to thank Alisa Levine for her research contributions to this manuscript.

REFERENCES

1. FLEGAL, K. M. & R. P. TROIANO. 1996. Shifts in the distribution of body mass index of adults in the US population. Obesity Res. 4(suppl 1): 68S.
2. NAJJAR, M. F. & M. ROWLAND. 1987. Anthropometric reference data and the prevalence of overweight, United States 1976-80. National Center for Health Statistics, Vital and Health Statistics, **11**(238):1-73, DHHS Pub. No. (PHS) 87-1688, US Government Printing Office. Washington, D.C.
3. GORTMAKER, S. L., W. H. DIETZ, A. M. SOBOL & C. A. WEHLER. 1987. Increasing pediatric obesity in the United States. Am. J. Dis. Child. **141**: 535.
4. HARLAN, W. R., J. R. LANDIS, K. M. FLEGAL, C. S. DAVIS & M. E. MILLER. 1988. Trends in body mass in the United States, 1960-1980. Am. J. Epidemiol. **128**: 1065.
5. FLEGAL, K. M., W. R. HARLAN & J. R. LANDIS. 1988. Trends in body mass index and skinfold thickness with socioeconomic factors in young adult women. Am. J. Clin. Nutr. **48**: 535.
6. NIH TECHNOLOGY ASSESSMENT CONFERENCE PANEL. 1992. Methods for voluntary weight loss and control. Ann. Int. Med. **116**: 942-949.
7. LEVY, A. S. & A. W. HEATON. 1993. Weight control practices of U.S. adults trying to lose weight. Ann. Int. Med. **119**: 661-666.
8. WILLIAMSON, D. F. 1993. Descriptive epidemiology of body weight and weight change in U.S. adults. Ann. Int. Med. **119**: 646-649.
9. HERMAN, P. C. & J. POLIVY. 1980. Restrained eating. In Obesity. A. J. Stunkard, Ed.: 208-225. H.B. Saunders. Philadelphia.
10. DREWNOWSKI, A. 1993. Low-calorie foods and the prevalence of obesity. In Low-Calorie Foods Handbook. A. M. Altschul, Ed.: 513-534. Marcel Dekker, Inc. New York.
11. DREWNOWSKI, A., D. K. YEE, C. L. KURTH & D. D. KRAHN. 1994. Eating pathology and DSM-IIIR bulimia nervosa: A continuum of behavior. Am. J. Psychiatry **151**: 1217-1219.
12. KRAHN, D. D., C. L. KURTH, M. A. DEMITRACK & A. DREWNOWSKI. 1922. The relationship of dieting severity and bulimic behaviors to alcohol and other drug use in young women. J. Subst. Abuse **4**: 341-352.
13. KURTH, C. L., D. D. KRAHN, K. NAIRN & A. DREWNOWSKI. 1995. The severity of dieting and bingeing behaviors in college women: Interview validation of survey data. J. Psychiatr. Res. **29**: 211-225.
14. GARNER, G. M., M. P. OLMSTED & J. POLIVY. 1983. The eating disorder inventory: A measure of cognitive-behavioral dimensions of anorexia nervosa and bulimia. In An-

orexia Nervosa: Recent Developments in Research. P. L. Darby, P. E. Garfinkel, D. M. Garner & D. V. Coscina, Eds.: 173-184. Alan R. Liss. New York.
15. HOEK, H. W. 1993. Review of the epidemiological study of eating disorders. Int. Rev. Psychiatr. **5**: 61-74.
16. DREWNOWSKI, A., S. A. HOPKINS & R. L. KESSLER. 1988. The prevalence of bulimia nervosa in the US college student population. Am. J. Public Health **78**: 1322-1325.
17. AMERICAN PSYCHIATRIC ASSOCIATION. 1994. Diagnostic and Statistical Manual of Mental Disorders, 4th Ed (DSM-IV), APA Press. Washington, D.C.
18. PRICE, A. R., A. J. STUNKARD, R. NESS, T. WADDEN, S. HESHKA, B. KANDERS & A. CORMILLOT. 1990. Childhood-onset (age <10) obesity has high familial risk. Int. J. Obesity **8**: 491.
19. DREWNOWSKI, A. 1991. Obesity and eating disorders: Cognitive aspects of food preference and food aversion. Bull. Psychon. Soc. **29**: 261-264.
20. DREWNOWSKI, A. 1996. The behavioral phenotype in human obesity. *In* Why We Eat What We Eat. E. D. Capaldi, Ed.: American Psychological Association. Washington D.C.
21. ROBERTS, S. B. & A. S. GREENBERG. 1996. The new obesity genes. Nutr. Rev. **54**: 41-49.
22. BOUCHARD, C. 1988. Inheritance of human fat distribution, fat distribution during growth and later health outcomes. C. Bouchard & F. E. Johnston, Eds: 103-125 Alan R. Liss. New York.
23. CARROLL, M. D., S. ABRAHAM & C. M. DRESSER. 1983. Dietary intake source data: United States, 1976-80, National Center for Health Statistics. Vital and Health Statistics Series 11-No 231, DHHS Pub No (PHS) 83-1681. U.S. Govt Printing Office. Washington, DC.
24. GLINSMAN, W. H., H. IRAUSQUIN & Y. K. PARK. 1986. Evaluation of health aspects of sugars contained in carbohydrate sweeteners. J. Nutr. **116**(11S): S1-216.
25. RODIN, J. 1981. Psychological factors in obesity. *In* Recent Advances in Obesity Research III. P. Bjorntorp, M. Cairella & A. N. Howard, Eds. 106-123. John Libbey. London.
26. DREON, D. M., B. FREY-HEWITT, N. ELLEWORTH, P. T. WILLIAMS, R. B. TERRY & P. D. WOOD. 1988. Dietary carbohydrate-to-fat ratio and obesity in middle-aged men. Am. J. Clin. Nutr. **47**: 995.
27. DREWNOWSKI, A. 1987. Sweetness and obesity. *In* Sweetness. J. Dobbing, Ed. ILSI-Nutrition Foundation Symposium. Springer-Verlag. Berlin.
28. WITHERLY, S. A., R. M. PANGBORN & J. STERN. 1980. Gustatory responses and eating duration of obese and lean adults. Appetite **1**: 53-63.
29. PANGBORN, R. M. & M. SIMONE. 1958. Body size and sweetness preference. J. Am. Diet. Assoc. **34**: 924-928.
30. PANGBORN, R. M., M. SIMONE & T. A. NICKERSON. 1957. The influence of sugar in ice cream: Consumer preferences for vanilla ice cream. Food Technol. **11**: 679-682.
31. DREWNOWSKI, A. & M. R. C. GREENWOOD. 1983. Cream and sugar: Human preferences for high-fat foods. Physiol. & Behav. **30**: 629-633.
32. DREWNOWSKI, A., J. D. BRUNZELL, K. SANDE, P. H. IVERIUS & M. R. C. GREENWOOD. 1985. Sweet tooth reconsidered: Taste responsiveness in human obesity. Physiol. & Behav. **35**: 617-622.
33. DREWNOWSKI, A., E. E. SHRAGER, C. LIPSKY, E. STELLAR & M. R. C. GREENWOOD. 1989. Sugar and fat: Sensory and hedonic evaluation of liquid and solid foods. Physiol. & Behav. **45**: 177-183.
34. DREWNOWSKI, A. & M. SCHWARTZ. 1990. Invisible fats: Sensory assessment of sugar/fat mixtures. Appetite **14**: 203-217.
35. DREWNOWSKI, A., C. L. KURTH & J. E. RAHAIM. 1991. Taste preferences in human obesity: Environmental and familial factors. Am. J. Clin. Nutr. **54**: 635-641.
36. MONNEUSE, M., F. BELLISLE & J. LOUIS-SYLVESTRE. 1991. Impact of sex and age on sensory evaluation of sugar and fat in dairy products. Physiol. & Behav. **50**: 1111-1117.
37. BACON, A., J. S. MILES & S. S. SCHIFFMAN. 1994. Effect of race on perception of fat alone and in combination with sugar. Physiol. & Behav. **55**(3): 603-606.

38. WARWICK, Z. & S. SCHIFFMAN. 1990. Sensory evaluations of fat-sucrose and fat-salt mixtures: Relationship to age and weight status. Physiol. & Behav. **48:** 633–636.
39. CRYSTAL, S., C. A. FRYE & R. B. KANAREK. 1995. Taste preferences and sensory perceptions in female varsity swimmers. Appetite **24:** 25–36.
40. MARTIN, C. & F. BELLISLE. 1989. Eating attitudes and taste responses in young ballerinas. Physiol. & Behav. **46:** 223–227.
41. FRYE, C. A., S. CRYSTAL, K. D. WARD & R. B. KANAREK. 1994. Menstrual cycle and dietary restraint influence taste preferences in young women. Physiol. & Behav. **55**(3):561–567.
42. DREWNOWSKI, A., K. A. HALMI, B. PIERCE, J. GIBBS & G. P. SMITH. 1987. Taste and eating disorders. Am. J. Clin. Nutr. **46:** 442–450.
43. DREWNOWSKI, A., F. BELLISLE, P. AIMEZ & B. REMY. 1987. Taste and bulimia. Physiol. & Behav. **41:** 621–626.
44. SIMON, Y., F. BELLISLE, M. O. MONNEUSE, B. SAMUEL-LAJEUNESSE & A. DREWNOWSKI. 1993. Taste responsiveness in anorexia nervosa. Br. J. Psychiatry **162:** 244–246.
45. DREWNOWSKI, A. & J. HOLDEN-WILTSE. 1992. Taste responses and food preferences in obese women: Effects of weight cycling. Int. J. Obesity **16:** 639–648.
46. MELA, D. J. & D. A. SACCHETTI. 1991. Sensory preferences for fats: Relationships with diet and body composition. Am. J. Clin. Nutr. **53:** 908–915.
47. FISHER, J. O. & L. L. BIRCH. 1995. Fat preferences and fat consumption of 3- to 5-year-old children are related to parental obesity. J. Am. Diet. Assoc. **95**(7): 759–764.
48. MEISELMAN, H. L., D. WATERMAN & L. E. SYMINGTON. 1974. Armed Forces Food Preferences, Technical Report 75-63-FSL. U.S. Army Natick Development Center. Natick, MA.
49. DREWNOWSKI, A., C. L. KURTH, J. HOLDEN-WILTSE & J. SAARI. 1992. Food preferences in human obesity: Carbohydrates versus fats. Appetite **18:** 207–221.
50. PRENTICE, A. M., A. E. BLACK, W. A. COWARD, H. L. DAVIES, G. R. GOLDBERG, P. R. MURGATROYD, J. ASHFORD, M. SAWYER & R. G. WHITEHEAD. 1986. High levels of energy expenditure in obese women. Br. Med. J. **292:** 983.
51. U.S. DEPARTMENT OF HEALTH AND HUMAN SERVICES. 1988. The Surgeon General's Report on Nutrition and Health. DHHS (PHS) Publication no. 88-50210. U.S. Government Printing Office. Washington D.C.
52. NATIONAL ACADEMY OF SCIENCES. 1989. Committee on Diet and Health. Food and Nutrition Board, Diet and Health. National Academy Press. Washington D.C.
53. DREWNOWSKI, A. 1987. Fats and food texture: Sensory and hedonic evaluations. *In* Food Texture. H. R. Moskowitz, Ed.: 217–250. Marcel Dekker. New York.
54. EADES, M. R. & M. D. EADES. 1996. Protein Power. Bantam Books. New York.
55. U.S. DEPARTMENT OF HEALTH AND HUMAN SERVICES. 1991. Healthy People 2000. U.S. Government Printing Office. Washington, D.C.
56. DREWNOWSKI, A., C. MASSIEN, J. LOUIS-SYLVESTRE, J. FRICKER, D. CHAPELOT & M. APFELBAUM. 1994. Comparing the effects of aspartame and sucrose on motivational ratings, taste preferences, and energy intakes. Am. J. Clin. Nutr. **59:** 338–345.
57. DREWNOWSKI, A., D. D. KRAHN, M. A. DEMITRACK, K. NAIRN & B. A. GOSNELL. 1995. Naloxone, an opiate blocker, reduces the consumption of sweet high-fat foods in obese and lean female binge eaters. Am. J. Clin. Nutr. **61:** 1206–1212.
58. LAITINEN, J. H., H. M. TUORILA & M. I. J. UUSITUPA. 1991. Changes in hedonic responses to sweet and fat in recently diagnosed non-insulin dependent diabetic patients during diet therapy. Eur. J. Clin. Nutr. **45:** 393–400.
59. DREWNOWSKI, A., C. MASSIEN, J. LOUIS-SYLVESTRE, J. FRICKER, D. CHAPELOT & M. APFELBAUM. 1994. The effects of aspartame versus sucrose on motivational ratings, taste preferences, and energy intakes in obese and lean women. Int. J. Obesity **18:** 570–578.

Dietary Fiber: Nutritional Lessons for Macronutrient Substitutes

KAY M. BEHALL[a]

Diet and Human Performance Laboratory
Building 308, BARC-East
Beltsville Human Nutrition Research Center
Agricultural Research Service
United States Department of Agriculture
Beltsville, Maryland 20705-2350

INTRODUCTION

Dietary fiber has generally been defined in the United States as plant material that is not readily digested by endogenous enzymes in the mammalian small intestine.[1,2] Dietary fiber is not one material, but a broad classification that encompasses a wide range of substantially different chemical structures.[1] Major components of plant fiber include cellulose, β-glucans, hemicelluloses, pectins, gums, and lignins. There is, however, still some discussion on what should be classified as a fiber. Starch that is resistant to digestion in the small intestine has been included in as well as excluded from the classification.[3] Fiber components have been classified by their ability to disperse in water (*e.g.,* polysaccharides that readily disperse in water have been described as soluble fibers).[1,3] Although isolated fibers can be either soluble or insoluble fiber, the fiber in most foods is a mixture of both types. The soluble fiber content of legumes averages 25% of the total dietary fiber; of cereals and vegetables, 32%; and of fruits, 38 percent. The total amount or percentage of soluble fiber in the total depends on the methodology used for analysis.[1,3,4]

Increased intake of carbohydrate as complex carbohydrates with a corresponding decrease in energy from fat has been recommended in Western countries.[4,5] Recommendations proposed by the National Academy of Sciences, American Heart Association, and American Diabetes Association[4-7] call for decreased fat intake in the U.S. diet to no more than 30% of total energy. Diets containing lower amounts of total fat, saturated fat, and cholesterol were shown to be an important dietary intervention for lowering plasma cholesterol concentrations in individuals at risk for coronary heart disease.[8,9] Increasingly, reduced-fat foods and high-fiber foods are being manufactured and used to reduce total fat intake. Low-fat or no-fat products are not without calories, however. The caloric value of the product depends on the carbohydrate used as the fat substitute: carbohydrates can provide little or no energy (*e.g.,* cellulose) up to the conventional 16.8 kJ (4 kcal)/g (*e.g.,* modified food starches).[10-13] The amount of energy reduction thus depends not only on how much fat is replaced, but on how much of which carbohydrate is used.[11-13] Intake of carbohydrate-based fat replacers is a small portion of the total energy intake. As more foods are manufactured

---

[a] Tel: (301) 504-8682; fax: (301) 504-9098; e-mail: behall@bhnrc.arsusda.gov.

with a reduced-fat content, substitutes could become a significant portion of the energy and fiber intake.

CARBOHYDRATE-BASED FAT SUBSTITUTES

A wide range of carbohydrate-based fat replacers exists, from modified starch to isolated plant fibers and other fiber sources: modified starches, dextrins, maltodextrins, starch polymers, microcrystalline cellulose, gums, and other fiber concentrates. TABLE 1 summarizes information about carbohydrate-based fat replacers, their sources, and some examples of their uses.

Starches used as fat replacers include dextrins and maltodextrins, produced primarily from partially hydrolyzed wheat, potato, corn, and tapioca starches; and modified starches, produced mainly from tapioca, corn, potato, and rice starches.[11-15] These materials provide bulking, texture, body, and resistance to caking; form films or oxygen barriers; give surface sheen; bind flavor and fat; and help solubilize or disperse other ingredients. These starch sources have been used to replace 50-100% of fat in a wide range of products, including frozen desserts, salad dressings, dips, sauces, gravies, cereals, snacks, bakery products and fillings, confectionary creams, chocolate candy, peanut butter, margarine, cheese, sour cream, yogurt, ice cream, and puddings.[11-15] The starch sources generally have a bland taste and are completely digestible, contributing 16.8 kJ (4 kcal)/g dry weight. However, they are usually used in a gel form, thereby diluting their caloric contribution by the amount of water added, the net result often being 4.2 kJ (1 kcal)/g.[11-13]

Polydextrose consists of glucose polymers, sorbitol, and citric acid in a 89 : 10 : 1 ratio.[12] Polydextrose is used to modify texture or mouthfeel, modify viscosity, decrease caking, and improve flowability.[11,12,14,15] It is used in bakery goods and mixes, salad dressing, chewing gum, frozen desserts, gelatins, puddings, candies, frostings, and confections. Polydextrose contributes 4.2 kJ (1 kcal)/g dry weight. Consumption of large amounts of polydextrose sometimes has a laxative effect, and products that contain more than 15 g per serving must be so labeled.[11-13]

Cellulose, microcrystalline cellulose, methyl cellulose, and carboxymethyl cellulose are fiber sources derived primarily from processed wood pulp that are used as fat replacers.[11,12,15] Powdered cellulose has been used to replace flour in bread, cookies, and cakes; the forms that gel have been used in salad dressings and frozen desserts. Cellulose is generally considered to be indigestible, contributing 0 kJ (0 kcal)/g dry material.[11,12] Z-trim is derived from corn and oat bran and other grain materials. It is primarily cellulose and assumed to contribute 0 kJ/g dry material but has not yet been incorporated into commercial food products.

Oatrim, produced from oat flour, is a mixture of amylodextrin and the soluble fiber, β-glucan.[11-13,15] It contains 5-10% β-glucan, depending on the processing, and is currently being used in dips, dressings, confections, bakery products, beverages, yogurt, ice cream, and frozen meals. Oatrim is considered to be mostly digestible carbohydrate, contributing nearly 16.8 kJ (4 kcal)/g dry weight.[11-13]

Ancient gums that are still being used in food preparation include plant exudates (such as gum arabic and gum tragacanth), plant extracts (such as pectin), seed gums (such as quince, psyllium, okra, and locust bean), and seaweed gums (first produced

TABLE 1. Sources and Examples of Fat Replacer/Substitute Uses

Material	Source	Energy kJ (kcal/g)	Examples of Use
Complex carbohydrates			
Maltodextrins	potato, cornstarch, tapioca	16.8 (4) when dry; 4.2–8.4 (1–2) when hydrated	frozen desserts, cheeses, sauces, dressings, spreads, baked products, processed meats
Modified food starch		(4) when dry; 4.2–8.4 (1–2) when hydrated	baked products, dressings, table spreads, sour cream, cream cheese, sauces, gravies, processed meats, frozen deserts
Oatrim	oats	16.8 (4) when dry (5–10% soluble fiber)	dressings, dips, ice cream, bakery products, beverages, yogurt, milk, frozen dinners
Polydextrose	starch polymer	4.2 (1)	frozen desserts, baked products, gelatins, puddings, salad dressings, candies, frostings, confections, chewing gum
Cellulose	wood pulp	0 (0)	salad dressings, frozen desserts
Fiber concentrates	sugar beet, apple	0–8.4 (0–2)	bakery products, cereals, frozen desserts
Brans	wheat, oats, rice	0–4.2 (0–1)	cereals, bread, bakery products
Gums and Gels			
Pectin	apple, citrus	< 8.4 (< 2)	yogurt, sour cream, cheese spread, salad dressings
Arabic	acacia tree	< 8.4 (< 2)	cream cheese, baked products, gravies, salad dressings
Guar gum	seeds	< 8.4 (< 2)	sauces, cheese, baked goods, gravies, frozen desserts, milk products, beverages
Locus bean gum	seeds	< 8.4 (< 2)	frozen desserts, cream cheese, dairy products, cheese, bakery products
β-glucan	oats, barley	< 8.4 (< 2)	dressings, dips, ice cream, bakery products, beverages, yogurt, milk, frozen dinners
Carrageenan	red seaweed	0 (0)	ground beef, processed cheese, cream cheese spread, salad dressings
Alginate	brown seaweed		processed cheese, cheese spread, salad dressings
Xanthan gum	microorganism	< 8.4 (< 2)	salad dressings, beverages, bakery fillings and products, dairy products, sauces, gravies
Cellulose gel	microcrystal	0 (0)	salad dressing, processed cheese, frozen dessert, frozen yogurt

in Asian countries).[16] Gums used in foods today include guar, locust bean, psyllium, karaya, arabic, tragacanth, gellan, curdlan, konjac, carrageenan, algin, xanthan, and pectin,[11,12,14,15] this wide range has some differences in viscosity, solubility, and taste. Isolated fibers are generally used in foods to modify textures by suspending, dispersing, or stabilizing other constituents and act as emulsifiers, gels, binders, or coagulants. Gums usually are used in small quantities (0.1–2%) in a food item and constitute less than 2% of the total fiber intake. Mixtures of gums, as well as single gums, have been used in processed cheeses, sour cream, yogurt, cream cheese, puddings, ice cream, milk, frozen desserts, salad dressings, sauces, gravies, ground beef, cereals, bakery products, and fillings.[11,12,14,15] These soluble fiber sources are generally not readily digested in the small intestine but are partially digested by colonic bacteria to short chain fatty acids. Some energy is recovered through colonic absorption of these acids. The net energy for the gums ranges from less than 4.2 kJ (1 kcal)/g to 13.9 (3.4 kcal)/g.[11–13]

Other fiber sources used include apple, sugar beet, and pea fiber, brans, toasted cereal defatted germ, and fruit pastes.[11] These fiber sources add bulk and flavor in low-fat or no-fat baked products. Brans and fiber concentrates are generally considered to be indigestible, usually contributing 0 kJ (0 kcal)/g dry material, but concentrated fruit pastes provide approximately 12.6 kJ (3 kcal)/g dry weight.[11]

HEALTH BENEFITS

Elevated blood lipid profiles have been listed as a major risk factor for atherosclerosis and coronary heart disease.[4–7] High-fiber diets containing whole foods (such as oats or legumes) or diets containing isolated soluble fibers incorporated into foods have been fed to normolipidemic or hyperlipidemic subjects to investigate the effect of fiber on blood lipids (TABLE 2). No decrease in cholesterol or triacylglycerols was observed after the addition of cellulose (an insoluble fiber) to the diet; cellulose has often been used as a control fiber for comparison with soluble fibers.[17–19] Pectin was among the first isolated dietary fibers that significantly reduced serum cholesterol in controlled experiments.[17–21] Decreases of 7–19% in total and low-density lipoprotein (LDL) cholesterol, but not triacylglycerols, were observed in normolipidemic and hyperlipidemic subjects consuming at least 12–15 g/d of pectin (doses were as high as 50 g/d). Guar gum was studied as a cholesterol-lowering agent more often than pectin was studied;[17–20,22–25] 13–19 g/d of guar gum was usual, although up to 40 g/d was fed as part of the diet. Decreases of 3–32% in total cholesterol were reported after guar gum consumption. Most of the decrease occurs in the LDL cholesterol fraction, with little of no change occurring in the high-density lipoprotein (HDL) cholesterol fraction. Total triacylglycerols were reduced in some studies, but the reduction was statistically significant only when guar gum was incorporated into very low-fat, starchy foods resulting in a low-fat diet. In one study, the form in which the guar gum powder was incorporated in the diet—added to fruit juices and soups baked into standard bread, or incorporated into a dry crisp bread—did not alter the effectiveness of the gum in decreasing cholesterol.[23] However, similar levels of guar gum have been reported in different studies to lower serum cholesterol to widely varying degrees, suggesting that different gum preparations are not equally effective.

TABLE 2. Effect of Different Kinds of Fiber on Lipid Metabolism in Humans[17-37]

Fiber Source	Cholesterol	LDL[a]	HDL[b]	TG[c]
Cellulose	U[d]	U	I[f]	U
Pectin	D[e]	U	U	U
Guar gum	D	D	U	D
Locust bean gum	D	D	U	ND
Psyllium	D	U	U	U
Carboxymethyl-cellulose	D	D	U	ND
Wheat grain	U	U	U	D
Wheat bran	D/U	ND[g]	ND	D
Oat bran	D	D	U	D
Legumes	D	U	U	D
Amylose starch	D/U	D/U	U	D
Beans	D	D	U	U
Carrot	U	U	U	ND
Cabbage	U	U	U	ND
Apple	U	U	U	ND

[a] LDL, low-density lipoproteins.
[b] HDL, high-density lipoproteins.
[c] TG, triacylglycerols.
[d] U, Unchanged.
[e] D, Decreased.
[f] I, increased.
[g] ND, not determined.

Locust bean, karaya, and xanthan gums used as the soluble fiber source in diets resulted in cholesterol reduction similar to that observed with pectin and guar gum.[17,19,25,26]

Consumption of wheat bran, similarly to consumption of cellulose, usually fails to significantly reduce blood lipid concentrations, and wheat bran is often used as the control fiber in crossover studies.[17] Little or no change in serum cholesterol was generally reported when vegetables and fruit fiber were consumed.[17,18] Oats and oat bran (containing both insoluble and soluble fiber) were used successfully to lower blood lipids and have been promoted as lipid-lowering foods.[17-20,27-33] The amount of oat bran (25-100 g/d, dry) and oatmeal (57-140 g/d, dry) in the diet required to decrease blood lipids varies greatly.[17,18,27-29] Total cholesterol,[17,18,27-30] LDL cholesterol,[17,18,27-31] and apolipoprotein B100[30] decrease significantly after oat bran, but not wheat bran, is added to the diet. Total plasma cholesterol concentrations were reduced from 3% to 22 percent. Triacylglycerols,[17-19,23,27-31] HDL cholesterol,[17,19,23,30,31] and apolipoprotein A-1[23,30,31] concentrations on average did not significantly decrease when oatmeal or oat bran were added to the diet, although significant decreases in triacylglycerols were reported in some studies.[17,23] Supplementation of 35-100 g/d of an oat source to self-selected diets was used successfully for up to two years to lower blood lipids in hyperlipidemic subjects.[9,32] One study, using various intakes of oatmeal or oat bran so that the subjects consumed approximately 0, 2, 4, or 6.0 g of β-glucan, observed a dose-dependent reduction in LDL-cholesterol concentrations from the β-

TABLE 3. Effect of Different Kinds of Fiber on Glycemic Response in Humans[23,25,38–42]

Fiber Source	Glucose	Insulin
Cellulose	U[a]	U
Pectin	D	D
Guar gum	D	D
Locust bean gum	D	D
Psyllium	D	D
Oatrim	D	D
Amylose/resistant starch	D/U	D

[a] For symbol definitions, See TABLE 2.

glucan in oat products, with the greatest percentage change from baseline after the higher β-glucan consumption.[33]

An average of 15% reduction from prestudy or maintenance values was observed in total cholesterol and LDL when 7.6 g/d of β-glucan from soluble oat extract (developed as a fat replacer) was added to the diet.[34] However, in another study, no statistically significant decrease in total cholesterol, LDL, or HDL concentrations occurred after the addition of 11.2 g of β-glucan concentrate per day to the diet.[35]

Cooked dried legumes, similar to oats, contain both insoluble and soluble fiber.[17–19] Consumption of 100 g/d of these foods resulted in decreases in cholesterol concentrations ranging from 7% to 23 percent. Triacylglycerol concentrations varied from an increase of 13% to a decrease of 21%; 18 subjects whose concentrations decreased were followed for one year and showed a 17% decrease. In another study, subjects consuming 100 g/d dry beans for two years maintained a 4% decrease in cholesterol and a 6% decrease in triacylglycerol concentrations.[17–19]

Amylose starch and resistant starch (retrograded starch produced from amylose during cooking, starch granules, and physically inaccessible starch) were suggested to function as both insoluble and soluble fiber. Plasma triacylglycerol and cholesterol concentrations decreased in subjects consuming a high-amylose diet.[36,37] Feeding amylose for five weeks resulted in a 16% and 8% greater decrease in fasting triacylglycerol and cholesterol concentrations, respectively, whereas there was no change after feeding a standard starch diet for five weeks.[36] In another study, triacylglycerol concentrations decreased 1% and cholesterol concentrations increased 2% from initial values after four weeks of amylose consumption; after 13 weeks of both amylose and standard starch, triacylglycerol values were 14% lower after amylose than after the standard starch, and no difference on cholesterol was observed between the two starches' effects.[37] If the effect of resistant starch was the same as that of soluble fiber, a greater difference in fasting lipids might have been expected after the high amylose than after the amylopectin diet.

As the U.S. population grows older, a higher percentage of people exhibits abnormal carbohydrate metabolism, as evidenced by elevated plasma glucose or insulin concentrations after a glucose tolerance test. Isolated fibers (TABLE 3) as well as whole foods (TABLE 4) have been used to study the affect of fiber on glucose and

TABLE 4. Representative Glycemic Indices of Foods[a]

Food	GI	Food	GI
White bread	100 (defined)	Apple	52
Whole wheat bread	99	Banana	76
Spaghetti	59	Peach	42
Oat bran bread	68	Pear	51
Pumpernickel bread	66	Grapes	62
Barley	36	Raisins	93
Rice, white	69	Apricot, dried	44
Cornflakes	119	Orange	62
Rice Krispies	117	Grapefruit	36
Shredded wheat	99	Rice	81
Oatmeal	78	Rice, instant	128
Cream of wheat	94	Potato, new boiled	80
Red lentils, dried	36	Potato, instant or baked	120
Kidney beans, dried	42	Carrot	101
Kidney beans, canned	74	Green peas	68
Lima beans	46	Corn	55
Peanuts	21	Popcorn	79

[a] Ratio of glucose response area to test meals containing 50 g (as calculated from food tables) carbohydrate portions in form of food indicated vs. white bread.[38]

insulin response in healthy hyperinsulinemic and diabetic subjects.[23,25,39–41] Consumption of glucose with an insoluble fiber, such as wheat bran, as a meal did not significantly decrease postprandial glucose or insulin responses; meals containing soluble fibers generally reduce the postprandial rise in blood glucose and insulin compared with that observed after glucose alone.[23,25,39–41] Soluble fiber appears to act by developing a gel containing the food inasmuch as postprandial reductions were greatest when the soluble fibers were consumed in a hydrated form with the carbohydrate source or meal rather than as a dry powder or before the test meal.[4,40] When the carbohydrates consumed in a tolerance test are mixed within the viscous gel resulting from hydrating soluble fiber, the rates at which nutrients leave the stomach and can be absorbed in the small intestine are reduced.[4] In a tolerance test, the percentage change in area under the curve (serum glucose plotted vs. time) varies greatly with the amount of fiber and carbohydrate consumed.[40,41]

Guar gum has been extensively used as the viscous fiber in tolerance test meals (2.5–15 g/tolerance) and long-term dietary consumption (9–26 g/d for 2–52 wk) studies.[23,39–41] When guar gum was consumed with glucose, decreases in the area under the response curve for glucose ranged from 27% to 68% (average 40%) and for insulin ranged from 37% to 68% (average 56%).[23,40,41] Guar has been mixed with bread, soup, mashed potato, pasta, and mixed meals for tolerance tests. Decreases in glucose ranged from 23% to 80% and in insulin from 6% to 59%, depending on the amount of guar and the nature of the meal. Guar consumed with the diet resulted in 0–39% reduction in glucose and a 0–28% reduction in insulin concentrations.[23,40,41] Reduction varied primarily with the form in which guar gum was added to the diet, granular guar and guar tablets having little or no effect on glucose and insulin response.[40] Six studies reported decreases of 11-55% in glucose and 2-76% in insulin response after consumption of pectin (9-14.5 g) mixed with glucose.[40] Fewer studies have been carried out with other isolated soluble fibers. The reduction in glucose and insulin concentrations after other gelling fibers, gum tragacanth, methyl cellulose, locust bean gum, agar, psyllium, xanthan gum, and konjac mannan, were added to a glucose tolerance test or meal was similar to that reported for guar gum and pectin.[25,40,41]

Consumption of oat extract (containing 10% β-glucan by weight) in pudding as a tolerance test or with glucose after consumption of the oat extract for five weeks resulted in a decrease of approximately 50% in glucose and 10% in insulin response.[42] This controlled feeding study used the oat extract to replace 5% of the fat in the subjects' diet. Consumption of high-amylose starch (in crackers or muffins) as part of a meal or a tolerance test also decreases insulin response (by approximately 75%) and glucose response (by approximately 50%) compared with standard starch.[36,37,43] After 13 weeks of high amylose or amylopectin consumption, glucose and insulin response averaged 35% and 48% less, respectively, after amylose and did not change after amylopectin.[37]

Diets supplemented with guar gum (to produce a high-fiber diet) and containing a carbohydrate content of more than 40% of total energy have been effective in decreasing blood glucose and lipid concentrations in diabetic subjects.[40,41] A glycemic index has been developed to compare the postprandial glucose response of different foods (portions containing 50 g of carbohydrate), using the response after white bread as the reference food.[38] High-carbohydrate, high-fiber diets using high-fiber food sources that are also low-glycemic-index food sources improved blood glucose control, reduced lipid concentrations, and reduced the insulin requirements of some diabetic subjects.[40,44,45] Diabetic subjects consuming the equivalent diet using high-glycemic-index foods with similar fiber content underwent a decrease in fasting glucose and cholesterol concentrations, but triacylglycerol and postprandial blood glucose concentrations were often increased.[40,44]

Obesity (along with the associated conditions of hypertriglyceridemia, hyperinsulinemia and insulin resistance, hypertension, and hypercholesterolemia) has been identified as a risk factor for cardiovascular disease, diabetes mellitus, respiratory problems, and gallbladder disease.[46,47] In addition, it was estimated that one-third of adults (over 20 years old) are overweight,[48] causing in a large percentage of the population to be at increased risk for other chronic health diseases. Reduction in some risk factors for the overweight or obese population may be achieved by either decreasing the fat content of the diet or by weight loss.[49,50] The ultimate goal in treating overweight individuals has been to normalize their body weight and then maintain the weight. Lowering total dietary fat intake with and without weight loss decreases the blood cholesterol concentration of hyperlipidemic subjects.[49]

A modeling study using a year-long study of dietary records of self-selected diets indicated that even in individuals without strong motivation to control macronutrient or energy intake, consumption of foods with fat replacers could be expected to decrease total fat intake whether or not total energy intake was reduced.[51] Weight loss alone was responsible for decreasing total cholesterol by approximately 50%, LDL cholesterol by approximately 60%, and triacylglycerols by approximately 70 percent. Combining weight loss and a low-fat diet appeared to be additive in reducing serum lipid concentrations.[49] In weight-loss programs fiber has been used to reduce energy intake, delay gastric emptying, increase gastric filling and satiety, and increase fecal energy excretion.[52] Low-fat and no-fat foods made with fat substitutes are promoted to this segment of the population. It is not clear whether the fat-substituted foods containing soluble fibers would be consumed in quantities sufficient to improve the lipid and glycemic values in overweight individuals, especially if no weight loss occurs.

Epidemiological studies indicate an inverse relationship between cancer development and consumption of fruits and vegetables, which are major sources of fiber in the United States.[53-55] Cruciferous vegetables, leafy green vegetables, and raw fruits and vegetables, as well as more than five servings of fruits and vegetables per day were most often mentioned as protective against colon cancer.[56,57] Food intake records of patients with cancer compared with those of control subjects indicated the cancer patients had a greater energy intake and consumed more fat, protein, and carbohydrate.[53] Per unit of energy intake, the self-selected diet of the colorectal cancer patients contained less cereal fiber, calcium, and phosphorus than did that reported by the control subjects.[54] In many animal studies, wheat bran was the most effective fiber source in decreasing the incidence of colon tumors.[57]

Dietary fiber is thought to protect against colorectal cancer through three mechanisms: by diluting fecal material and shortening transit time, thus reducing contact of potential carcinogens with the intestinal mucosa;[54] by modifying bile acid metabolism;[54] and by producing butyric acid, which is used as the main energy source of colonocytes during colonic fermentation of soluble fibers.[57,58] Short-chain fatty acids (butyrate, acetate, and propionate produced as by-products of fermentation) used as colonic infusions or enemas have potential healing benefits in patients with diversion colitis and distal ulcerative colitis.[58]

POTENTIAL ADVERSE CONDITIONS

Cell hyperproliferation was noted in some studies with fiber-supplemented diets, particularly fermentable fibers.[57-59] In rats, colon carcinogens appears to depend on both the fat and fiber content of the diet.[57] Wasan and Goodlad[59] reviewed seven rat studies that used pectin as the fiber source, four reported enhanced tumor development, two reported no fiber effect, and one reported a protective effect. Guar, carrageenan, and agar had similar effects on colon cancer. Of the seven studies using psyllium as the fiber source, four reported a protective effect, two reported no fiber effect, and only one reported enhanced tumor development. Hyperproliferation was proposed as an important early change in the development of colorectal cancers.[59] Whether the observations on cell proliferation and tumor enhancement in rats fed soluble fibers are directly applicable to human colonic cancer is unresolved and remains an important question for future research.

Other potential problems resulting from large intakes of fiber include intestinal gas production, diarrhea, and mineral loss. Although consumption of large quantities of legumes, amylose starch, or soluble fibers, such as guar, pectin, or oatrim, can beneficially decrease glycemic response to a meal and decrease blood lipids after prolonged consumption, increased bloating and flatulence may also result from more nutrients reaching the bacteria in the large intestine. The fat substitute polydextrose also has a laxative effect and must be so labeled when used in quantity.[11,12] Discomfort usually is reported during the first week of a study when the diet changes from low to high fiber. With a slower transition, less flatulence, bloating, and abdominal discomfort are noted.

In some studies, high intakes of dietary fiber resulted in a negative balance for some minerals, particularly when a single fiber source was used to achieve the high-fiber diet.[25,60,61] Decreased transit time could also contribute to decreased mineral absorption in the small intestine.[61] However, other studies, especially those using soluble fibers, reported no effect from added fibers.[25,60,61] Addition of guar gum to the diet of adults with noninsulin-dependent diabetes was beneficial to some of the diabetic subjects, lowering their blood glucose and lipid concentrations without apparently changing mineral balance from prestudy levels.[25] Studies longer than 3-4 weeks generally did not report significant negative mineral balances with high fiber consumption.[60,61] Vegetarians, who habitually consume a higher fiber diet than the general population, do not usually have a negative mineral balance.[60]

SUMMARY AND CONCLUSIONS

The wide array of low-fat foods containing soluble fibers have the potential for helping in weight loss or weight control. Consumption of soluble fibers in sufficient quantities has been shown to lower serum lipid concentrations[17-20] and to improve glycemic response.[23,25,38,39] Some individuals could, eventually, consume a significant portion of their soluble dietary fiber from processed foods containing soluble-fiber fat substitutes. Changes in dietary fiber and starch sources increase the amount of fermentable material reaching the colon. Short-chain fatty acids thus produced[17,19] are used as an energy source by colonocytes and may inhibit hepatic cholesterol synthesis.[4,17,58] However, colonic fermentation can also result in flatulence or diarrhea. In addition, some diets high in soluble fiber have been shown to change intestinal cell morphology in rats. The possible benefits from consumption of a diet high in soluble fiber fat substitutes in serum lipid reduction, glycemic response improvement, and/or weight reduction as well as potential problems in flatulence, mineral absorption, and colonic cell hyperproliferation should be investigated.

REFERENCES

1. SPILLER, R. C. 1994. Pharmacology of dietary fibre. Pharm. Ther. **62:** 407-427.
2. ASP, N. G., I. BJORCK & M. NYMAN. 1993. Physiological effects of cereal dietary fibre. Carbohydr. Polym. **21:** 183-187.
3. ENGLYST, H. N., H. TROWELL, D. A. T. SOUTHGATE & J. H. CUMMINGS. 1987. Dietary fiber and resistant starch. Am. J. Clin. Nutr. **46:** 873-874.
4. SCHNEEMAN, B. O. & J. TIETYEN. 1994. Dietary fiber. In Modern Nutrition in Health and Disease. M. E. Hills, J. A. Olson & M. Shike, Eds.: 85-100. Lea and Febiger. Baltimore, MD.
5. TRUSWELL, A. S. 1987. Evolution of dietary recommendations, goals, and guidelines. Am. J. Clin. Nutr. **45:** 1060-1072.

6. U.S. DEPARTMENT OF AGRICULTURE, U.S. DEPARTMENT OF HEALTH AND HUMAN SERVICES. 1990. Nutrition for your health. Dietary guidelines for Americans. 3rd ed.: 273-293. U.S. Government Printing Office. Washington D.C.
7. NATIONAL CHOLESTEROL EDUCATION PROGRAM. 1990. Report of the Expert Panel on Population Strategies for Blood Cholesterol Reduction. U.S. Department of Health and Human Services, Public Health Service, National Institutes of Health, National Heart, Lung, and Blood Institute. NIH Publication No. 90-3046.
8. STORY, L., J. W. ANDERSON, W. J. L. CHEN, D. KAROUNOS & B. JEFFERSON. 1985. Adherence to high-carbohydrate, high-fiber diets: Long-term studies of non-obese diabetic men. J. Am. Diet. Assoc. **85:** 1105-1110.
9. ANDERSON, J. W., B. M. SMITH & N. J. GUSTAFSON. 1994. Health benefits and practical aspects of high-fiber diets. Am. J. Clin. Nutr. **59:** 1242S-1247S.
10. MIRAGLIO, A. M. 1995. Nutrient substitutes and their energy values in fat substitutes and replacers. Am. J. Clin. Nutr. **62:** 1175S-1179S.
11. WARSHAW, H. S. & M. A. POWERS. 1993. Ingredients that replace fat: Their role in today's foods and challenges in educating people with diabetes. Diabetes Educ. **19:** 419-430.
12. SETSER, C. S. & W. L. RACETTE. 1992. Macromolecule replacers in food products. Crit. Rev. Food Sci. Nutr. **32:** 275-297.
13. SCHLICKER, S. A. & C. REGAN. 1990. Innovations in reduced-calorie foods: A review of fat and sugar replacement technologies. Top. Clin. Nutr. **6:** 50-60.
14. GERSHOFF, S. N. 1995. Nutrition evaluation of dietary fat substitutes. Nutr. Rev. **53:** 305-313.
15. HUDNALL, M. J., S. L. CONNOR & W. E. CONNOR. 1991. Position of the American Dietetic Association: Fat replacements. J. Am. Diet. Assoc. **91:** 1285-1288.
16. WHISTLER, R. L. 1984. Factors influencing gum costs and applications. *In* Starch: Chemistry and Technology. R. L. Whistler, J. N. BeMiller & E. F. Paschall. Eds.: 26-79. Academic Press. New York, NY.
17. JENKINS, D. J. A., P. J. SPADAFORA, A. L. JENKINS & C. G. RAINEY-MACDONALD. 1993. Fiber in the treatment of hyperlipidemia. *In* CRC Handbook of Dietary Fiber in Human Nutrition. G. A. Spiller, Ed.: 419-438. CRC Press. Ann Arbor, MI.
18. TRUSWELL, A. S. 1995. Dietary fibre and plasma lipids. Eur. J. Clin. Nutr. **49:** S105-S109.
19. GLORE, S. R., D. VAN TREECK, A. W. KNEHANS & M. GUILD. 1994. Soluble fiber and serum lipids. A literature review. J. Am. Diet Assoc. **94:** 425-436.
20. HOPEWELL, R., R. YEATER & I. ULLRICH. 1993. Soluble fiber: Effect on carbohydrate and lipid metabolism. Prog. Food & Nutr. Sci. **17:** 159-182.
21. BEHALL, K. M. & S. REISER. 1986. Effects of pectin on human metabolism. *In* Recent Advances in the Chemistry and Function of Pectin. M. L. Fishman & J. J. Jen, Eds.: 248-265. American Chemical Society, Washington, D.C.
22. SPILLER, G. A., J. W. FARQUHAR, J. E. GATES & S. F. NICHOLS. 1991. Guar gum and plasma lipoproteins and cholesterol in hypercholesterolemic adults. Arteriosclerosis Thrombosis **11:** 1204-1208.
23. JENKINS, D. J. A., A. L. JENKINS, T. M. S. WOLEVER, V. VERKSAN, A. V. RAO, L. U. THOMPSON & R. G. JOSSE. 1995. Effect of reduced rate of carbohydrate absorption on carbohydrate and lipid metabolism. Eur. J. Clin. Nutr. **49:** S68-S73.
24. MCIVOR, M. E., C. C. CUMMINGS, M. A. VAN DUYN, T. A. LEO, S. MARGOLIS, K. M. BEHALL, J. E. MICHNOWSKI & A. I. MENDELOFF. 1986. Long-term effects of guar gum on blood lipids. Atherosclerosis **60:** 7-13.
25. BEHALL, K. M. 1990. Effect of soluble fibers on plasma lipids, glucose tolerance and mineral balance. *In* New Developments in Dietary Fiber. I. Furda & C. J. Brine, Eds.: 7-16. Plenum Press, New York, NY.
26. OSILESI, O., D. L. TROUT, E. E. GLOVER, S. M. HARPER, E. T. KOH, K. M. BEHALL, T. M. O'DORISIO & J. TARTT. 1985. Use of xanthan gum in dietary management of diabetes mellitus. Am. J. Clin. Nutr. **42:** 597-603.

27. SACKS, F. M. 1991. The role of cereals, fats, and fibers in preventing coronary heart disease. Cereal Foods World **36:** 822–826.
28. RIPSIN, C. M., J. M. KEENAN, D. M. JACOBS, P. J. ELMER, R. R. WELCH, L. VAN HORN, W. H. TURNBULL, F. W. THYE, M. KESTIN, M. HEGSTED, D. M. DAVIDSON, M. H. DAVIDSON, L. D. DUGAN, W. DEMARK-WAHNEFRIED & S. DELING. 1992. Oat products and lipid lowering. J. Am. Med. Assoc. **267:** 3317–3325.
29. SCHINNICK, F. L., R. MATHEWS & S. INK. 1991. Serum cholesterol reduction by oats and other fiber sources. Cereal Foods World **36:** 815–821.
30. KESTIN, M., R. MOSS, P. M. CLIFTON & P. J. NESTEL. 1990. Comparative effects of three cereal brans on plasma lipids, blood pressure, and glucose metabolism in mildly hypercholesterolemic men. Am. J. Clin. Nutr. **52:** 661–666.
31. ANDERSON, J. W., N. H. GILINSKY, D. A. DEAKINS, S. F. SMITH, D. S. O'NEAL, D. W. DILLON & P. R. OELTGEN. 1991. Lipid responses of hypercholesterolemic men to oat-bran and wheat-bran intake. Am. J. Clin. Nutr. **54:** 678–683, 1991.
32. DAVIDSON, M. H., L. D. DUGAN, J. H. BURNS, K. BOVA, K. STORY & K. B. DRENNAN. 1991. The hypocholesterolemic effects of β-glucan in oatmeal and oat bran. J. Am. Med. Assoc. **265:** 1833–1839.
33. ANDERSON, J. W., L. STORY, B. SIELING, W. J. L. CHEN, M. S. PETRO & J. STORY. 1984. Hypocholesterolemic effects of oat-bran or bean intake for hypercholesterolemic men. Am. J. Clin. Nutr. **40:** 1146–1155.
34. BEHALL, K. M., D. J. SCHOLFIELD & J. HALLFRISCH. 1997. Effect of beta-glucan level in oat fiber extracts on blood lipids in men and women. J. Am. Coll. Nutr. **16:** 46–51.
35. TÖRRÖNEN, R., L. KANSANEN, M. UUSITUPA, O. HANNINEN, O. MYLLYMAKI, H. HARKONEN & Y. MALKKI. 1992. Effects of an oat bran concentrate on serum lipids in free-living men with mild to moderate hypercholesterolaemia. Eur. J. Clin. Nutr. **46:** 621–627.
36. BEHALL, K. M., D. J. SCHOLFIELD, I. YUHANIAK & J. J. CANARY. 1989. Diets containing high amylose vs. amylopectin starch: Effects on metabolic variables in human subjects. Am. J. Clin. Nutr. **49:** 337–344.
37. BEHALL, K. M. & J. C. HOWE. 1995. Effect of long term consumption of amylose vs. amylopectin starch on metabolic parameters in human subjects. Am. J. Clin. Nutr. **61:** 334–40.
38. FOSTER-POWELL, K. & J. B. MILLER. 1995. International tables of glycemic index. Am. J. Clin. Nutr. **62:** 871S–893S.
39. MANN, J. 1985. Diabetes mellitus: Some aspects of aetiology and management of non-insulin-dependent diabetes. *In* Dietary Fibre, Fibre-Depleted Foods and Disease. H. Trowell, D. Burkitt & K. Heaton, Eds.: 263–287. Academic Press. New York, NY.
40. WOLEVER, T. M. S. & D. J. A. JENKINS. 1993. Effect of dietary fiber and foods on carbohydrate metabolism. *In* CRC Handbook of Dietary Fiber in Human Nutrition. G. A. Spiller, Ed.: 111–152. CRC Press. Ann Arbor, MI.
41. ANDERSON, J. W. & A. O. AKANJI. 1993. Treatment of diabetes with high fiber diets. *In* CRC Handbook of Dietary Fiber in Human Nutrition. G. A. Spiller, Ed.: 349–360. CRC Press. Ann Arbor, MI.
42. HALLFRISCH, J., D. J. SCHOLFIELD & K. M. BEHALL. 1995. Diets containing soluble oat extracts improve glucose and insulin responses of moderately hypercholesterolemic men and women. Am. J. Clin. Nutr. **61:** 379–384.
43. BEHALL, K. M., D. J., SCHOLFIELD & J. J. CANARY. 1988. Effect of starch structure on glucose and insulin responses in adults. Am. J. Clin. Nutr. **47:** 428–432.
44. BRAND, J. C., S. COLAGIURI, S. CROSSMAN, A. ALLEN & A. S. TRUSWELL. 1991. Low glycemic index carbohydrate foods improve glucose control in non-insulin dependent diabetes mellitus (NIDDM). Diabetes Care **14:** 95–101.
45. ANDERSON, J. W., D. S. O'NEAL, S. RIDDELL-MASON, T. L. FLOORE, D. W. DILLON & P. R. OETTGEN. 1995. Postprandial serum glucose, insulin and lipoprotein responses to high- and low-fiber diets. Metabolism **44:** 848–854.

46. PI-SUNYER, F. X. 1994. Obesity. *In* Modern Nutrition in Health and Disease. Vol. 2. 8th edition. M. E. Shils, J. A. Olson & M. Shike, Eds.: 984–1006. Lea & Febiger. Philadelphia, PA.
47. RAVUSSIN, E., A. M. FONTVIEILLE, B. A. SWINBURN & C. BOGARDUS. 1993. Risk factors for the development of obesity. Ann. N.Y. Acad. Sci. **683:** 141–150.
48. KUCZMARSKI, R. J., K. M. FLEGAL, S. M. CAMPBELL & C. L. JOHNSON. 1994. Increasing prevalence of overweight among U.S. adults. The national health and nutrition examination surveys, 1960–1991. J. Am. Med. Assoc. **272:** 205–211.
49. LEENEN, R., K. VAN DER DOOY, S. MEYBOOM, J. C. SEIDEL, P. DEURENBERG & J. A. WESTSTRATE. 1993. Relative effects of weight loss and dietary fat modification on serum lipid levels in the dietary treatment of obesity. J. Lipid Res. **34:** 2183–91.
50. DATTILO, A. M. & P. M. KRIS-ETHERTON. 1992. Effects of weight reduction on blood lipids and lipoproteins: A met-analysis. Am. J. Clin. Nutr. **56:** 320–328.
51. BEATON, G. H., V. TARASUK & G. H. ANDERSON. 1992. Estimation of possible impact of non-caloric fat and carbohydrate substitutes on micronutrient intake in the human. Appetite **19:** 87–103.
52. ROSSNER, S. 1992. Dietary fibre in the prevention and treatment of obesity. *In* Dietary Fibre—A Component of Food. T. F. Schweizer, C. A. Edwards, Eds.: 265–277. Springier-Verlag. New York, NY.
53. BYERS, T. 1995. Dietary fiber and colon cancer risk: The epidemiologic evidence. *In* Dietary Fiber in Health and Disease. D. Kritchevsky & C. Bonfield, Eds.: 183–190. Eagun Press. St. Paul, MN.
54. KAAKS, R. & E. RIBOLI. 1995. Colorectal cancer and intake of dietary fibre. A summary of the epidemiological evidence. Eur. J. Clin. Nutr. **49:** S10–S17.
55. VERNIA, P. & M. CITTADINI. 1995. Short-chain fatty acids and colorectal cancer. Eur. J. Clin. Nutr. **49:** S18–S21.
56. GREENWALD, P. & C. CLIFFORD. 1995. Fiber and cancer: Prevention research. *In* Dietary Fiber in Health and Disease. D. Kritchevsky & C. Bonfield, Eds.: 159–173. Eagun Press. St. Paul, MN.
57. SHANKAR, S. & E. LANZA. 1991. Dietary fiber and cancer prevention. Hematol. Oncol. Clin. N. Am. **5:** 25–41.
58. ROMBEAU, J. L. & J. A. ROTH. 1995. Short-chain fatty acids—Research and clinical updates. *In* Dietary Fiber in Health and Disease. D. Kritchevsky & C. Bonfield, Eds.: 441–449. Eagun Press. St. Paul, MN.
59. WASAN, H. S. & R. A. GOODLAD. 1996. Fibre-supplemented foods may damage your health. Lancet **348:** 319–320.
60. GORDON, D., D. STOOPS & V. RATLIFF. 1995. Dietary fiber and mineral nutrition. *In* Dietary Fiber in Health and Disease. D. Kritchevsky & C. Bonfield, Eds.: 267–293. Eagun Press. St. Paul, MN.
61. FROLICK, W. 1993. Bioavailability of minerals from cereals. A Review. *In* CRC Handbook of Dietary Fiber in Human Nutrition. 2nd edition. G. A. Spiller, Ed.: 209–245. CRC Press, Inc. Boca Raton, FL.

Appropriate Animal Models for Clinical Studies

RUTH B. S. HARRIS [a]

Pennington Biomedical Research Center
Louisiana State University
6400 Perkins Road
Baton Rouge, Louisiana 70808

The objective of this presentation is to review the role of animal studies in determining the nutritional and physiological impact of dietary components, specifically macronutrient substitutes. Animal experiments are an integral part of the process for demonstrating safety of a new ingredient or additive, but as the specifics of these studies are defined by federal agencies they will not be discussed here. However, animal experiments have applications other than toxicology and can provide the basic information needed to determine appropriate dietary manipulations and meaningful end point measures for human studies.

JUSTIFICATION FOR ANIMAL STUDIES

The advantages and disadvantages of animal studies over pilot clinical trials vary according to the animal model that is selected. The greatest advantage, applicable to all animal models, is the ability to manipulate a single dietary component while controlling all other variables. Animals are fed diets of uniform and defined composition, and intake measures are made as frequently and precisely as desired. Errors associated with the measurement of food intake of human subjects by recall, food diaries, or food-frequency questionnaires[1] are avoided, and the labor and cost of providing food and measuring intake is minimal compared with that involved when human subjects are provided with meals as inpatients or as outpatients fed in an institutional dining room. Voluntary drop-out rate in an animal study is zero, and compliance with the study protocol is 100%. The subjects are not tempted to deviate from the experimental diet by easy availability of more appetizing foods, participation in social events, or peer pressure. One criticism of testing dietary manipulations in the extremely controlled environment associated with animal studies is that the test conditions are not representative of the human environment in which the diet would normally be consumed. However, any indication of a relationship between the dietary intervention and an end-point measure in an animal study provides justification for further investigation. This may result in a continuation of animal studies to examine the mechanism of response, to determine whether it was relevant to the human situation, or data from the animal studies may be enough to justify initiation of clinical trials.

---

[a] Tel: (504) 763-2521; fax: (504) 763-2525; e-mail: harrisrb@mhs.pbrc.edu.

A second advantage that is common to all animal models is the ability to take invasive, or fatal, end-point measures. This is especially relevant when measuring physiological or metabolic responses to a dietary intervention. Invasive measurements are required to demonstrate how a substance is metabolized at a cellular level, which organs are involved in the metabolism, and whether specific tissues show morphological changes in response to the diet. Similarly, animal studies facilitate extreme levels of dietary manipulation, resulting in a deficit of an essential nutrient or potentially toxic concentrations of a fat-soluble substance. These types of manipulations either would not be tolerated by human subjects or could involve unacceptable health risks. Finally, animal models allow measurement of response in subpopulations that are at increased risk for a negative response, such as older individuals with multiple chronic diseases or very young children in which there is the potential for a long-lasting impact on growth and development.

Other advantages of animal studies are speed, uniformity of experimental subjects, availability of subjects, and cost-effectiveness. However, the size of these advantages is determined by which animal model is used. Cost and subject number are more limited in experiments involving nonhuman primates than those using rodent models. Speed is determined by a combination of end point of interest and animal model selected. For example, studies examining the impact of dietary restriction on parameters of aging in rodents last 2 or 3 years.[2] Similar studies with nonhuman primates may take decades,[3] losing the advantage of speed, but environmental control, retention of subjects in the study, and compliance with prolonged caloric restriction are overwhelming advantages of this animal model, compared with attempting a similar human trial.

Despite these advantages, extrapolation of results from animal models to human trials should be approached cautiously. A majority of nutritional studies in animals involve a single dietary manipulation. Consumption of a purified diet is not representative of a human diet and excludes the effects of potential nutrient interactions and the intermittent, or erratic, consumption of the dietary component of interest that will most likely occur in a human population that has a continuously expanding variety of foods from which to select their diets. Another confounding behavioral factor is that small experimental animals live in an unenriched environment, receiving few of the environmental queues or social stimuli that influence food intake and selection in humans. Due to the nature of animal experiments, a laboratory rodent is exposed to a limited number of food choices and is unlikely to be influenced by preconceptions about specific food items or to have developed learned preferences, or aversions, that are apparent even in young children.[4] Additionally, when food choices of an animal model appear to reflect those made by humans, it cannot be assumed that sensory properties of a food are detected in a similar manner. Although rats may demonstrate a taste preference for a solution that humans also find pleasant, it is impossible to confirm that both species are responding to similar sensory stimuli.

An essential aspect of animal studies is that the model selected is appropriate for the clinical end-point measure. Digestive processes, metabolism of nutrients, and feedback control of regulatory mechanisms should be very similar, if not identical. For example, rats and pigs are reasonable models for studying regulation of food intake and energy balance in humans, as digestive processes, nutrient metabolism, and central mechanisms regulating food intake are similar to those of humans.[5–7]

Hamsters, guinea pigs, rabbits, or monkeys are more appropriate models for examining the effects of diet composition on human lipid metabolism.[8-10] Finally, it is essential that the dietary manipulation tested in animal studies is relevant to humans and that novel additives or ingredients could realistically be incorporated into the human diet.

APPLICATION OF ANIMAL STUDIES

The advantages of speed, cost, and control that are associated with animal studies justify their use for screening potential dietary manipulations in clinical trials. However, there are limitations on the end-point measures made in animal studies that can be extrapolated to human responses. As mentioned above, although animals may show preferences and aversions for food or solutions of particular flavor, it is impossible to translate these measurements into a meaningful human response. Alternatively, animals may not respond to a taste or flavor in the same way as humans. A good example of this difference in hedonic response is aspartame. Although humans find aspartame solutions sweet, rats show little or no preference for aspartame, presumably because it does not deliver a taste similar to that of sucrose.[11]

Due to these limitations animal studies can only provide useful preclinical information in specifically defined areas. Animal models can be used to determine the effect of diet composition on basic physiological responses, such as nutrient requirement, energy balance, growth, and longevity. Results from these studies can be used to determine both the appropriate level of an ingredient or supplement in a diet for measurement of a biological effect and the maximum level of intervention that would be considered safe to use in human trials. Alternatively, animal studies may be used to investigate cellular mechanisms underlying a physiological response that is observed in humans but that requires tissue samples that cannot be obtained from human subjects. Identification of peripheral and central mechanisms that initiate a negative physiological response to a change in diet composition facilitates identification of subpopulations that are at especially high risk, or may provide insight into strategies that can be used to prevent the negative health effects of a specific dietary component.

ANIMAL MODELS AND MACRONUTRIENT SUBSTITUTES

The objectives of this volume are threefold: to enhance understanding of the impact of macronutrient substitutes on energy and nutrient intake, food selection, and dietary patterns; to evaluate the effect of macronutrient-modified foods on dietary goals and food selection; and to identify knowledge gaps and research opportunities related to the nutritional implications of macronutrient substitutes. The current commercial status of fat substitutes, fat mimetics, and artificial sweeteners is such that there are few opportunities for animal studies to provide information that is relevant to consumer response to foods containing macronutrient substitutes. Animal models cannot evaluate the effect of fat-modified foods on food choices of specific subsets of consumers. Nor will they provide any insights into how consumers substitute and trade off full fat foods when they incorporate fat-modified foods into their diets.

However, review of the development of fat-modified foods shows that animal studies provided information on aspects of fat substitutes and mimetics that are either the subject of postmarketing surveillance, now that foods containing nondigestible fat substitutes are being introduced, or that are being replicated and confirmed in human studies.

Fat-modified Foods

Fat-modified foods were developed largely in response to consumer demand for food items that facilitated compliance with recommendations from health professionals that fat intake be reduced to 30%, or less, of calories.[12,13] Consumers wanted to reduce their fat intake in order to reduce the risk for a number of chronic diseases, such as cardiovascular disease, hypertension, diabetes, and obesity, without sacrificing the preferred organoleptic properties of high-fat foods. There are a wealth of animal and epidemiological studies to show that consumption of a low-fat diet is associated with decreased risk for chronic diseases prevalent in Western society.[12] Fat substitutes, ingredients that have similar physical properties as fat but have no nutritional value, and fat mimetics, processed proteins and carbohydrates that provide physical and sensory properties typically associated with fat, provided the opportunity to develop foods that had similar organoleptic properties as high-fat foods but that delivered the health benefits associated with a low-fat diet.[14]

Early rat studies with sucrose polyester (olestra: Olean™, Procter & Gamble, Cincinnati, OH), a nondigestible fat substitute, confirmed that it was not absorbed,[15] that it did reduce the availability of fat-soluble vitamins,[16] but that it also had the beneficial effect of reducing plasma cholesterol concentration.[17] These studies were confirmed in humans[18] and ultimately led to the supplementation of Olean™ with fat-soluble vitamins. In addition, further animal studies were carried out to confirm the mechanisms by which plasma cholesterol was reduced and vitamin A absorption was inhibited.[19,20] This series of investigations illustrate the utility of animal models in providing information on appropriate end-point measures for clinical trials and in elucidating mechanisms involved in a physiological response to dietary manipulation.

Although animal studies will not predict human food choices or their ability to incorporate fat-modified foods into their daily diet, the rat preference studies reported by Sclafani et al.[21-23] demonstrate that energy balance status can impact preference for nutritional fats versus nonnutritive fats. Acroff et al.[21] showed that nonfood-deprived rats had equal preferences for nutritive 30% corn oil emulsions and nonnutritive 30% mineral oil emulsions, measured in short, three-minute, two-bottle preference tests. When the preference tests were extended to 30 minutes, the rats showed a small preference for the corn oil emulsion. However, when the rats were food deprived to less than 90% of their ad libitum weight, they had 85% preference for the corn oil emulsion over the mineral oil emulsion. These results indicate that rats learn to prefer solutions that deliver a postabsorptive benefit, and that when they are hungry they greatly prefer solutions associated with calories. Similar results were obtained in a study that examined preference of rats for full-fat and fat-free commercially available pound cake (Entenmanns™, Bayshore, NY).[23] When ad libitum-fed rats were offered full-fat and fat-free cake in 30 minute/day two-jar preference tests for

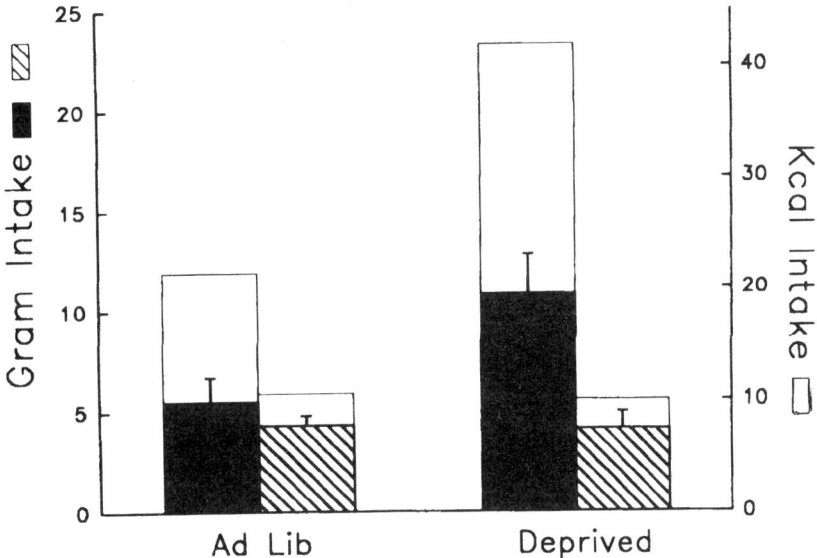

FIGURE 1. Preference for full-fat or fat-free pound cake in rats fed ad libitum or deprived to less than 90% of ad libitum body weight. Female Sprague Dawley rats were tested in 30 minute/day 2-jar preference tests on six days. Ad libitum fed rats ate similar amounts of the full-fat and fat-free cake, whereas food-deprived rats preferred full-fat cake. ■, high fat; ▨, no fat. (Sclafani et al.[23] With permission from *Obesity Research.* Copyright © 1993 NAASO.)

six days, they had similar preferences for the two cakes, resulting in greater energy intake from the high-fat cake. When the rats had been food deprived to 85% of their ad libitum body weight, they showed a much greater preference for the full-fat cake over the fat-free cake (see FIG. 1), suggesting that the rats selected the food that was associated with a greater caloric density. Although results from rat preference tests cannot be directly translated to human food choices, these studies suggest that although fat-modified foods have similar organoleptic properties as high-fat counterparts, preference for the low-fat foods can be influenced by whether an individual is reducing fat-intake independent of calorie intake or as part of a weight-loss diet. The relevance of this observation in animals to humans is demonstrated by a study in which human subjects were assigned to a low-fat diet that excluded discretionary fat sources, a low-fat diet that included fat-reduced foods, or to a normal diet. During the 12 weeks of the study, pleasantness ratings of high-fat foods declined only in the subjects that did not consume any discretionary fats. Preference for high-fat foods did not change in the subjects consuming fat-modified foods, even though their fat intake was significantly reduced.[24]

There are a limited number of animal studies examining the physiological impact of fat mimetics. This may be due to mimetics being composed of carbohydrates and proteins that are already a part of the food supply. As there are no safety issues associated with the ingredients, studies investigating behavioral and physiological

TABLE 1. Body Weight, Energy Intake, and Serum Insulin of Rats Fed Diets of Similar Texture but Different Fat Content[a]

	63% kcal Fat	51% kcal Fat	30% kcal Fat
Body weight (g)	252 ± 6[a]	246 ± 5[a]	231 ± 2[b]
Body fat (g)	43 ± 5[a]	35 ± 1[b]	26 ± 1[c]
Energy intake (kcal/14 d)	731 ± 20[a]	671 ± 16[ab]	671 ± 22[b]
Serum insulin (pmol/L)	352 ± 43[a]	222 ± 7[b]	201 ± 7[b]
Serum glucose (nmol/L)	5.9 ± 0.3	6.2 ± 0.2	6.0 ± 0.2

[a] Female Sprague Dawley rats were fed diets containing different amounts of fat. The two lower fat diets included a carbohydrate-based fat mimetic that conferred similar texture to all diets. After 64 days of the experimental diet, body-fat content and serum insulin concentrations were inversely proportional to dietary fat content. Groups that have a different superscript for a particular parameter are significantly different at p < 0.05, determined by one-way ANOVA and calculation of $lsd_{0.05}$. Data are means ± SEM for groups of 10 rats.[25]

responses to diets containing fat mimetics have been carried out in humans. However, there are a few animal studies that provide information on the potential beneficial effects of reduced-fat foods.

Three studies have demonstrated improved insulin responsiveness and reduced body fat content in rats fed diets containing fat mimetics.[25–27] In the first study rats were fed either a very high-fat diet (63% kcal fat), a 51% kcal fat diet, or a 30% kcal fat diet.[25] The two lower fat diets contained fat mimetics to maintain a similar texture to that of the high-fat diet. Energy intake of the rats was significantly reduced on the 30% fat diet compared with the 63% fat diet, and both body fat content and serum insulin decreased progressively with the reduction in dietary fat content (see TABLE 1). The levels of dietary fat used in this study were abnormally high compared with a human diet but were typical for rodent studies examining the mechanism of response to high-fat diets.[28] In the second study rats were fed one of three diets: a high-fat diet containing 38% kcal fat, a control diet containing 21% kcal fat, or a very low-fat diet containing only essential fatty acids (2% kcal) and fat mimetics to maintain dietary texture.[26] After 36 days rats fed the very low-fat diet had consumed more energy than rats fed the 21% fat diet, but less than those fed the high-fat diet. They had the same body fat content as the rats fed the 21% kcal fat diet, and adipocytes from these two groups were equally insulin responsive. The rats fed the 38% fat diet were fatter than the two other groups (Table 2), and their adipocytes were insulin resistant. Both of these animal studies used diet compositions that are not representative of human diets; however, they demonstrated that reducing fat intake causes a progressive improvement in body composition and insulin sensitivity that plateaus once fat intake is reduced to 20% of energy. Reduction of fat intake to very low levels in humans is extremely difficult to achieve, even with fat-modified foods, and these results suggests that extreme reductions in dietary fat have little effect on body composition or insulin responsiveness beyond that achieved with a 20% kcal fat diet.

A third study with rats compared the effects of reducing dietary fat from 40 to 30% kcal of fat, a manipulation relevant to humans, using either carbohydrate or a

TABLE 2. Body Weight, Energy Intake, and Serum Insulin of Rats Fed Diets Containing Fat Mimetics[a]

	38% kcal Fat	21% kcal Fat	2% kcal Fat
Body weight (g)	256 ± 8	243 ± 10	257 ± 6
Inguinal fat (g)	3.5 ± 0.3	3.3 ± 0.3	3.3 ± 0.3
Energy intake (kcal/28 d)	433 ± 23[a]	363 ± 11[a]	415 ± 9[b]
Serum insulin (pmol/L)	316 ± 36[a]	244 ± 29[b]	208 ± 7[a]
Serum glucose (mmol/L)	7.0 ± 0.3	6.9 ± 0.4	6.8 ± 0.4

[a] Measurements made in rats fed diets of different fat content for 30 days. The 2% kcal fat diet contained a carbohydrate-based fat mimetic (5.9% cellulose, 0.3% xanthan, 93.8% water) to give it a similar texture to the 38% fat diet. Groups that have a different superscript for a particular parameter are significantly different at $p < 0.05$, determined by one-way ANOVA and calculation of $lsd_{0.05}$. Data are means ± SEM for 5 female Sprague Dawley rats.[26]

fat mimetic consisting of cellulose and water.[27] There were four treatment groups in the experiment: rats fed the high-fat diet, rats fed a control 30% kcal fat diet in which carbohydrate replaced fat, rats fed the high-fat diet for 10 weeks and switched to the control diet, and rats fed the high-fat diet for 10 weeks and switched to a 30% kcal fat diet in which fat mimetics replaced fat. The high-fat diet caused insulin resistance, which was reversed within three days of switching to a lower fat diet, irrespective of the diet containing fat mimetics or carbohydrate. Serum insulin also normalized within seven days in rats fed the 30% kcal fat diets (see FIG. 2), even though body fat was still elevated. This study demonstrated that the controlled conditions associated with animal experiments allow identification of diet-induced changes that may not be measurable in human studies; however, the study can be criticized for not replicating the food choices encountered in human studies.

A "cafeteria" study[29] came a little closer to mimicking the variety of foods available to humans in clinical trials. Rats were offered a basal 30% kcal fat diet supplemented with a variety of either high-fat or fat-free snack foods. A third group of rats had no snack food supplements. Rats offered snack food consumed significantly more energy than those with only a control diet available; however, rats fed the low-fat snack foods consumed a greater proportion of their energy as carbohydrate than those fed the control diet. This resulted in a reduction in body-fat content, despite a higher total energy intake. By contrast, rats fed the high-fat snack foods had elevated energy intakes, gained significant amounts of body fat, and were insulin resistant (see TABLE 3). Similar results were found by Sclafani et al.[23] when they offered rats chow plus either a full-fat cake or a fat-free cake. The availability of cake in addition to chow caused an increase in total energy intake and weight gain, but the full-fat cake promoted greater overeating and weight gain than the fat-free cake (see FIG. 3). The results from these two animal studies suggest that although low-fat and fat-free foods provide more choices to consumers who wish to reduce their fat intake, these fat-modified foods will need to be eaten in moderation if they are intended to contribute to a reduction in energy intake.

Although there have been a number of studies with adult humans investigating the impact of fat substitutes on energy intake, nutrient intake, and energy balance

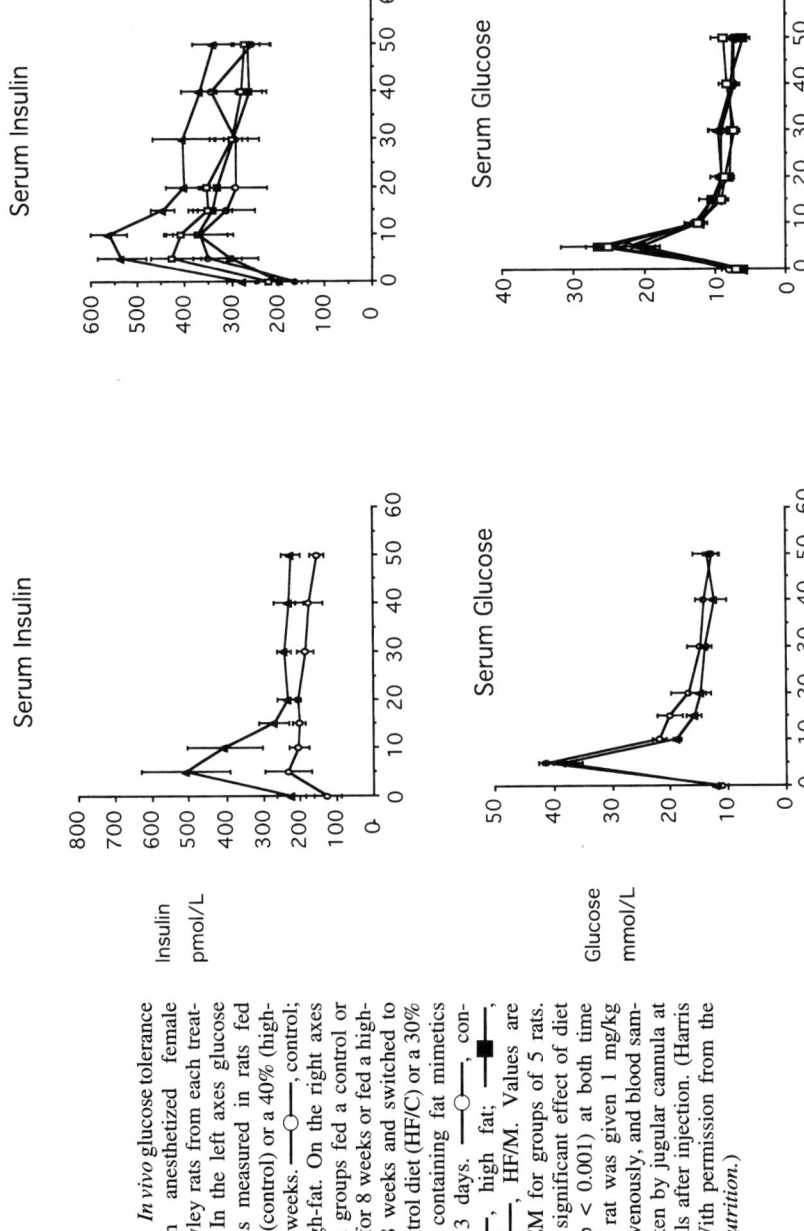

FIGURE 2. *In vivo* glucose tolerance measured in anesthetized female Sprague Dawley rats from each treatment group. In the left axes glucose tolerance was measured in rats fed either a 30% (control) or a 40% (high-fat) diet for 8 weeks. ———, control; ———▲———, high-fat. On the right axes are rats from groups fed a control or high-fat diet for 8 weeks or fed a high-fat diet for 8 weeks and switched to either the control diet (HF/C) or a 30% kcal fat diet containing fat mimetics (HF/M) for 3 days. ———●———, control; ———▲———, high fat; ———■———, HF/C; ———□———, HF/M. Values are means ± SEM for groups of 5 rats. There was a significant effect of diet on insulin ($p < 0.001$) at both time points. Each rat was given 1 mg/kg glucose intravenously, and blood samples were taken by jugular cannula at timed intervals after injection. (Harris and Kor.[27] With permission from the *Journal of Nutrition*.)

TABLE 3. Body Weight, Energy Intake, and Body Composition of Rats Fed Low- or High-fat Cafeteria Foods[a]

	Control	Low-fat Cafeteria	High-fat Cafeteria
Start weight (g)	312 ± 4	311 ± 4	313 ± 5
End weight (g)	432 ± 10	449 ± 8	444 ± 10
Energy intake (kcal/36 d)	2965 ± 44[a]	3193 ± 16[b]	4354 ± 26[c]
Gain in body fat (g)	3.0 ± 3.4	0.9 ± 3.1	10.9 ± 5.3
Gain in body protein (g)	39.1 ± 3.6	44.5 ± 3.0	38.0 ± 3.0
Serum glucose (mmol/L)	7.7 ± 0.4	7.2 ± 0.2	7.6 ± 0.2
Serum insulin (pmol/L)	363 ± 42[a]	348 ± 32[a]	437 ± 56[b]

[a] Groups of 7 or 8 male Sprague Dawley rats were fed either a 30% kcal fat control diet or a control diet plus low-fat or high-fat cafeteria foods for 38 days. The rats offered cafeteria foods consumed more energy than those given only the control diet. The rats fed high-fat cafeteria foods tended to gain more fat than the other groups and were insulin resistant.

for periods as long as 20 days,[30–32] studies with children have, so far, only included manipulation of three meals and monitoring macronutrient and energy intake during the subsequent 48 hours,[33] or monitoring children offered a fat-free ice cream in place of a premium ice cream every day for seven days.[34] The ability to investigate the effect of fat replacement on growth in young animals demonstrates the utility of animal models for studying subpopulations that would be considered at high risk if exposed to prolonged dietary intervention. Growth and body composition was measured in rats offered very low-fat diets, containing only 4% kcal essential fatty acids combined with a fat mimetic made of cellulose, xanthan, and water.[35] Low-fat diets containing fat mimetics were compared with control (17% kcal fat) and high-fat (36% kcal) diets. Addition of the mimetic to the low-fat diets made them palatable, and normal growth was supported. Rats on the low-fat diets had more lean body mass than those on the control or high-fat diets (see TABLE 4). This degree of fat replacement could not be replicated in the human diet; however, these results suggest that reducing the fat intake of young children without reducing calorie intake is unlikely to inhibit normal growth and may promote deposition of lean tissue.

Artificial Sweeteners and Energy Intake

There are two types of artificial sweeteners available: intensely sweet compounds used as food additives, and bulk nonnutritive sweeteners. Aspartame, the methyl ester of aspartylphenylalanine, is an example of the first type of sweetener added to foods in very small amounts, delivering sweet taste without addition of carbohydrate calories. Rat studies with aspartame provided an example of the need to use an appropriate animal model for an end-point measure relevant to humans. Aspartame, 1.0 g/kg given orally, caused hypothalamic lesions in neonatal rats, but there was no effect when higher doses of 2.0 g/kg were given to nonhuman primates.[36] These results indicate differences in the abilities of rodents and primates to either metabolize

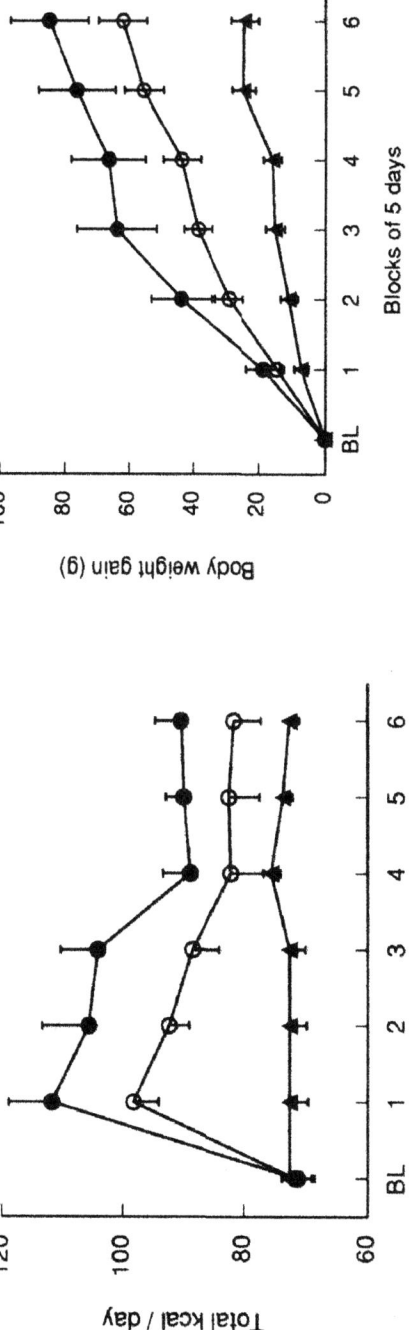

FIGURE 3. Energy intake and body weight gain of female Sprague Dawley rats offered chow (control), chow plus full-fat cake (high-fat) or chow plus fat-free cake (no fat) for 30 days. Rats offered cake had higher energy intakes and gained more weight than those offered only chow. High-fat rats gained more weight than no-fat rats. ●——●, high fat; ○——○, no fat; ▲——▲, control. (Sclafani *et al.*[23] With permission from *Obesity Research.* Copyright © 1993 NAASO.)

TABLE 4. Growth of Young Rats Fed Very Low-fat Diets Containing Fat Mimetics[a]

	Control	Low-fat I	High fat	Low-fat II
Energy intake (kcal/2 rats/26 days)	3110 ± 90	3162 ± 33	3104 ± 60	2924 ± 58
Weight gain (g/2 rats/26 day)	297 ± 4[a]	328 ± 8[b]	285 ± 6[a]	322 ± 6[b]
Carcass protein (g)	51 ± 0.4[a]	54 ± 0.8[b]	51 ± 1.2[a]	54 ± 0.8[b]
Carcass fat (g)	14 ± 0.8	16 ± 0.8	14 ± 0.4	14 ± 0.8

[a] Groups of 10 young male Sprague Dawley rats were fed either the control diet (17% kcal fat), a high-fat diet (36% kcal fat), or low-fat diets containing only essential fatty acids (4% kcal) with added fat mimetics (0.3% xanthan, 5.9% cellulose, 93.8% water) to give textures similar to either the control diet (low-fat I) or the high-fat diet (low-fat II). Rats fed the low-fat diets gained as much weight as those fed either the control or high-fat diets. The low-fat diets resulted in a greater accretion of carcass protein than did the two higher-fat diets.[35]

high concentrations of amino acids or to control transport across the blood brain barrier. As mentioned previously, rodents do not indicate a preference for aspartame over water in a two-bottle preference test,[11] demonstrating a difference in organoleptic responses between rodents and humans. As with any other new food additive, initial studies investigating the metabolism of aspartame were performed in rodents, rabbits, and monkeys[37] and demonstrated that the ester was hydrolyzed in the intestine to a dipeptide that was split into free amino acids that were absorbed and metabolized in the same way as natural constituents of the diet. The effect of noncaloric sweeteners on hunger, appetite, energy intake, and body weight continue to be investigated;[38-40] however, these issues can only be addressed in clinical studies in which all of the sensory and motivational factors that impact human food intake and selection are in place.

The second type of artificial sweetener is the low-calorie, or noncaloric, bulk sweetener. Included here are the sugar alcohols, such as sorbitol (ADM, Decatur, IL); inversion sugars, such as D-Tagatose (Biospherics Inc., Beltsville, MD); and fructooligosaccharides, such as Neosugar (Meiji Seika, Japan).[41,42] These agents supply the orosensory properties of sucrose at a reduced caloric intake. Animal studies have demonstrated that bulk sweeteners provide little metabolizable energy,[43,44] and chronic pair feeding of sucrose and D-Tagatose-containing diets results in a reduced fat gain in D-Tagatose rats compared with those fed sucrose.[43] Other studies have shown that bulk sweeteners can increase intestinal bifidobacteria, which may reduce risk for colon cancer.[41,45] The beneficial effects of bulk sweeteners on energy balance and gastrointestinal health have yet to be confirmed in humans trials.

SUMMARY

Results from experiments with animal models can provide useful information relevant to human diet studies. They may indicate approximate levels of supplementation required to see an effect on the end-point measure of interest. They also allow investigation of metabolic responses that require invasive tissue sampling inappropriate for human studies. Animal studies carry the advantages of cost-effectiveness, speed, and control of potential confounding variables. However, results from animal studies cannot be directly extrapolated to clinical trials due to the absence of potential nutrient interactions, environmental stimuli, and learned food preferences and aversions that are experienced by human subjects.

REFERENCES

1. THE AMERICAN SOCIETY FOR CLINICAL NUTRITION. 1994. Dietary assessment methods. Am. J. Clin. Nutr. **59:** 1575–2665 (Suppl).
2. MCCARTER, R. J. & J. PALMER. 1992. Energy metabolism and aging: A lifelong study in Fischer 344 rats. Am. J. Physiol **263:** E448–E452.
3. LANE, M. A., A. Z. REZNICK, E. M. TILMONT, A. LANIR, S. S. BALL, V. READ, D. K. INGRAM, R. G. CUTLER & G. S. ROTH. 1995. Aging and food restriction alters some indices of bone metabolism in male rhesus monkeys *(Macaca mulatta)*. J. Nutr. **125:** 1600–1610.
4. BIRCH, L. L. 1992. Children's preferences for high-fat foods. Nutr. Rev. **50:** 249–255.
5. FULLER, R. W. & T. T. YEN. 1987. The place of animal models and animal experimentation in the study of food intake regulation and obesity in humans. Ann. N.Y. Acad. Sci. **499:** 167–178.
6. HOUPT, K. A., T. R. HOUPT & W. G. POND. 1979. The pig as a model for the study of obesity and control of food intake. A review. Yale J. Biol. Med. **52:** 307–327.
7. GALLAHER, D. D. 1992. Animal models in human nutrition research. Nutr. Clin. Practice **7:** 37–39.
8. WEINGAND, K. W. & B. P. DAGGY. 1991. Effects of dietary cholesterol and fasting on hamster plasma lipoprotein lipids. Eur. J. Clin. Chem. Clin. Biochem. **29:** 425–428.
9. BROUSSEAU, M. E., J. M. ORDOVAS, R. J. NICOLOSI & E. J. SCHAEFER. 1994. Effects of dietary fat saturation on plasma lipoprotein (a) and hepatic apolipoprotein (a) mRNA concentrations in cynomolgus monkeys. Atherosclerosis **106:** 109–118.
10. LIN, E. C., M. L. FERNANDEZ, M. A. TOSCA & D. J. MCNAMARA. 1994. Regulation of hepatic LDL metabolism in the guinea pig by dietary fat and cholesterol. J. Lipid Res. **35:** 446–457.
11. SCLAFANI, A. & M. ABRAMS. 1986. Rats show only a weak preference for the artificial sweetener aspartame. Physiol. & Behav. **37:** 253–256.
12. SURGEON GENERAL. 1988. The Surgeon General's report on Nutrition and Health. Department of Health and Human Services. Publication No. 88-50210. U.S. Government Printing Office. Washington, DC.
13. NATIONAL RESEARCH COUNCIL. 1989. Diet and Health: Implications for reducing chronic disease risk. National Academy of Science Press. Washington D.C.
14. DREWNOWSKI, A. 1990. The new fat replacements. A strategy for reducing fat consumption. Postgrad. Med. **87:** 111–121.
15. MATTSON, F. H. & G. A. NOLAN. 1972. Absorbability by rats of compounds containing from one to eight ester groups. J. Nutr. **102:** 1171–1176.
16. MATTSON, F. H., E. J. HOLLENBACH & C. M. KUEHLTHAU. 1979. The effect of a non-absorbable fat, sucrose polyester, on the metabolism of vitamin A by the rat. J. Nutr. **109:** 1688–1693.
17. MATTSON, F. H., R. J. JANACEK & M. R. WEBB. 1976. The effect of a non-absorbable lipid, sucrose polyester, on the absorption of dietary cholesterol by the rat. J. Nutr. **106:** 747–752.
18. FALLAT, R. W., C. J. GLUECK, R. LUTMER & F. H. MATTSON. 1976. Short-term study of sucrose polyester: A nonabsorbable fat-like material as a dietary agent for lowering plasma cholesterol. Am. J. Clin. Nutr. **29:** 1204–1215.

19. SLETTEN, E. G., D. HOLLANDER & V. DADUFALZA. 1985. Does the non-absorbable fat (sucrose polyester), interfere with the intestinal absorption of vitamin A? Acta Vitaminol. Enzymol. **7:** 49–53.
20. MATTSON, F. H. & R. J. JANDACEK. 1985. The effect of a non-absorbable fat on turnover of plasma cholesterol in the rat. Lipids **20:** 273–277.
21. ACKROFF, K., M. VIGORITO & A. SCLAFANI. 1990. Fat appetite in rats: The response of infant and adult rats to nutritive and non-nutritive oil emulsions. Appetite **15:** 171–188.
22. ELIZADE G. & A. SCLAFANI. 1990. Fat appetite in rats: Flavor preferences conditioned by nutritive and non-nutritive oil emulsions. Appetite **15:** 189–197.
23. SCLAFANI, A., K. WEISS, C. CARDIERI & K. ACKROFF. 1993. Feeding response of rats to no-fat and high-fat cakes. Obesity Res. **1:** 173–178.
24. MATTES, R. D. 1993. Fat preference and adherence to a reduced-fat diet. Am. J. Clin. Nutr. **57:** 373–381.
25. HARRIS, R. B. S. & W. K. JONES. 1991. Physiological response of mature rats to replacement of dietary fat with a fat substitute. J. Nutr. **121:** 1109–1116.
26. HARRIS, R. B. S. 1992. Adipocyte insulin responsiveness in female Sprague Dawley rats fed a low fat diet containing a fat mimetic carbohydrate. J. Nutr. **122:** 1802–1810.
27. HARRIS, R. B. S. & H. KOR. 1992. Insulin insensitivity is rapidly reversed in rats by reducing dietary fat from 40% to 30% of energy. J. Nutr. **122:** 1811–1822.
28. HILL, J. O., S. K. FRIED & M. DIGIROLAMO. 1983. Effects of a high fat diet on energy intake and expenditure in rats. Life Sci. **33:** 141–149.
29. HARRIS, R. B. S. 1993. The impact of high- or low-fat cafeteria foods on nutrient intake and growth of rats consuming a diet containing 30% energy as fat. Int. J. Obesity **17:** 307–315.
30. ROLLS, B. J., P. A. PIRRAGLIA, M. B. JONES & J. C. PETERS. 1992. Effects of olestra, a noncaloric fat substitute, on daily energy and fat intakes in lean men. Am. J. Clin Nutr. **56:** 84–92.
31. COTTON, J. R., J. A. WESTRATE & J. E. BLUNDELL. 1996. Replacement of dietary fat with sucrose polyester: Effects on energy intake and appetite control in nonobese males. Am. J. Clin. Nutr. **63:** 891–896.
32. GLUECK, C. J., M. M. HASTINGS, C. ALLEN, E. HOOG, L. BAEHLER, P. S. GARSIDE, D. PHILLIPS, M. JONES, E. J. HOLLENBACH, B. BRAUN & J. V. ANASTASIA. 1982. Sucrose polyester and covert caloric dilution. Am. J. Clin. Nutr. **35:** 1352–1359.
33. BIRCH, L. L., S. L. JOHNSON, M. B. JONES & J. C. PETERS. 1993. Effects of non-energy fat substitute on children's energy and macronutrient intake. Am. J. Clin. Nutr. **58:** 326–333.
34. WIDHAM, K., W. W. STARGEL, T. S. BURNS & C. TSCHANZ. 1994. Evaluation of clinical and biochemical parameters in children after consumption of microparticulated protein fat substitute (Simplesse). J. Am. Coll. Nutr. **13:** 392–396.
35. HARRIS, R. B. S. 1991. Growth measurements in Sprague Dawley rats fed diets of very low fat concentration. J. Nutr. **121:** 1075–1080.
36. REYNOLDS, W. A., V. BUTLER & N. LEMKEY-JOHNSTON. 1976. Hypothalamic morphology following ingestion of aspartame or MSG in the neonatal rodent and primate: A preliminary report. J. Toxicol. Environ. Health **2:** 471–480.
37. RANNEY, R. E., J. A. OPPERMANN, E. MULDOON & F. G. MCMAHON. 1976. Comparative metabolism of aspartame in experimental animals and humans. J. Toxicol. Environ. Health **2:** 441–451.
38. BLUNDELL, J. E. & S. M. GREEN. 1996. Effect of sucrose and sweeteners on appetite and energy intake. Int. J. Obesity **20** (Suppl 2): S12–S17.
39. DREWNOWSKI, A., C. MASSIEN, J. LOUIS-SYLVESTRE, J. FRICKER, D. CHAPELOT & M. APFELBAUM. 1994. Comparing the effects of aspartame and sucrose on motivational ratings, taste preferences, and energy intakes in humans. Am. J. Clin. Nutr. **59:** 338–345.

40. ROGERS, P. J., V. J. BURLEY, L. A. ALIKHANIZADEH & J. E. BLUNDELL. 1995. Postingestive inhibition of food intake by aspartame: Importance of interval between aspartame administration and subsequent eating. Physiol. & Behav. **57:** 489–493.
41. BORNET, F. R. J. 1994. Undigestible sugars in food products. Am. J. Clin. Nutr. **59** (Suppl): 763S–769S.
42. LEVIN, G. V., L. R. ZEHNER, J. P. SAUNDERS & J. R. BEADLE. 1995. Sugar substitutes: Their energy value, bulk characteristics, and potential health benefits. Am. J. Clin. Nutr. **62** (Suppl): 1161S–1168S.
43. LIVESEY, G. & J. C. BROWN. 1996. D-Tagatose is a bulk sweetener with zero energy determined in rats. J. Nutr. **126:** 1601–1609.
44. TOKUNAGA, T., T. OKU & N. HOYSOYA. 1986. Influence of chronic intake of new sweetener fructooligosaccharide (Neosugar) on growth and gastrointestinal function in the rat. J. Nutr. Sci. Vitaminol. **32:** 111–121.
45. KOO, M. & A. V. RAY. 1991. Long-term effects of bifidobacteria and Neosugar on precursor lesions of colonic cancer in CF1 mice. Nutr. Cancer **16:** 249–257.

Nutritional Aspects of Macronutrient-substitute Intake

JOHN C. PETERS [a]

The Procter & Gamble Company
Winton Hill Technical Center
6071 Center Hill Avenue
Cincinnati, Ohio 45224

DIET COMPOSITION AND HEALTH

Obesity has become a significant health concern in the U.S. today. The last National Health and Nutrition Examination Survey (NHANES III) found that one-third of adult Americans are now overweight, as defined by a body mass index (BMI) of over 27.8 for men and over 27.3 for women.[1] This represents a 33% increase in the incidence of overweight, compared to the health survey taken just a decade earlier—a jump that has alarmed many public health experts and that has led to obesity in America being termed an epidemic. An even stricter definition of overweight (BMI over 25) was recommended by the 1995 Dietary Guidelines for Americans. By this criteria, over half of adult Americans would be considered too heavy. The prevalence of childhood obesity has risen just as dramatically. The last national health survey also found that approximately 22% of the children ages 6-17 in the U.S. are now overweight. Unfortunately, it has been estimated that about 80% of overweight adolescents become obese adults.[2]

Excessive body weight is linked to a variety of undesirable medical conditions, including cardiovascular disease, diabetes, hypertension, cancer, stroke, osteoarthritis, and gallbladder disease. Although Americans are increasingly concerned with diet and weight control, the convenience and plenitude of palatable energy-dense foods, combined with the relatively sedentary nature of the typical American lifestyle, makes maintaining weight, for most Americans, an ongoing battle. Obesity, by nature, results from a cumulative energy imbalance in which total energy intake exceeds energy expenditure over some period of time. New food technologies, especially substitution of the major energy-contributing macronutrients, fat and carbohydrates, may be a promising strategy for limiting excess energy intake, and, thus, for preventing the development of obesity.

MACRONUTRIENT SUBSTITUTION

Macronutrient substitutes are ingredients added to food in place of the normal macronutrients to achieve a desired end, generally a reduction in energy content. The two most common types of macronutrient substitutions are carbohydrate replace-

---

[a] Tel: (513) 634-4600; fax: (513) 634-4600; e-mail: peters.jc.1@pg.com.

ment and fat replacement. Carbohydrate replacement usually aims to retain sweetness or bulk while reducing energy content. The most common sweetening carbohydrate, for example, sucrose, may be replaced by either a slightly less calorically dense sweetening carbohydrate, like fructose, or may be replaced by an intense sweetener plus a low or noncaloric bulking agent. Bulking agents basically fall into two categories: low-molecular-weight bulking agents, and complex carbohydrate polymers. Low-molecular-weight bulking agents are hydrogenated analogues of simple sugars called polyols or sugar alcohols. Sorbitol and mannitol are two of the most common. Polyols are typically used in hard candies and chewing gum. Complex carbohydrate polymers, commonly known as dietary fiber, include cellulose, pectins, and gums. These carbohydrates provide very little energy value because they are largely indigestible. They can be used in a variety of applications, including bakery products, dairy products, desserts, and frozen foods.

Replacements for the fat content of foods fall into four main categories: protein-based substitutes, carbohydrate-based substitutes, fat-based substitutes, and synthetic fat substitutes. Protein-based fat substitutes are part of a group of fat replacers that are also called fat mimetics, because microparticulation of the protein produces microscopic micelles that give the smooth mouthfeel associated with fat. These substitutes are fully digestible but highly hydrated, which significantly reduces the caloric contribution. The most common commercial example of protein-based substitutes is Simplesse (NutraSweet®), a product of milk and egg albumin that replaces, for example, 27 kcal of fat in ice cream with 4 kcal of protein. Protein-based substitutes are suitable mainly for frozen desserts and dairy products, in as much as the proteins are denatured by cooking temperatures.

Carbohydrate-based substitutes can be either caloric or noncaloric. The noncaloric substitutes are based on cellulose, seaweed, and gums, and include such substances as carrageenan, cellulose gel, guar gum, and xanthan gum. These substitutes are largely indigestible and contribute very little energy content to food in which they are included. Calorie-containing carbohydrate-based substitutes are modified forms of naturally occurring starches. These products are fat mimetics also, and because they are highly hydrated, their energy density is reduced compared to natural fat or pure carbohydrate. These carbohydrate-based substitutes include such commercial products as Amalean®, Leanmaker®, Litese®, Maltrin®, N-oil®, Oatrim®, and Staslim®. Carbohydrate-based substitutes can be used in a variety of products, including baked goods, meat products, chips, spreads, soups, and salad dressings, but cannot withstand high temperature frying.

Fat-based substitutes are true triacylglycerols, so-called "tailored triglycerides" that provide less than the traditional 9 kcal/g. Two main commercial products exist: Caprenin®, a triglyceride containing caprylic, capric, and behenic acids; and Salatrim®, a group of triglycerides containing acetic, propionic, butyric, and stearic acids. Both products have a digestible energy value of about 5 kcal/g. Caprenin is designed as a cocoa butter substitute; Salatrim is used primarily in baking and dairy products.

Synthetic fat substitutes are artificially produced molecules designed to be physically similar to fats and oils and to theoretically replace fat on a one-to-one weight basis in foods. They can be either low-calorie or noncaloric and are formulated to be heat stable. One class of low-calorie synthetic substitutes to be recently produced are the carboxy/carboxylate esters; they provide 1–3 kcal/g. Noncaloric synthetic

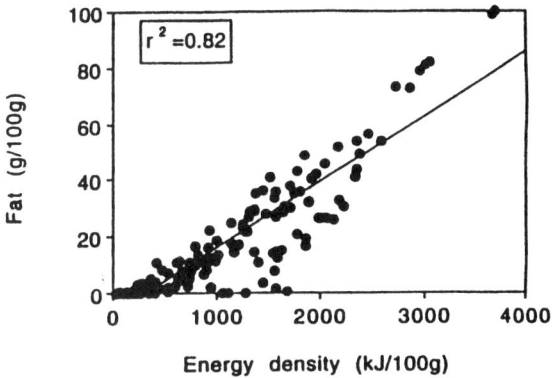

FIGURE 1. Scatter plot showing high correlation between fat content and energy density of 170 randomly chosen food items.[17] (Popitt.[17] With permission from the *International Journal of Obesity*).

substitutes developed include dialkyl dihexadecylmalonate (DDM), esterifed propoxylated glycerol (EPG), and trialkoxytricarballate (TATCS). The most widely studied synthetic substitute, however, is olestra (Olean®), a specific composition of lipids from the category of molecules referred to as sucrose polyesters. Olestra is a mixture of hexa-, hepta-, and octaesters formed from the reaction of fatty acids with sucrose. It is neither digested nor absorbed and therefore contributes no energy to the foods in which it is used. Because it is made up of naturally occurring fatty acids, its physical and sensory properties are essentially identical to regular fat. Olestra is heat stable and can thus be used in a wide range of cooked and uncooked products, including fried foods, producing foods that are virtually indistinguishable from their high-fat counterparts.

Both carbohydrate and fat replacers lower the energy content of the foods in which they are included and so have the potential to lower total energy intake and help prevent the development of obesity. Much recent research has focused on the effects of reducing dietary fat content, including the use of fat substitutes, on energy balance. The relatively greater recent interest in dietary fat manipulation may stem from the dietary guidelines that continue to emphasize fat reduction. In addition, there may be increasing recognition that replacement of dietary fat with a low-calorie or zero calorie substitute generally has a greater impact on the energy density of the food than does replacement of carbohydrate. This is because fat has the greatest energy density of the three major energy-yielding nutrients (protein, carbohydrate, and fat), and the energy density (kcal/g) of a particular food is closely tied to its fat content (see FIG. 1). In addition, a variety of studies, mainly in experimental animals, suggest that, in general, calorie for calorie, foods high in carbohydrate tend to be more satiating than foods high in fat, especially under conditions of positive energy balance. Therefore, manipulating the energy content of food by changing the carbohydrate content is more likely to lead to compensation for energy intake.[3] Conversely, high-fat foods appear to be more weakly satiating than high-carbohydrate foods under ad libitum food intake conditions, and reduction in dietary fat content has been observed to lead to reductions in both fat and energy intakes.[4–6] Based on these observations, substitution of dietary fat would appear to have greater promise for modifying macronutrient and energy intake compared to substitution of carbohydrate.

The fact that Americans eat a substantial proportion of total energy as fat (up to 37% of daily intake, on the average, compared to a recommended 30%) and that the incidence of obesity in America is steadily increasing is likely more than a coincidence. Fat intakes have resoundingly been shown to be associated with obesity, as well as with obesity's descendants: cardiovascular disease and diabetes. Laboratory studies show that animals and humans, allowed to eat ad libitum on high-fat diets, eat the same amounts of food as when allowed to eat ad libitum on low-fat diets.[7–10] Due to the fact that people tend to eat for volume and that high-fat foods are high in energy density, this leads to excess energy intake and weight gain. Numerous epidemiological studies, as well, have demonstrated that the percentage of fat in the diet correlates positively with the prevalence of obesity.[9,11–13]

Because of the potentially greater importance of dietary fat (versus carbohydrate or protein) as a permissive factor in the development of obesity, the discussion from this point on will concentrate on fat substitutes and the effects that they might have on energy balance, weight control, and obesity. To better understand the potential role that fat substitutes may play in this area, however, it is necessary to consider some aspects of the effects of diet composition on energy intake and energy expenditure.

EFFECTS OF ALTERING DIETARY MACRONUTRIENT COMPOSITION ON ENERGY BALANCE

Effect on Energy Intake

Numerous studies have shown that fat intake and energy density of the diet correlate positively with total energy intake. For example, in one two-week study a group of women were allowed to eat ad libitum, from diets having low-, medium- or high-energy density, as determined by fat content (see FIG. 2). Total energy intake and body weight changes closely mirrored the percentage of fat in the available diet. Similar results were obtained when the period of dietary manipulation was extended to 11 weeks.[14] A similar study conducted in lean young men examining covert manipulation of dietary fat under ad libitum feeding conditions also found that total energy intake was directly proportional to the percentage of fat the available diet contained.[15,16]

The tendency for people to consume excess energy on high-fat diets has been termed "passive overconsumption," a phenomenon that may be related to the palatability of high-fat foods, the tendency for people to eat relatively fixed amounts of food (even when the energy density of the food has been manipulated), and to the relatively weaker action of fat on satiety compared to carbohydrate, at least under some circumstances. High-fat foods are generally very palatable, which may serve to stimulate excessive intake in the short term (*i.e.,* within a meal). In addition, high-fat foods are generally much more energy dense than high-carbohydrate foods; thus, if individuals consume a similar volume of a high-fat food compared to a high-

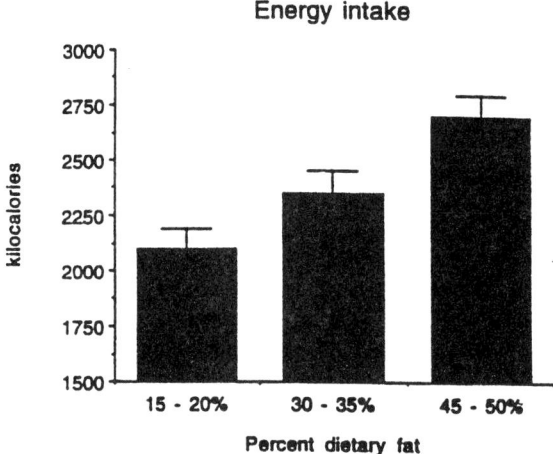

FIGURE 2. Mean daily energy intake per 14 d dietary treatment ± SEM in 24 women consuming in random order either a low-, moderate-, or high-fat diet. (Lissner et al.[4] With permission from the *American Journal of Clinical Nutrition*).

carbohydrate food (*e.g.,* consume to the same level of "fullness"), they will consume substantially more energy when eating the high-fat food.[17,18] Finally, although the data in humans are not definitive, under some conditions, high-fat foods appear to be less satiating, calorie for calorie, than foods high in protein or carbohydrate. For example, in one study, meals with a high-fat content were shown to suppress hunger less often than meals with proportionately lower fat.[19] In another study, intravenous infusion of energy as fat suppressed subsequent oral energy intake less than the same amount of energy infused as amino acids and carbohydrates.[20]

Effect on Energy Expenditure

The amount and composition of the diet consumed generally have little impact on total energy expenditure in the short term. The impact of diet composition on energy expenditure is generally seen as a secondary consequence of the effect of altering diet composition on body weight, which is the major determinant of energy expenditure in sedentary individuals. However, diet composition can have a pronounced effect on the composition of the fuel mixture burned, which in turn can provide insight into how the composition of the diet may affect the steady state body weight and body composition achieved and maintained by an individual over the longer term.

The most pronounced effect of diet composition on energy metabolism is seen under conditions of positive energy balance, whether driven by ad libitum consumption (passive overconsumption) of a high-energy (high-fat) diet or by forced overfeeding. Under these conditions it has repeatedly been observed that ingestion of dietary fat does not stimulate a greater degree of fat oxidation by the body.[15,21] For example, a

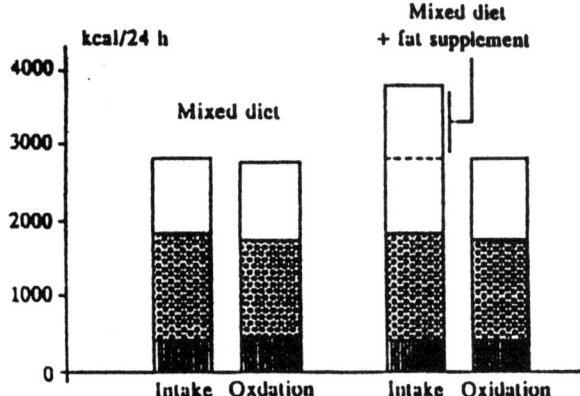

FIGURE 3. Effect of fat supplement on nutrient oxidation. The first column shows the nutrient intake, and the second shows nutrient oxidation. On the first day subjects were in energy and nutrient balance. On the second day subjects received a 106 g fat supplement above the first day. □, fat; ▨, carbohydrate; ■, protein. (Jequier.[21] With permission from Raven Press).

study by Jequier and colleagues[21] measured nutrient oxidation in several subjects on two different days. On the first day the subject consumed a mixed diet, with 15% protein, 50% carbohydrates, and 35% fat. Measurement of nutrient oxidation revealed that the subjects achieved energy balance. On the second day the diet was duplicated, except that the subjects received a large fat supplement as well. Nutrient oxidation rates were identical to the first day; essentially all of the excess fat consumed was stored (see FIG. 3).

The weak relationship between fat consumption and its oxidation is exemplified by a study that looked at individuals in a whole-body calorimeter on three different diets, composed of 20%, 40%, and 60% fat. Fat balance was determined on each diet, measured as the cumulative difference between fat intake and fat oxidation (see FIG. 4). Fat balance increased steadily with the percentage of fat in the available diet, demonstrating that fat oxidation was insufficient to offset fat intake. Fat oxidation was constant over time; excess fat consumed was not oxidized but was stored.[22]

Under these conditions of mandatory consumption or ad libitum intake, the excess ingested fat is stored during the immediate postprandial period. In order to achieve fat balance and prevent this storage from becoming permanent, the stored fat must be subsequently released from adipose tissue and oxidized. The extent to which this oxidation occurs in different individuals is important in determining the liklihood of whether or not a permanent increase in the fat mass will occur over time.

In contrast to the sluggish metabolic response to fat consumption, ingestion of either protein or carbohydrate is accompanied by a prompt increase in the oxidation of each, such that the balances of these macronutrients are generally achieved and maintained over the short term.[15,21] The reason for the different response to carbohydrate and protein may relate to the body's relatively limited storage capacity for these nutrients. There is no readily accessible storage pool for excess protein (amino acids), and the ability to efficiently store excess carbohydrate is limited. The glycogen

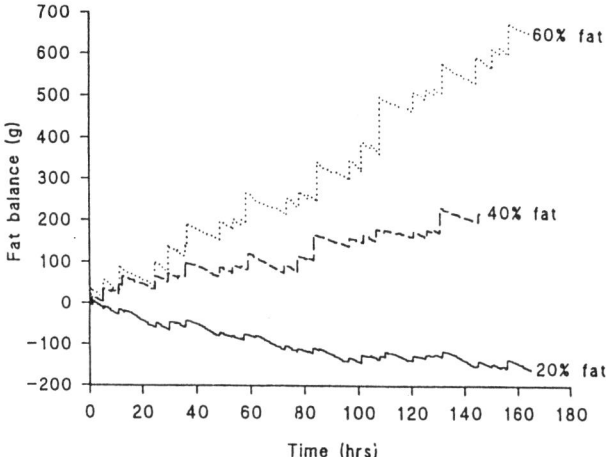

FIGURE 4. Effect of diet composition (20%, 40%, or 60% fat content) on nutrient balance. Fat balance was computed as the difference between fat intake (ascending lines) and oxidation (descending lines) calculated from respiratory gas exchange measured in a whole-body calorimeter over three 7-day periods. (Stubbs et al.[15] With permission from the *BNF Nutrition Bulletin*).

storage pool represents only about a days intake of carbohydrate. Many successive days of carbohydrate overfeeding can lead to net conversion of carbohydrate into fat, but the nutritional circumstances necessary to achieve this do not occur in most free-living humans consuming typical Western diets.

The consequences of this metabolic hierarchy of fuel oxidation (protein > carbohydrate > fat) is that excess dietary fat consumed is more likely to be stored as fat (and with greater efficiency), compared to excesses of the other macronutrients. By nature then, of the main dietary macronutrients, consumption of fat has the potential to lead to greater energy deposition and hence is more promoting towards obesity. Whether or not positive energy balance and increased fat storage occurs on a given diet then depends on the degree to which individuals "overeat" the particular diet. As was discussed earlier, foods high in fat are energy dense and are often associated with passive overconsumption. Fat may therefore be considered a permissive factor for the development of obesity.

The body's preference for fat storage seems to be enhanced in some obesity-prone individuals and in those who have lost weight. One investigator looked at 24 obese women before and after weight-reduction programs; subjects were at stable body weight and on a controlled diet providing 22% of energy as protein, 55% as carbohydrate, and 23% as fat. An examination of fuels metabolized showed that after weight loss, fat oxidation dropped significantly; a high proportion of the fat consumed was preferentially stored (see FIG. 5).[23] Similar studies by Astrup and colleagues have also demonstrated impaired fat oxidation and preferential fat storage both in individuals with a genetic predisposition for obesity and in the formerly obese.[24-26]

Considering the tendency for high-fat, energy-dense diets to stimulate excess energy intake and the relative efficiency of weight gain when excess fat is consumed,

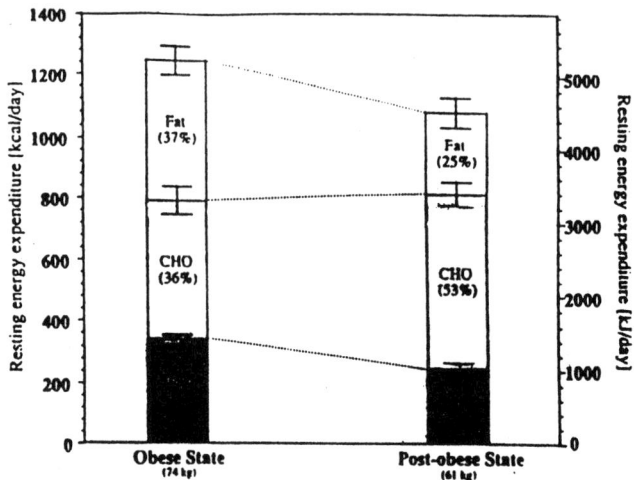

FIGURE 5. Resting energy expenditure and substrate oxidation in 24 women before (mean weight 74 kg) and after weight reduction (mean weight 61 kg), measured with subjects in a weight-stable state on a diet providing 22% of energy as protein, 55% as carbohydrate (CHO), and 23% as fat. SEM shown. (Schutz et al.[23] With permission from the *American Journal of Clinical Nutrition*).

it may not be surprising that many studies examining fat intake and weight control have found that when subjects were provided ad libitum access to food with a relatively low percentage of energy from fat, the total weight of food consumed was maintained, but total energy intake was reduced, and many of the subjects lost weight.[4-6,27-29]

In considering the overall impact of diet on energy balance, it is also necessary to understand the role of physical activity and its effects on macronutrient oxidation and total energy expenditure. Stubbs *et al.* investigated intake and expenditure in two different studies of normal-weight men. The first studied men in a whole-body calorimeter (physical activity severely restricted); the second studied men resident in a hotel suite. Subjects were fed ad libitum on low-, medium-, or high-fat diets for one week. Energy intake increased with the percentage of fat in the available diet, but intakes of the same fat content diet were identical when subjects were housed in the calorimeter or in the hotel where increased physical activity was possible. Although energy expenditure was 2.8 MJ/d higher in those housed in the hotel, subjects did not compensate for the greater energy expenditure by consuming more energy. Thus, physical activity was shown to play a pivotal role in determining the overall energy balance in all groups studied. Activity ameliorated the negative affects of the high-fat diet and promoted weight loss in the medium- and low-fat groups. Conversely, the sedentary group maintained a positive energy balance on the medium- and high-fat diets, but maintained energy balance on the low-fat diet[15,30] (see FIG. 6).[31] In sedentary individuals, therefore, diet plays a major role in determining the overall energy balance.

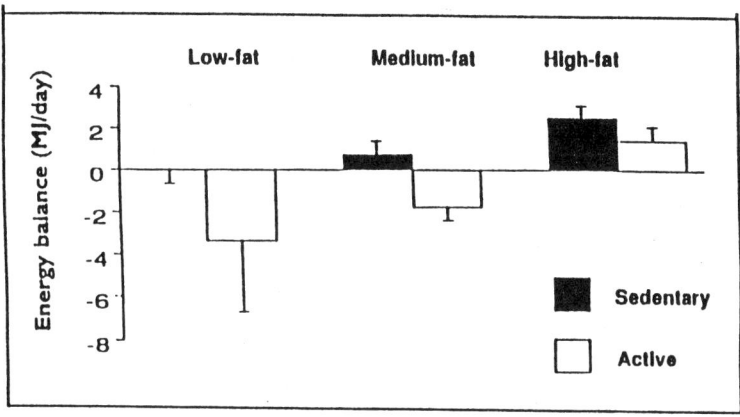

FIGURE 6. The combined effect of diet composition and physical activity in determining overall energy balance in normal-weight men feeding ad libitum. (Stubbs.[31] With permission from the *BNF Nutrition Bulletin*).

THE IMPACT OF MACRONUTRIENT SUBSTITUTES IN THE REAL WORLD

In the real world, of course, the situation gets even more complex. People do not eat controlled percentages of nutrients nor do they live in whole-body calorimeters. One's overall diet is determined by a host of factors apart from nutrient value or hunger, including appearance or aroma of food, social environment in which it is available, cultural expectations, and mood. These factors need to be addressed when considering macronutrient substitutes in food, as well as other issues specific to macronutrient substitution. That is, What nutrient is being replaced? Is it being replaced by a caloric or noncaloric substitute? and Will the substitute stimulate hunger or other compensatory intake? The specific effect of macronutrient substitution on food intake and energy balance depends on many factors, including product use and acceptance, the composition of energy intake, and the amount of physical activity. Real-life studies, however, demonstrate that adoption of low-fat diets, including the use of fat-modified foods, can be helpful in weight loss and in long-term maintenance of weight loss.[6,32,33] The data outlined briefly here provide a framework for assessing the influence of changing diet composition on energy balance and suggest a potentially beneficial role for macronutrient substitutes, especially fat substitutes, in limiting the occurrence of positive energy balance, positive fat balance, and obesity.

CONCLUSION

The results of the studies discussed suggest that with fat intakes in developed countries consistently exceeding recommended levels, replacement of fat with fat substitutes could help reduce daily fat intake. However, macronutrient substitutes are only one tool to manage energy intake and should not supplant efforts to improve eating habits and increase activity levels in our society. In a largely sedentary society, however, with convenient access to a wide and tempting array of high-fat and energy-dense foods, fat substitutes hold promise as a means to reduce passive excess-energy intake and hence reduce the incidence of positive energy balance and obesity.

REFERENCES

1. KUCZMARSKI, R. J., K. M. FLEGAL, S. M. CAMPBELL & C. L. JOHNSON. 1994. Increasing prevalence of overweight among US adults. The National Health and Nutrition Surveys 1960-1991. J. Am. Med. Assoc. **272:** 205-211.
2. KOLATA, G. 1986. Obese children: A growing problem. Science **232**(4746): 20-21.
3. FLATT, J. P. 1996. Glycogen levels and obesity. Int. J. Obesity **20**(Suppl 2): S1-S11.
4. LISSNER, L., D. A. LEVITSKY, B. J. STRUPP, H. J. KALKWARF & D. A. ROE. 1987. Dietary fat and the regulation of energy intake in human subjects. Am. J. Clin. Nutr. **46:** 886-892.
5. HILL, A. J., P. D. LEATHWOOD & J. E. BLUNDELL. 1987. Some evidence for short-term caloric compensation in normal weight human subjects: The effects of high- and low-energy meals on hunger, food preference and good intake. Hum. Nutr. Appl. Nutr. **41A:** 244-257.
6. SIGGAARD, R., A. RABEN & A. ASTRUP. 1966. Weight loss during 12 weeks' ad libitum carbohydrate-rich diet in overweight and normal-weight subjects at a Danish work site. Obesity Res. **4**(4): 347-356.
7. RABEN A. & A. ASTRUP. 1996. Manipulating carbohydrate content and sources in obesity prone subjects: Effect on energy expenditure and macronutrient balance. Int. J. Obesity **20**(Suppl. 2): S24-S30.
8. ASTRUP, A. & A. RABEN. 1995. Carbohydrate and obesity. Int. J. Obesity **19**(Suppl. 5): S27-S37.
9. WARWICK, Z. S. & S. S. SCHIFFMAN. 1992. Role of dietary fat in calorie intake and weight gain. Neurosci. Biobehav. Rev. **16:** 585-596.
10. LISSNER, L. & B. L. HEITMANN. 1995. Dietary fat and obesity: Evidence from epidemiology. Eur. J. Clin. Nutr. **49:** 79-90.
11. WESTRATE, J. A. 1995. Fat and obesity. Int. J. Obesity **19**(Suppl. 5): S38-S43.
12. ASTRUP, A., B. BUEMANN, P. WESTERN, S. TOUBRO, A. RABEN & N. J. CHRISTENSEN. 1994. Obesity as an adaptation to a high-fat diet: Evidence from a cross-sectional study. Am. J. Clin. Nutr. **59:** 350-355.
13. TURNER, L. A. & M. J. KANO. 1992. Dietary fat and body fat: A multivariate study of 205 adult females. Am. J. Clin. Nutr. **56:** 616-622.
14. KENDALL, A., D. A. LEVITSKY, B. J. STRUPP & L. LISSNER. 1991. Weight loss on a low-fat diet: Consequences of the imprecision of the control of food intake in humans. Am. J. Clin. Nutr. **53:** 1124-1129.
15. STUBBS, R. J., C. G. HARBRON, P. R. MURGATROYD & A. M. PRENTICE. 1995. Covert manipulation of dietary fat and energy density: Effect on substrate flux and food intake in men feeding ad libitum. Am. J. Clin. Nutr. **62:** 316-329.
16. STUBBS, R. J., P. RITZ, W. A. COWARD & A. M. PRENTICE. 1995. Covert manipulation of the ratio of dietary fat to energy density: Effect on food intake and energy balance in free-living men feeding ad libitum. Am. J. Clin. Nutr. **62:** 330-338.
17. POPPITT, S. D. 1995. Energy density of diets and obesity. Int. J. Obesity **19**(Suppl 5): S20-S26.
18. TREMBLAY, A., G. PLOURDE, J. P. DESPRES & C. BOUCHARD. 1989. Impact of dietary fat content and fat oxidation on energy intake in humans. Am. J. Clin. Nutr. **49:** 799-805.
19. VAN AMELSVOORT, J. M. M. 1989. Effects of varying the carbohydrate:fat ratio in a hot lunch on postprandial variables in male volunteers. Br. J. Nutr. **61:** 267-283.

20. FRIEDMAN, M. I. 1990. Body fat and the metabolic control of food intake. Int. J. Obesity **14**(Suppl 3): S3-S7.
21. JEQUIER, E. *et al.* 1992. In Energy Metabolism: Tissue Determinants and Cellular Corollaries. J. M. Kinney, & H. N. Tucker, Eds. Raven Press. New York.
22. PRENTICE, A. M. & S. D. POPPITT. 1996. Importance of energy density and macronutrients in the regulation of energy intake. Int. J. Obesity **20**(Suppl 2): S18-S23.
23. SCHUTZ, Y., A. TREMBLAY, R. L. WEINSIER & K. M. NELSON. 1992. Role of fat oxidation in the long-term stabilization of body weight in obese women. Am. J. Clin. Nutr. **55**: 670-674.
24. ASTRUP, A. 1993. Dietary composition, substrate balances and body fat in subjects with a predisposition to obesity. Int. J. Obesity **17**(Suppl. 2): 532-536.
25. ASTRUP, A., B. BUEMANN, N. J. CHRISTENSEN & S. TOURBRO. 1994. Failure to increase lipid oxidation in response to increasing dietary fat content in formerly obese women. Am. J. Physiol. **266**: E592-E599.
26. RABEN, A., H. B. ANDERSEN, N. J. CHRISTENSEN, J. MADSEN, J. J. HOLST & A. ASTRUP. 1994. Evidence for an abnormal postprandial response to a high-fat meal in women predisposed to obesity. Am. J. Physiol. **267**: E549-E559.
27. DUNCAN, K. H., J. A. BACON & R. L. WEINSIER. 1983. The effects of high and low energy density diets on satiety, energy intake, and eating time of obese and nonobese subjects. Am. J. Clin. Nutr. **37**: 763-767.
28. SHEPPARD, L., A. R. KRISTAL & L. H. KUSHI. 1991. Weight loss in women participating in a randomized trial of low-fat diets. Am. J. Clin. Nutr. **54**: 821-828.
29. PREWITT, T. E., D. SCHMEISSER, P. E. BOWEN, P. AYE, T. A. DOLOCEK, P. LANGENBERG, T. COLE & L. BRACE. 1991. Am. J. Clin. Nutr. **54**: 304-310.
30. STUBBS, R. J., P. R. MURGATROYD, G. R. GOLDBERG & A. M. PRENTICE. 1993. Carbohydrate balance and the regulation of day-to-day food intake in humans. Am. J. Clin. Nutr. **57**: 897-903.
31. STUBBS, R. J. 1994. Macronutrients, appetite and energy balance in humans: Human appetite regulation—a multidisciplinary challenge. British Nutrition Foundation. Nutr. Bull. **19**(Suppl): 53-68.
32. KRISTAL, A. R., E. WHITE, A. L. SHATTUCK, S. CURRY, G. L. ANDERSON, A. FOWLER & N. URBAN. 1992. Long-term maintenance of a low-fat diet: Durability of fat-related dietary habits in the Women's Health Trial. J. Am. Diet Assoc. **92**: 553-559.
33. URBAN, N., E. WHITE, G. L. ANDERSON, S. CURRY & A. R. KRISTAL. 1992. Correlates of maintenance of a low-fat diet among women in the Women's Health Trial. Prev. Med. **21**: 279-291.

Fat and Sugar Substitutes and the Control of Food Intake[a]

BARBARA J. ROLLS [b]

Nutrition Department
226 Henderson Building
The Pennsylvania State University
University Park, Pennsylvania 16802-6501

In this review we will consider how sugar and fat substitutes influence appetite, hunger and satiety, food and nutrient intakes, and body weight. We will limit the discussion to laboratory-based studies that examine effects of macronutrient substitutes in adults (comprehensive reviews of this topic are available[1-6]). This approach is reductionist in that the goal is usually to isolate and manipulate one variable and then to characterize the influence of that variable on food-intake behaviors. Many of the studies have concentrated on the biological effects of macronutrient substitutes, and thus have covertly manipulated foods. To examine how these biological effects interact with beliefs about the nutrient or energy content of foods, other studies have overtly used macronutrient substitutes. The goal of some investigations has been to determine the influence of the sensory properties of macronutrient substitutes, that is, the sweet or fatty taste. This review of the effects of sugar and fat substitutes is divided into three sections: effects on satiety, effects on satiation, and long-term effects.

EFFECTS OF MACRONUTRIENT SUBSTITUTES ON SATIETY

Satiety refers to the effects of a food or meal after eating has ended. A technique for studying satiety is to administer a fixed amount of a given food or nutrient as a preload and, after a predetermined delay, measure the effects on subsequent food intake (the test meal).[7] The aim of a preloading study is to determine whether intake in the test meal is varied in relation to the calories in the preload. That is, is there caloric compensation? As indicators of satiety, ratings of subjective sensations, such as hunger and fullness, are usually made before and after the preload and in the interval before the test meal. Although subjective ratings provide a useful indicator of what the test subjects are experiencing, they do not always accurately predict subsequent food intake.

The influence of a preload on subsequent food intake depends upon a number of variables that often differ between studies, such as macronutrient composition or caloric content of the preloads and subject characteristics. For example, we have conducted a series of studies in which the carbohydrate and fat content of yogurt

---

[a] This work was supported by NIDDK Grants DK39177 and DK50156.
[b] Tel: (814) 863-8572; fax: (814) 863-8574; e-mail: BJR4@PSU.edu.

were varied through the incorporation of sugar or fat substitutes. We found that caloric compensation following the yogurt was influenced by the interval between the preload and test meal[8] and by the characteristics of the study participants. For example, older men,[9] as well as obese individuals and those concerned with their body weight,[10] showed less accurate caloric compensation than younger participants of normal weight. It is important to note that variables such as these could account for differences between studies. Attempts to apply the results of a particular study to broad generalizations about the effects of sugar and fat substitutes may be inappropriate.

Sugar Substitutes

Intense sweeteners, such as aspartame, saccharin, and acesulfame-K, provide sweet tastes that are inherently pleasant and that can improve the palatability of a variety of foods. Sweetness can therefore affect the appetite for or desire to eat particular foods. Before the introduction of intense sweeteners, the sweet taste was invariably provided by sugars and therefore was associated with the ingestion of energy. Consumption of energy in the form of carbohydrates, such as sugar, would usually be associated with a reduction in hunger, increased satiety, and a suppression of further intake. Through experience, individuals can learn that particular foods are associated with these changed sensations.[11,12] A key question in recent debates about the actions of intense sweeteners has been what happens to hunger, satiety, and food intake when the sweet taste is dissociated from the ingestion of energy.

In preloading studies using intense sweeteners, two different designs can be used. In one, an intense sweetener is substituted for sucrose so that the foods or drinks are equally sweet but have different calorie levels. The advantage of this design is that it is similar to the situation in which many consumers might use sweeteners. However, it has been argued that this design obscures any effects of sweetness on intake because of the caloric differences.[13] The effect of sweetness per se can be studied in a design that employs isocaloric foods or drinks that are either sweet or not. Of course, this design is potentially confounded by differences in palatability between the test foods or drinks.

There have been a number of studies in which the sweeteners in flavored drinks have been manipulated covertly in order to study both the effects of sweetness and manipulation of calories. We conducted a study comparing the effects of water and of aspartame- and sucrose-sweetened lemonades on hunger ratings and food intake.[14] The subjects, who were normal weight, nondieting males, consumed 8 or 16 ounces of aspartame- or sucrose-sweetened lemonade, plain water, or no drink, either with a self-selection lunch, or 30 or 60 minutes before the lunch. When drinks were taken with the meal, more overall calories (lunch plus the drink) were consumed when subjects received the sucrose-sweetened lemonade. This trend remained when the drinks were consumed 30 and 60 minutes before the meal, but it was not statistically significant. In all of the conditions, calories from the food consumed at lunch remained relatively constant so that the additional calories from the sucrose-sweetened drinks increased total energy intake. Hunger ratings were similar following the different drinks.

Studies from a number of other laboratories have confirmed that flavored drinks sweetened with aspartame or saccharin have effects similar to water consumption on hunger and food intake.[15-17] Furthermore, preceding or accompanying a meal with a noncaloric drink was associated with a reduction in total energy intake (drink plus meal) compared to consumption of a sugar-sweetened drink. However, one laboratory has reported different results, in that unflavored solutions of aspartame, saccharin, or acesulfame-K increased hunger ratings compared with water, but there was no increase in food intake following consumption.[18] Although this study lead to the suggestion that consumption of intense sweeteners can lead to a loss of control over appetite and increased food intake because of the dissociation of the sweet taste from ingestion of calories,[19] this claim has not been supported by experimental evidence from the other laboratories investigating the effects of sugar substitutes in drinks. In addition, well-controlled studies in which intense sweeteners were incorporated into foods reinforce this conclusion.

In some studies, in order to determine whether the sweet taste per se can influence food intake, calories in a preload were held constant, and the level of sweetness was varied by the addition of an intense sweetener. For example, Mattes[20] compared isocaloric breakfasts of unsweetened cereal, or cereal sweetened with either sugar or aspartame on subsequent hunger and food intake. Again in this study it was found that there were no significant differences in hunger ratings, in intake of the next meal, or in total daily intake. The breakfasts were tested both in subjects who knew and those who did not know the type of sweetener used. Although informing the subjects about the sweetener did not significantly affect intakes, there was a nonsignificant trend for the subjects who knew they had consumed aspartame to eat more during the rest of the day, perhaps because they mistakenly believed that aspartame-sweetened cereal had fewer calories. It should be noted that in two separate studies, one with food[21] and one with drinks (unpublished), we have failed to find an effect of informing the subjects about the sweetener content on subsequent intake. Nevertheless, it is possible, that the value of intense sweeteners in weight management will depend on the responses to the expected energy savings they provide.

A thorough study by Drewnowski and colleagues[22] has controlled for effects of both sweetness and calories by employing four test conditions. The food used in the preloads was fromage blanc (a creamy white cheese). Because this cheese is consumed both sweetened and unsweetened in France where the study was conducted, maintaining palatability of the unsweetened cheese was not a problem. The four versions of this test food were (A) sugar-sweetened, 700 kcal; (B) aspartame-sweetened with maltodextrin, 700 kcal; (C) aspartame-sweetened, 300 kcal; and (D) unsweetened, 300 kcal. Twenty-four normal-weight young men and women consumed the test foods at breakfast, and the effects on hunger ratings and intakes at the meals over the rest of the day were determined. The results showed that intake over the rest of the day was similar following all of these breakfasts. Therefore, a comparison of conditions C and D, the isocaloric sweet and unsweetened cheese, indicated that the sweetness per se did not influence hunger ratings or food intake. Also, the effects of sugar and aspartame in isocaloric test meals did not differ, in that intakes and hunger ratings following conditions A and B were similar. Despite the relatively large caloric difference between conditions, there was no significant caloric compensation over the day following the test breakfasts. Thus, consumption of the lower calorie breakfasts (C and D) was associated with a significant decrease in daily energy intake. This lack of compensation was confirmed in a similar study conducted in 12 lean and 12 obese women.[23]

These short-term studies indicate clearly that intense sweeteners in foods or drinks do not cause paradoxical increases in subsequent food intake; indeed in some studies sugar substitutes were associated with a decrease in energy intake. The issue of whether sweetener use is associated with a reduction in energy intake will be discussed further when we consider longer-term studies.

Fat Substitutes

Researchers have shown that taste is the primary determinant of the foods we choose to eat. Fats contribute heavily to the richness of food flavor and overall palatability of foods, and therefore foods high in fat are often selected and preferred. However, to reduce the risk of diseases associated with high-fat consumption, we are being urged to reduce fat intake. In response to consumer demand for reduced-fat products that are still high in taste, a number of fat substitutes have been developed and incorporated into a variety of foods. As with sugar substitutes, it is important to assess the impact that these fat substitutes will have on hunger, satiety, and food intake.

The fat substitute most often used in studies of human food intake is olestra, a sucrose polyester (SPE), because it can readily replace dietary fat, gram-for-gram, while providing no calories but similar sensory properties. Preloading studies have tested whether olestra consumption is associated with reductions in energy intake and changes in macronutrient composition.

The first studies on the effects of olestra on satiety were conducted simultaneously in the United States[24] and the United Kingdom.[25] At each site, olestra was used covertly to replace 20 or 36 g of fat at a compulsory breakfast in 24 lean, nondieting young male subjects. When intakes at lunch, dinner, and the evening snack were analyzed, the data showed that the consumption of olestra did not affect daily energy intake; that is, subjects compensated for the reduction in calories associated with the olestra. However, subjects did not eat more fat to compensate for the reduction in calories from fat. The substitution led to a significant dose-dependent reduction in daily fat intake and a reciprocal increase in carbohydrate intake. There were no systematic differences in ratings of hunger or fullness between conditions.

Several laboratories in Europe have recently reported on the effects of incorporation of a different form of SPE on food intake. This SPE is also calorie free but is more liquid at body temperature than the form used in the United States. Unless direct comparisons are made we cannot assume that different forms of fat substitutes have the same effects. In a study from the Netherlands,[26] SPE was incorporated into croissants, and the effects on subsequent intake were determined after different intervals between the preload and the test meal. At all intervals the subjects showed incomplete compensation for the calorie reduction associated with SPE, so that there was an overall decrease in energy intake. However, no compensation was seen for the reduction in fat intake, so that the daily proportion of calories consumed as fat was reduced.

In another study conducted in the United Kingdom,[27] the incorporation of SPE in either meals or snacks across the day was associated with a decrease in energy intake on that day, and compensation was not seen through the next day. As in all other studies, SPE was associated with a reduction in calories from fat. This same laboratory has, however, also reported that caloric compensation can occur following SPE consumption.[28] In another study, they used SPE to reduce fat intake well below habitual levels (down from 32% to 20% of calories) and found that subjects compensated for 74% of the caloric reduction associated with the SPE. They hypothesize that whereas reductions in fat intake within the normal range of consumption (*i.e.*, from 40% down to 30% of calories) may lead to reductions in fat and energy intake, restriction of fat intake below normal levels may be associated with caloric compensation, so that there will be no decrease in energy intake.

The substitution of olestra for fat was associated consistently with a reduction in the percentage of calories from fat. However, more studies are needed to clarify the effects of fat substitutes on energy intake. The available data indicate that in some circumstances SPE may be associated with a reduction in energy intake; but this may not always occur. The reasons for these different results are not understood, but could relate to differences in subject characteristics, or the magnitude or timing of the fat manipulation. Although the effects of SPE on energy intake may be variable, the availability of fat substitutes in food is likely to aid in the reduction of fat intake if reduced-fat foods are chosen instead of the full-fat versions of the same foods.

An issue not yet discussed is whether the sensory properties imparted by fat substitutes could interfere with energy intake regulation when low-fat foods are consumed. That is, if a low-energy, low-fat food has the taste and texture of a high-fat food, will some people compensate for the food as if it were high in fat and energy? This question follows from evidence that humans can make physiologic associations between the sensory cues provided by a food and its energy content.[11,12] The use of an energy-free fat substitute, like olestra, could potentially alter this regulatory process. A study conducted in our laboratory tested this hypothesis. Soups were developed in three versions: fat-free, fat-free plus olestra (33 g olestra), and high-fat (33 g of fat).[29] The olestra soup had the nutrient composition of the fat-free soup, but the sensory properties (thickness, creaminess) of the high-fat soup. Lean or obese men and women consumed either no preload or a fixed amount of one of the soups before lunch. Intake over the rest of the day was similar following all three soups. The subjects compensated completely for the energy in the fat-free and olestra soups, in that total intake (soup plus lunch) was equivalent to intake in the no preload condition. However, total intake was significantly greater when the high-fat soup was consumed than in the other conditions (Fig. 1). Because there were no differences in the response to the two low-fat conditions, one with the taste of fat and one without, it appears that the sensory properties of fat alone, that is, apart from the physiological effects of fat, do not disturb energy intake regulation.

Most of the research discussed thus far has focused on the physiologic effects of fat reduction, but cognitive factors also play an important role in determining food intake. Today, people are constantly bombarded with information about the fat content of foods, and they may assume that a low-fat food is also lower in calories. However, some low-fat products, such as yogurt and cake, may contain more energy in a given portion than the full-fat versions. In order to test the hypothesis that the perceived

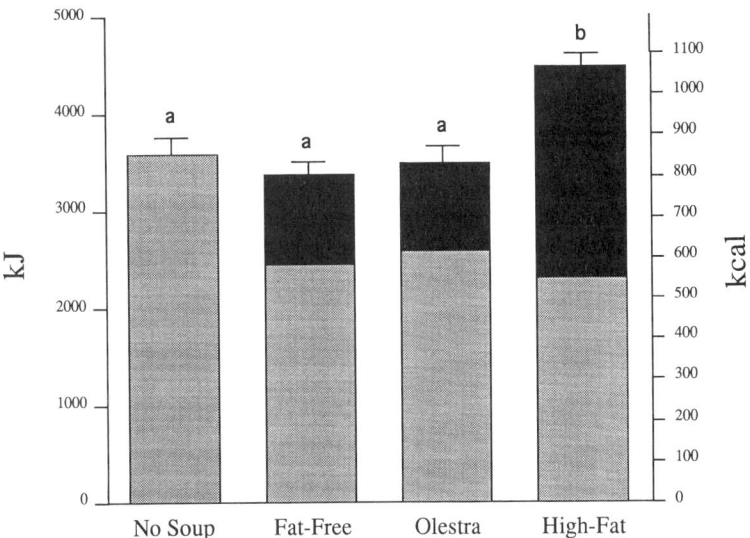

FIGURE 1. Mean energy (± SEM) intake at lunch following preloads of soup made with regular fat, no fat, or with olestra as a replacement for fat. Means with different letters are significantly different. ■, soup; ▨, test lunch.

fat content of a preload affects subsequent food intake, normal-weight, nondieting women were given preloads of three different yogurts (low-fat/low-calorie; low-fat/high-calorie; high-fat/high-calorie), or no yogurt, followed by lunch and dinner.[30] The fat reduction in this study was achieved by adding gums and emulsifiers to the yogurt. Half of the subjects received, in the form of a label, accurate information concerning the fat content of the yogurts, but were not told the energy content; the other half received no information. Subjects informed of the fat content consumed significantly more calories following the preload labeled "low-fat" than after the *isocaloric* preload labeled "high-fat." The opposite response was seen in the condition in which subjects were not given information about the content of the yogurts; subjects ate more following the high-fat/high-calorie yogurt than after the low-fat/high-calorie preload. Overall intake was still significantly higher in the informed low-fat condition when energy consumed at dinner was included in the analyses, implying that the effect of the low-fat label persisted over the rest of the day. These results suggest that the low-fat label may have given the women license to eat more during the rest of the day, perhaps because they perceived the low-fat message to be synonymous with low-energy content.

EFFECTS OF MACRONUTRIENT SUBSTITUTES ON SATIATION

Most of the studies on macronutrient substitutes have required subjects to eat a fixed amount of the manipulated food items. In two studies, we have offered subjects free access to foods incorporating either a sugar or a fat substitute to determine whether satiation, or the amount consumed in a meal, is affected by a reduction in the energy density of foods. Inasmuch as palatability could affect food intake, the regular and substituted versions of foods were shown to be similar in palatability.

Sugar Substitutes

We examined the effects of consumption of commercially available foods sweetened with either sucrose or aspartame on appetite ratings and food intake.[21] Normal-weight, nondieting males and females, given large portions of either a high- or low-calorie pudding or jello, were instructed to eat as much as they liked. Because all subjects ate similar weights of the different caloric versions of each food, energy intake differed significantly between conditions. Ratings of hunger and fullness were affected similarly by consumption of the foods with the different sweeteners. Information about the caloric content of the foods did not influence intake or appetite, in that both informed and uninformed subjects responded similarly in the tests.

Fat Substitutes

To determine how changes in the fat content of foods affect satiation, we offered snacks of regular or fat-free potato chips. Habitual consumers of potato chips (lean and obese men and women) were given free access to either regular potato chips (5.3 kcal/g, 60% energy from fat) or chips made with olestra (2.8 kcal/g, 0% fat).[31,32] The palatability of the chips did not differ. Participants came to the laboratory every afternoon for 10 successive weekdays to eat one type of chip. All participants were tested with both types of chips, but 50 subjects were given information about the energy and fat content of the chips and 46 subjects were not. When no nutritional information was given, the subjects had to rely on physiological cues if they were to adjust intake in relation to calorie content. We found that all subjects ate similar amounts of both the no-fat and regular chips over the 10-day period (FIG. 2), indicating that they were not responsive to caloric differences. Because of the fat and calorie reduction in the olestra chips, all participants ate less fat and fewer calories in the snack when eating the olestra chips than when eating the regular chips. The results were similar when participants were given nutritional information about the chips (FIG. 2), in that amounts consumed of both types of chips were similar. However, some individuals who were concerned about their body weight ate significantly more (10 g) of the no-fat chips. Because the no-fat chips contained only half the calories of the regular chips, this slight increase in amount consumed did not negate the reductions in fat and energy intakes.

In these studies of satiation, when offered two equally palatable foods, the strategy that subjects employed was to eat the same amount in grams regardless of the energy content of the foods. This implies that, at least in the short term, the energy density (calories per gram) was the most important determinant of energy intake. Even knowing the caloric content of the foods, or repeatedly eating them for 10 days, did not alter this strategy of eating a particular portion size. Thus, energy intake decreased

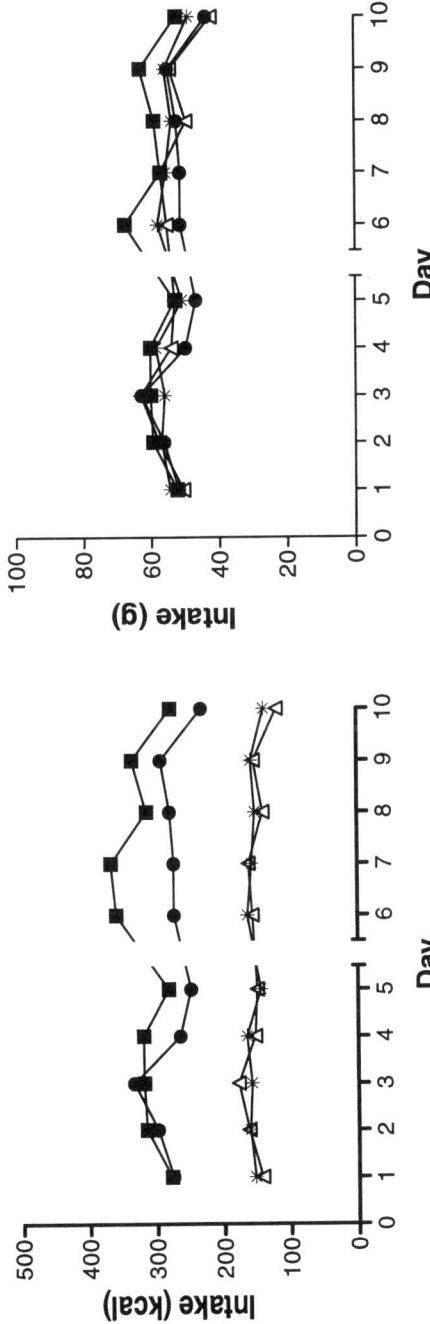

FIGURE 2. Left: Intake of potato chips (kcal) offered as a snack for 10 days. Caloric intake was significantly higher with the regular chips than with the no-fat chips, because, as shown on the right, the amount consumed (g) did not differ between conditions or over time. ■——, regular/no information; ●——, regular/information; ✳——, olestra/no information; △——, olestra/information.

when the caloric content of the foods was reduced through the use of macronutrient substitutes.

EFFECTS OF LONG-TERM USE OF MACRONUTRIENT SUBSTITUTES

Although manipulations of the energy density, or the sugar or fat content of single foods or meals shed light on the short-term controls of food intake, long-term studies of caloric manipulations over days or weeks are required to determine whether the use of intense sweeteners or fat substitutes is associated with persistent alterations in food or nutrient intakes.

Sugar Substitutes

There have been several studies in which aspartame replaced sugar throughout the day over a number of days. Porikos and colleagues studied both normal weight and obese individuals who were confined to a hospital room for the duration of the study.[33] Subjects were not told that food intake was being measured and that the caloric content of the foods and drinks was being manipulated. Foods were served from platters with large portions available, and subjects were encouraged to consume sweet drinks (they were required to drink at least two sodas a day). In these studies hospitalized obese and lean subjects ate fewer calories during a 6- or 12-day period when all sucrose was covertly replaced with aspartame, compared to their intake on a high-sucrose diet (first 6 days of study, which represented baseline). After 4-6 days of dilution, subjects compensated for 40% of the missing calories; however, total caloric intake remained significantly below baseline levels (approximately 15%) during the rest of the dilution period. When, at the end of the study, sucrose was again consumed, energy intake increased to the level eaten in the baseline period. Porikos and colleagues suggest that aspartame may have some efficacy in weight control. This conclusion is supported by data from a controlled clinical trial that showed that aspartame use was associated with increased weight loss and satisfaction with the diet, and better long-term maintenance of reduced body weight.[34]

The types of drinks consumed could also have an impact on total energy intake and body weight. Tordoff and Alleva[35] compared the effects of consumption of sodas sweetened with high-fructose corn syrup or aspartame. Over three successive three-week periods, subjects received daily, 40 ounces of aspartame-sweetened soda, 40 ounces of high-fructose corn syrup-sweetened soda, or no soda in a counterbalanced order. Consumption of the high-fructose corn syrup-sweetened soda was associated with higher daily caloric intakes and significantly higher weight gains than in the other conditions. Consumption of the aspartame-containing soda decreased daily caloric intake in both sexes compared with the no-drink condition and was associated with decreased body weight in the males and no change in weight in the females. One of the most interesting findings in this study was that consumption of both types of sweet drinks was associated with a reduction in intake of refined sugar from other sources. This suggests that sweetness does not maintain and promote the consumption of sweet foods. On the contrary, as has been suggested by theories of both alliesthesia[36] and sensory-specific satiety,[37] consumption of sweet foods or drinks decreases the consumption of other sweet foods and drinks. Although these data imply that aspartame may be of some benefit in weight control, the authors are cautious about extrapolating their findings too broadly. Their study involved the covert substitution of aspartame for large volumes of high-fructose corn syrup-sweetened soda. Clearly, more naturalistic studies in which normal quantities of diet foods or drinks are knowingly substituted for sugar-sweetened products are required.

Fat Substitutes

Although there have been a number of studies comparing the effects of low- and high-fat diets on weight loss,[38] there are few data on the long-term effects of fat substitutes. The relevant studies have examined the effects of incorporation of olestra into diets for up to 20 days. In the first study,[39] conducted in 1982, an early version of SPE was incorporated into hypocaloric weight-loss diets in obese persons. In one 20-day period an average of 60 g of SPE was incorporated into various foods daily, whereas during the other 20-day period only foods made with regular fat were offered. Neither caloric nor fat-specific compensation was seen over the test period with olestra, so there was a significant reduction in energy and fat intakes. The participants lost weight in both conditions inasmuch as they were asked to diet during both phases of the protocol; however, they did lose significantly more weight when consuming SPE. Although the results of this study indicate that SPE may be useful in limiting energy and fat intakes, and may be useful for weight loss, the results should be interpreted with caution. Subjects were given only a limited opportunity to make up missing calories in that they were only offered free access to foods without SPE in the evening.

More recently, the effects of incorporating various levels of olestra into diets for two-week periods have been examined at three different sites. In a study carried out in the Netherlands[40] using the more liquid form of SPE, fat in the dinner meal was replaced with SPE (52 g) in normal-weight men and women. Half the participants were told about the use of the fat replacer and half were not told. The SPE and the regular fat conditions each lasted for 12 days. Both energy intake and the proportion of fat in the diet were reduced by the incorporation of SPE into the diet. Informing the subjects of the manipulation had little effect on the results. The authors conclude that the use of SPE helps in reducing fat and energy intake in normal-weight people; however, the study was not long enough to adequately assess effects on body weight.

In the two other studies that investigated the longer-term use of olestra, reductions in both energy and fat intakes were also reported. In one,[41] the covert substitution of a third of the dietary fat with olestra in six men over a 12-day period was associated with compensation for only 35% of the caloric reduction. In the other study,[42,43] which consisted of two 14-day periods, olestra covertly replaced approximately 20-35 g of fat for an 8% reduction in daily energy intake. Both energy and fat intakes were significantly reduced in the olestra condition in the 53 obese and lean men and women tested.

Thus, in four separate studies in which olestra was incorporated into the diet over a period of 12 to 20 days, the data consistently showed a reduction in both fat and energy intakes associated with consumption of the fat substitute. Two of the studies determined whether caloric compensation improved as a function of the number of days on the reduced-fat diet and found no change with time.[40,43] Although these studies suggest that fat substitutes could aid weight loss, longer studies are required to determine whether, as the energy deficit accumulates, compensation will occur.

CONCLUSIONS

In this chapter we have considered data from laboratory-based studies on the effects of sugar and fat substitutes on food intake. Such new food technologies provide excellent tools for the investigation of basic mechanisms underlying human ingestive behavior. For example, in some situations caloric compensation for covert reductions in the energy content of foods has been demonstrated; however, in a number of studies in which fat or sugar substitutes were incorporated into a single food or a number of meals for several days, there was a significant reduction in energy intake. In a number of studies, it has been shown that when given free access to a particular type of food, subjects eat a constant weight of food regardless of the energy content. This indicates that energy density, or the calories in a given weight of food, will be a major determinant of energy intake. These data imply that if macronutrient substitutes are used to reduce the caloric density of foods, they could provide a useful addition to diet therapies for weight management. Furthermore, the availability of low-calorie foods that are palatable may aid in compliance to diets by increasing food choices. Fat and sugar substitutes may also help to shift the nutrient composition of the diet to one with lower proportions of fat or sugar. None of the studies conducted in the laboratory have shown that more sugar or fat is consumed to compensate for changes in the nutrient composition of the diet associated with consumption of macronutrient substitutes.

However, more research in needed to determine how individuals incorporate macronutrient substitutes into their diets. Research shows that in some situations the consumption of foods using macronutrient substitutes, particularly those labeled low fat, may be used as an excuse to eat more of other foods. Consumers may assume that macronutrient substitutes are always associated with a reduction in the calorie content of foods, although some foods are of equivalent energy density. The key to the use of macronutrient substitutes is likely to depend upon the motivation of the consumer to bring about dietary change and to incorporate new food technologies into a balanced and varied diet.

Future studies should continue to explore how macronutrient substitutes affect food and nutrient intakes and body weight. For example, more information is needed about the effects of different types of sugar and fat substitutes and about combinations of these in foods and drinks. Laboratory-based studies should also clarify why caloric compensation is sometimes seen following consumption of sugar or fat substitutes and what characteristics of the consumers predict this behavior. Other critical issues are whether the amounts of the substitutes ingested and the timing of this consumption affect energy and nutrient intakes. Long-term studies are needed to assess whether over time, as the energy deficit associated with macronutrient substitute intake accumulates, compensation will occur and thereby negate effects on body weight. However, even if such physiological compensatory mechanisms are engaged, foods with macronutrient substitutes can be effectively used for weight management if they are reduced in calories, consumed as direct replacements for the regular version of the food, not used as an excuse to eat more of other foods, and incorporated into a healthy long-term diet and exercise program.

REFERENCES

1. Anderson, H. G. 1995. Sugars, sweetness, and food intake. Am. J. Clin. Nutr. **62:** 195S–202S.
2. Drewnowski, A. 1995. Intense sweeteners and the control of appetite. Nutr. Rev. **53:** 1–7.
3. Miller, D. L. & B. J. Rolls. 1996. Implications of fat reduction in the diet. *In* Handbook of Fat Replacers. S. Roller & S. A. Jones, Eds.: 27–44. CRC Press. Boca Raton, FL.
4. Rolls, B. J. 1991. Effects of intense sweeteners on hunger, food intake and body weight: A review. Am. J. Clin. Nutr. **53:** 872–878.
5. Rolls, B. J. 1996. Role of fat substitutes in obesity prevention and treatment. *In* Progress in Obesity Research: 7. A. Angel, H. Anderson, C. Bouchard, D. Lau, L. Leiter & R. Mendelson, Eds.: 459–464.: John Libbey & Company LTD./7th International Congress on Obesity. London, England.
6. Rolls, B. J. & D. J. Shide. 1996. Evaluation of hunger, food intake, and body weight. *In* Clinical Evaluation of a Food Additive: Assessment of Aspartame. C. Tschanz, H. H. Butchko, W. Stargel & F. N. Kotsonis, Eds.: 275–287. CRC Press. Boca Raton, FL.
7. Rolls, B. J. & V. A. Hammer. 1995. Fat, carbohydrate and the regulation of energy intake. Am. J. Clin. Nutr. **62:** 1086–1095S.
8. Rolls, B. J., S. Kim, A. L. McNelis, M. W. Fischman, R. W. Foltin & T. Moran. 1991. Time course of effects of preloads high in fat or carbohydrate on food intake and hunger ratings in humans. Am. J. Physiol. **260:** R756–R763.
9. Rolls, B. J., K. A. Dimeo & D. J. Shide. 1995. Age-related impairments in the regulation of food intake. Am. J. Clin. Nutr. **62:** 923–931.
10. Rolls, B. J., S. Kim-Harris, M. W. Fischman, R. W. Foltin, T. H. Moran & S. A. Stoner. 1994. Satiety after preloads with different levels of fat and carbohydrate: Implications for obesity. Am. J. Clin. Nutr. **60:** 476–487.
11. Booth, D. A., P. Mather & J. Fuller. 1982. Starch content of ordinary foods associatively conditions human appetite and satiation, indexed by intake and eating pleasantness of starch-paired flavours. Appetite **3:** 163–184.
12. Birch, L. L., L. McPhee, L. Steinberg & S. Sullivan. 1989. Conditioned flavor preferences in young children. Physiol. & Behav. **47:** 501–505.
13. Blundell, J. E., P. J. Rogers & A. J. Hill. 1988. Uncoupling sweetness and calories: Methodological aspects of laboratory studies on appetite control. Appetite **11** (Suppl. 1): 54–61.
14. Rolls, B. J., S. Kim & I. C. Fedoroff. 1990. Effects of drinks sweetened with sucrose or aspartame on hunger, thirst and food intake in men. Physiol. & Behav. **48:** 19–26.
15. Rodin, J. 1990. Comparative effects of fructose, aspartame, glucose, and water preloads on calorie and macronutrient intake. Am. J. Clin. Nutr. **51:** 428–435.
16. Black, R. M., P. Tanaka, L. A. Leiter & H. G. Anderson. 1991. Soft drinks with aspartame: Effect on subjective hunger, food selection, and food intake of young adult males. Physiol. & Behav. **49:** 803–810.
17. Canty, D. J. & M. M. Chan. 1991. Effects of consumption of caloric vs. noncaloric sweet drinks on indices of hunger and food consumption in normal adults. Am. J. Clin. Nutr. **53:** 1159–1164.
18. Rogers, P. J., J. Carlyle, A. J. Hill & J. E. Blundell. 1988. Uncoupling sweet taste and calories: Comparison of the effects of glucose and three intense sweeteners on hunger and food intake. Physiol. & Behav. **43:** 547–552.

19. BLUNDELL, J. & A. J. HILL. 1986. Paradoxical effects of an intense sweetener (aspartame) on appetite. Lancet **1:** 1092-1093.
20. MATTES, R. 1990. Effects of aspartame and sucrose on hunger and energy intake in humans. Physiol. & Behav. **47:** 1037-1044.
21. ROLLS, B. J., L. J. LASTER & A. SUMMERFELT. 1989. Hunger and food intake following consumption of low-calorie foods. Appetite **13:** 115-127.
22. DREWNOWSKI, A., C. MASSIEN, J. LOUIS-SYLVESTRE, J. FRICKER, D. CHAPELOT & M. APFELBAUM. 1994. Comparing the effects of aspartame and sucrose on hunger ratings, taste preferences and energy intakes in humans. Am. J. Clin. Nutr. **59:** 338-345.
23. DREWNOWSKI, A., C. MASSIEN, J. LOUIS-SYLVESTRE, J. FRICKER, D. CHAPELOT & M. APFELBAUM. 1994. The effects of aspartame versus sucrose on motivational ratings, taste preferences, and energy intakes in obese and lean women. Int. J. Obesity **18:** 570-578.
24. ROLLS, B. J., P. A. PIRRAGLIA, M. B. JONES & J. C. PETERS. 1992. Effects of olestra, a non-caloric fat substitute, on daily energy and fat intake in lean men. Am. J. Clin. Nutr. **56:** 84-92.
25. BURLEY, V. J. & J. E. BLUNDELL. 1991. Evaluation of the action of a non-absorbable fat on appetite and energy intake in lean, healthy men. Int. J. Obesity **15** (suppl. 1): 8.
26. HULSHOF, T., C. DE GRAAF & J. A. WESTRATE. 1995. Short-term effects of high-fat and low-fat/high SPE croissants on appetite and energy intake and three deprivation periods. Physiol. & Behav. **57:** 377-383.
27. COTTON, J. R., V. J. BURLEY, J. A. WESTRATE & J. E. BLUNDELL. 1996. Fat substitution and food intake: Effect of replacing fat with sucrose polyester at lunch or evening meals. Br. J. Nutr. **75:** 545-556.
28. COTTON, J. R., J. A. WESTRATE & J. E. BLUNDELL. 1996. Replacement of dietary fat with sucrose polyester: Effects on energy intake and appetite control in nonobese males. Am. J. Clin. Nutr. **63:** 891-896.
29. ROLLS, B. J., V. H. CASTELLANOS, D. J. SHIDE, D. L. MILLER, C. L. PELKMAN, M. L. THORWART & J. C. PETERS. 1997. Sensory properties of a non-absorbable fat substitute did not affect regulation of energy intake. Am. J. Clin. Nutr. **65:** 1375-1383.
30. SHIDE, D. J. & B. J. ROLLS. 1995. Information about the fat content of preloads influences energy intake in healthy females. J. Am. Dietetic Assn., **95:** 993-998.
31. MILLER, D. L., V. A. HAMMER, D. J. SHIDE, J. C. PETERS & B. J. ROLLS. 1995. Consumption of fat-free potato chips by obese and restrained males and females. FASEB J. **9:** A190.
32. MILLER, D. L., V. A. HAMMER, J. C. PETERS & B. J. ROLLS. 1995. Effects of substituting fat-free (olestra) potato chips on 24-hour fat and energy intake. Obesity Res. **3:** 327S.
33. PORIKOS, K. P. & F. X. PI-SUNYER. 1984. Regulation of food intake in human obesity: Studies with caloric dilution and exercise. Clin. Endocrinol. Metab. **13:** 547-561.
34. BLACKBURN, G. L., B. S. KANDERS, P. T. LAVIN, S. D. KELLER & J. WHATLEY. 1997. The effect of aspartame as part of a multidisciplinary weight-control program on short- and long-term control of body weight. Am. J. Clin. Nutr. **65:** 409-418.
35. TORDOFF, M. G. & A. M. ALLEVA. 1990. Effect of drinking soda sweetened with aspartame or high-fructose corn syrup on food intake and body weight. Am. J. Clin. Nutr. **51:** 963-969.
36. CABANAC, M. & R. DUCLAUX. 1970. Specificity of internal signals in producing satiety for taste stimuli. Nature **227:** 966-967.
37. ROLLS, B. J. 1986. Sensory-specific satiety. Nutr. Rev. **44:** 93-101.
38. HAMMER, V. A. & B. J. ROLLS. 1996. Diet composition and the regulation of food intake and body weight. *In* Obesity and Weight Control, The Health Professional's Guide to Understanding and Treatment. S. Dalton, Ed., Aspen Publishers, Inc. Gaithersberg, MD. In press.
39. GLUECK, C. J., M. M. HASTINGS, C. ALLEN, E. HOGG, L. BAEHLER, P. S. GARTSIDE, D. PHILLIPS, M. JONES, E. J. HOLLENBACH, B. BRAUN & J. V. ANASTASIA. 1982. Sucrose polyester and covert caloric dilution. Am. J. Clin. Nutr. **35:** 1352-1359.

40. DE GRAAF, C., T. HULSHOF, J. A. WESTSTRATE & J. G. A. J. HAUTVAST. 1996. Nonabsorbable fat (sucrose polyester) and the regulation of energy intake and body weight. Am. J. Physiol. **270:** R1386–R1393.
41. BRAY, G. A., A. SPARTI, M. M. WINDHAUSER & D. A. YORK. 1995. Effect of two weeks' fat replacement by olestra on food intake and energy metabolism. FASEB J. **9:** A439.
42. JOHNSON, S. L., D. A. COOPER, M. STONE, H. SEAGLE, S. SMITH, F. WYATT, K. RICCARDI, Z. TRAN, J. C. PETERS & J. O. HILL. 1996. Effects of covert substitution of olestra on self-selected food intake. FASEB J. **10:** A550.
43. JOHNSON, S. L., G. W. REED, D. A. COOPER, M. STONE, H. M. SEAGLE, J. C. PETERS & J. O. HILL. 1996. Time course effects of covert substitutions of olestra on adults' ad libitum food intake. Obesity Res. **4:** 33S.

Food Intake Regulation in Children

Fat and Sugar Substitutes and Intake

LEANN L. BIRCH [a,c] AND JENNIFER O. FISHER [b,d]

[a]*Department of Human Development and Family Studies*
[b]*Graduate Program in Nutrition*
110 Henderson Building South
The Pennsylvania State University
University Park, Pennsylvania 16802

A wide abundance of reduced-fat and reduced-energy foods are increasingly available on supermarket shelves across the United States. Although not marketed for children, these types of products are purchased by families with children, are frequently available to children, and can be incorporated into children's diets. Public health messages regarding the prevalence of obesity and the relationship between dietary fat intake and chronic disease may provide the impetus for concerned parents to incorporate reduced-calorie or reduced-fat foods into the diets of their children. Although current dietary fat intakes are around 35% of dietary energy, the American Academy of Pediatrics recommends that dietary fat intakes constitute no more than 30% of dietary energy for children over the age of 2.[1] Controversy exists regarding dietary fat intake recommendations for children because although maintaining positive energy balance is critical to sustain children's growth and health, overnutrition among children is a pervasive problem in the United States today, and the prevalence of childhood obesity is high and still increasing.[2]

Although the appropriateness of dietary fat recommendations for children has been questioned, this issue has generated much discussion on the viability of various strategies to reduce fat intake in pediatric populations. In a recent paper, using computer simulation, Sigman-Grant and colleagues were able to show how reductions in the percent of energy from fat in children's diets can be accomplished without the use of macronutrient substitutes.[3] The efficacy of reducing children's fat intakes by reducing the percentage of energy from fat in diets offered to children, however, is not clear. In a recent experiment,[4] when we offered children menus, where 32% of energy came from fat, the diets they actually selected ranged from 28% to 42% of energy from fat, and these individual differences in the percentage of fat in the diet were related to the children's preferences for high-fat foods.

As foods containing macronutrient substitutes become more available, they may have an increasing role in modifying children's diets. With an increase in reduced-fat and reduced-calorie foods, parents may turn to the use of these types of foods in attempting to modify both children's dietary fat and energy intakes. In considering the impact of macronutrient substitutes in pediatric nutrition, a primary issue is

---

[c]Tel: (814) 863-0053; fax: (814) 863-7963; e-mail: llb15@psu.edu.
[d]Tel: (814) 865-1447; fax: (814) 863-7963; e-mail: jaf7@psu.edu.

whether the use of a fat substitutes or other low-energy alternatives reduce children's energy intake or alters the macronutrient composition of their diets. Given the importance of maintaining growth and health while avoiding obesity, determining whether and under what conditions children adjust their food and energy intake to compensate for reductions in the fat and energy of their diets is essential in understanding the consequences of reduced-fat and reduced-calorie foods in children's diets. At this point, the impact of macronutrient substitutes on children's macronutrient and energy intake is not known. The limited data relevant to this issue will be presented below. From a practical standpoint, the evidence on this issue is certainly relevant to developing healthy diets of moderate fat content that children will accept and consume, and to the design of prevention and treatment programs for childhood obesity.

MACRONUTRIENT SUBSTITUTES: TOOLS FOR INVESTIGATING THE ROLE OF ENERGY CONTENT IN BEHAVIORAL CONTROL OF HUMAN FOOD INTAKE

Macronutrient substitutes alter the macronutrient composition and the energy density of foods; if they are good substitutes, they also keep the sensory characteristics of the food relatively unaltered. Given these characteristics, macronutrient substitutes provide excellent tools for investigating how human eating behavior is affected by the energy and macronutrient composition of foods in the diet. One caveat: the research we have reviewed has been conducted in order to understand how manipulations of the macronutrient and energy content of food affect children's food and energy intake. The research has not investigated the impact of macronutrient substitutes per se, and no systematic series of experiments comparing and contrasting the effects of various macronutrient substitutes on children's food intake has been conducted.

The experiments included in this review are presented in summary form in TABLE 1, and the review includes a discussion of each of these experiments in turn. The experiments share a focus: they examine how children's food acceptance patterns are influenced by alterations in the macronutrient and energy content of foods. In most, but not all, of the manipulations of macronutrient and energy content, macronutrient substitutes are used. Several contrasts that do not involve comparing conditions with and without macronutrient substitutes, or that do not use macronutrient substitutes at all, are also presented. In a few cases, findings from contrasts that do not use macronutrient substitutes to alter energy density are included, as their inclusion allows us to draw conclusions about whether there is something unique about the alterations in energy density of foods brought about by way of the use of fat and sugar substitutes.

When we shift the focal research question from "How do alterations in the macronutrient and energy content of food affect children's food intake?" to "What is the impact of macronutrient substitutes on children's food intake?", we see that the research designs used to answer the first question do not include the contrasts necessary to answer the second question. For example, designs have not included conditions that allow us to tease apart the confounding of energy density and macronutrient composition. In many of these designs, foods presented in different treatment conditions vary simultaneously on several dimensions, including macronutrient and energy content, and the presence of other nutrients. No direct comparisons of the

TABLE 1. Summary of the Research Investigating Children's Responses to Manipulations of the Energy Density and Macronutrient Content of Foods

Publication	Participants	Design	Preload–ad-lib Delay (min)	(Preload) Energy Difference	Compensation for energy?
Anderson et al.[5]	9- to 10-yr-olds	P[a]	90	asp[c]/sucrose 200–300 kcal	No
Birch et al.[7]	3- to 5-yr-olds	P	20–30	asp/sucrose, LGM 100 kcal/100 mL	Yes
	adults	P	20–30	same	No
Birch et al.[10]	3- to 5-yr-olds	P		asp/sucrose, LGM 110 kcal/100 mL	Yes
Birch et al.[15]	3- to 5-yr-olds	P	30	LGM addition 90 kcal/100 g	Yes
Birch et al.[11]	Expt. 1: 4- to 5-yr-olds	P	0, 30, 60	asp/sucrose, LGM 90 kcal/200 mL	Yes
	Expt. 2: 2- to 3-yr-olds	P	0, 30, 60	67 kcal/150 mL	Yes
Birch et al.[12]	3- to 5-yr-olds	P	30	asp/fructose LGM 150 kcal/100 mL	Yes
Fomon et al.[22]	1 1/2–4 mo	D, AL	NA[b]	fat 67 vs. 133 kcal/dL	Yes
Fomon et al.[23]	1 1/2–4 mo	D, AL	NA	fat 54 vs. 100 kcal/dL	Yes
Johnson et al.[18]	Expt. 1: 4- to 5-yr-olds	P	60	fat 120 kcal/100 g	Yes
	Expt. 2: 2- to 3-yr-olds	P	90	120 kcal/100 g	Yes
Birch et al.[20]	3- to 5-yr-olds	P	120	1, 12, 18 g fat fat/olestra 14 g	No
Birch et al.[20]	2- to 5-yr-olds	D, AL	NA		Yes
Johnson et al.[16]	3- to 5-yr-olds	P	20	asp/sucrose, LGM 150 kcal	Yes, but (45%)

[a] P, preload; D, dilution; ad-lib, AL.
[b] Not applicable.
[c] Aspartame.

relative effects of different macronutrient substitutes on children's intake have been conducted. For this reason, the experiments conducted to answer the question "How do alterations in the macronutrient and energy content of foods affect children's food and energy intake?" are presented, and we will attempt to draw conclusions pertinent to the issue of the impact of macronutrient substitutes.

Research from our laboratory has focused on understanding the development of the behavioral controls of food intake in children. In particular, we have examined the effects of alterations in the energy and macronutrient content of foods on children's food selection and energy intake. A secondary question guiding our research concerns what children learn from eating foods with varying energy density that may affect how children regulate their energy intakes in response to the energy density of the foods. In this research, we have manipulated energy density, through fat and sugar substitutes, to investigate whether children learn to differentially associate food's sensory cues with postingestive consequences of foods consumed as a function of differences in energy and macronutrient composition of those foods. Findings reveal that children can learn preferences for energy-dense foods, and children can learn to anticipate how they will feel after eating familiar foods (conditioned satiety). These investigations have been integral in understanding how children regulate food intake, as this type of associative learning provides a mechanism by which children regulate their intakes based upon the energy density of the foods they consume.

As shown in TABLE 1, with a few exceptions in which 24-h intake data are available, the research is limited to experiments using protocols involving single meal preloading designs. These designs involve diluting the energy/macronutrient content of foods, typically through the use of macronutrient substitutes, including aspartame and olestra to replace carbohydrate or fat in foods. Energy density is varied using manipulations that have included varying carbohydrate (CHO) content by the use of aspartame, sucrose, fructose, or low-glucose maltodextrin (LGM); and varying fat content through the use of reduced-fat or fat-free, normal-fat, or fat-added foods containing fat substitutes (olestra) or other substances to produce similar sensory characteristics across foods differing in energy and fat. The predominant design appearing in TABLE 1 is the single-meal preloading protocol, in which fixed volumes or weights of a first course, varying in energy density, are consumed. Following a delay, ad libitum consumption is measured in a self-selected meal, and intake in this meal provides the data of interest.

We begin with a review of those experiments in which CHO was manipulated to alter energy density, and then move to a review of those that have manipulated fat content to alter energy density. Taken together, the results indicated that, in general, young children adjust their food intake in response to alterations of the energy content of foods produced by the use of sugar and fat substitutes. These adjustments in intake in response to manipulations of energy density are termed caloric compensation. Results reveal that while children can compensate for energy, this compensation is usually partial and incomplete, and that there are individual differences in how responsive children are to manipulations of the energy density of foods.

TABLE 2. The Effect of a Drink Containing Either Sucrose or Aspartame on Lunchtime Food Intake of Children

	Treatment		
	Aspartame	Sucrose	$F(1,19)$[b]
Energy (kcal)	777 (58)[a]	765 (67)	0.04
Protein (%)	15.2 (1.2)	15.2 (0-9)	0.06
Fat (%)	37.9 (1.6)	38.4 (1.2)	0.09
Carbohydrate (%)	48.8 (1.7)	48.3 (1.1)	0.11

[a] Mean (standard error).
[b] F value (df).

CALORIC COMPENSATION I: USING ASPARTAME AND CARBOHYDRATES TO ALTER ENERGY DENSITY

Evidence for Caloric Compensation in Older Children

Anderson and colleagues[5] conducted research to investigate the effects of aspartame on subsequent food intake, appetite, and hedonic response in children. This experiment included comparisons of the effects of preloads containing aspartame and saccharin, and in a second experiment, compared the effects of preloads on subsequent intake, when the preloads were sweetened either with aspartame or sucrose. In a double-blind, within subjects, crossover design, 9- and 10-year-olds were given 300 mL of either an aspartame-sweetened drink or a sucrose-sweetened drink (1.75 g/kg) on two different days, containing between 200 and 300 kcal. A similar design was used to compare the effects of the sugar substitutes. Prior food intake was controlled by bringing the children to the laboratory after an overnight fast and feeding them a standard breakfast at a fixed time. The preload was consumed midmorning (10:30), and lunch was served at noon after a 90-min delay. Children were encouraged to self-select a meal from an array of foods well accepted by children. The results revealed no differences in subsequent intake between the aspartame and saccharin conditions; the results shown in TABLE 2 reveal no differences in intake following the aspartame- and sucrose-sweetened drinks. There was no evidence that children adjusted their subsequent energy intake at lunch in response to the differences in the energy content of the previously consumed preload drink: children's intake at lunch was 777 kcal following the aspartame-sweetened drink, and 765 kcal following the sucrose-sweetened drink. This experiment reveals no evidence for caloric compensation; children ate nearly identical lunches despite the differences in the preload drinks' macronutrient and energy content, and the presence or absence of aspartame. As shown in TABLE 1, these results differ from those typically obtained with younger children in our laboratory. The children participating in the research of Anderson et al.[5] were considerably older than our 3- to 5-year-olds, and a 90-min delay between the preload and the meal was used.

One issue that arises in attempting to review the literature using preloading protocols is that different delays have been used across experiments and across laboratories. Given that the effects of ingested nutrients will differ over time, differences in the delay interval can be critical to obtaining effects on subsequent intake. With respect to the time delay, this 2-h interval is considerably longer than that which has consistently yielded clear effects of CHO manipulations on subsequent food intake. Work from our laboratory reviewed below suggests that shorter delays of about 20 to 30 minutes are more optimal for detecting the effects of CHO on children's intake. Research with adult participants using similar preloading protocols[6] suggests that 30-min delays are optimal to observe the maximal effect of CHO preloads on subsequent intake.

Evidence for Caloric Compensation in Young Children

In one of the first investigations from our laboratory designed to explore children's ability to show caloric compensation in response to differences in the energy density of foods, we used preloads containing aspartame or sucrose plus LGM to manipulate the energy density of the preloads (see TABLE 1). Participants were preschool children (n = 21 3 to 5-year-olds) and a group of young adults (n = 26 25 to 35-year-olds).[7] Two preloads of differing energy density (100 kcal/3.5 oz) were used. Low- and high-energy preloads were created using aspartame or sucrose plus LGM, respectively. Fat and protein content of the preloads did not differ. As in nearly all the subsequent preloading experiments, a within-subjects design was employed with all participants consuming each preload manipulation on separate occasions. Prior to lunch on different days, about one week apart, participants consumed the high- or low-energy preload, followed by lunch. Ad libitum consumption of the self-selected lunch, consisting of a selection of sandwiches and other typical lunch items, followed the preload after a 25-min delay. Also, to minimize the effects of child-feeding practices on children's intake, all the adults present while the children were consuming the self-selected meals were instructed and monitored to avoid the use of coercive child-feeding practices, and to avoid discussions of food and eating as a topic of conversation at meals. This control was employed in all the preloading experiments conducted in our laboratory and presented in TABLE 1, except for the research that investigated the impact of child-feeding practices on caloric compensation. This aspect of the experimental procedure provided children the opportunity to exert control over their intake and to minimize effects of external, social factors on their eating. These social factors have subsequently been shown to have clear effects on children's eating, especially their responsiveness to energy density.

Results are shown in FIGURE 1 and revealed clear evidence for caloric compensation by children: energy intake at lunch was 237 kcal following low-energy preload and 128 kcal following the high-energy density preload; 20 of 21 kids showed evidence of caloric compensation. In the same protocol, individual differences in caloric compensation were greater among adults; 16 of 26 adults showed some evidence of compensation, as indicated by eating more following the low-energy preload. For the total sample of adults, there was no effect of preload-energy density on subsequent lunch intake; intake following the high-energy preload was 390 kcal, following the low-energy preload of 390 kcal. Thus, whereas young children showed caloric compensation, reflecting their responsiveness to energy density, the adult

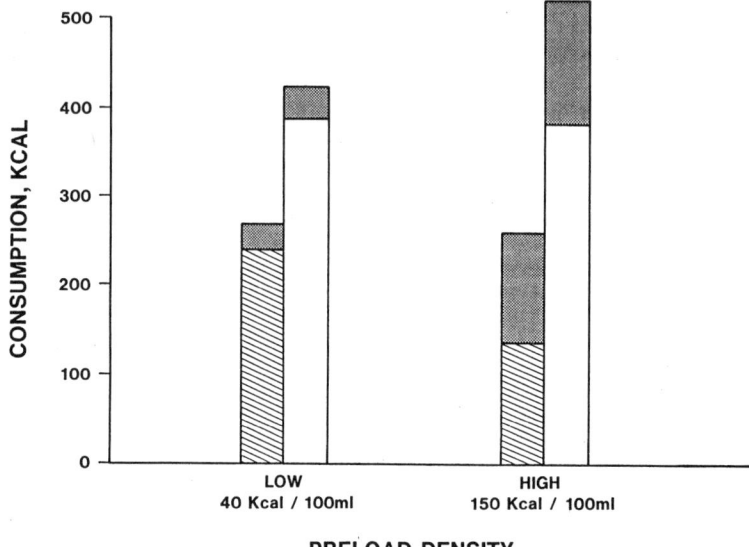

FIGURE 1. Ad libitum lunch consumption and high- and low-caloric density preload consumption (kcal) by children and adults. ■, preload; ▨, lunch (children, n = 21). ■, preload; □, lunch (adults, n = 26).

sample did not. The data obtained for 3- to 5-year-olds in this experiment are also inconsistent with those from the Anderson et al.[5] experiments presented above.

As shown in TABLE 1, there are a number of experiments that replicate the basic finding that young children show caloric compensation in preloading protocols, using different preload preparations and different delay intervals; these findings will be reviewed below. There are also a number of experiments indicating that adults are not always responsive to energy-density differences in preloading protocols. Although we would not classify them as adults, the lack of responsiveness to energy density and macronutrient content of preloads that Anderson observed in 9- and 10-year-olds was very similar to those we have observed for adults. The patterns of findings presented here as well as additional evidence beyond the scope of this chapter has led us to suggest that this pattern of age differences in caloric compensation may reflect true developmental differences in responsiveness to energy density.

The Developing Controls of Food Intake: Declining Responsiveness to Energy Density?

The age differences we have seen in responsiveness to energy density in combination with subsequent research has led us to hypothesize about the development of the control of food intake. We describe these developmental hypotheses here because they account for age differences in the data, but more importantly, because they can provide a framework for interpreting the seemingly inconsistent results obtained in research investigating responsiveness to energy density as a control of food intake in humans. This view indicates that there are age differences in responsiveness to energy density, and there are also individual differences in the extent to which we continue to be responsive to the energy density of foods in controlling our food intake. With respect to the question of the impact of fat and sugar substitutes, this view suggests that these effects will differ for different age groups, and among adults, depending on the extent to which they remain responsive to the energy density of the diet in controlling intake.

Developmentally, we all begin life as depletion-driven eaters who are responsive to the energy density of the diet, and we eat in response to hunger and satiety cues.[8] As we grow and develop, factors other than hunger and satiety also begin to influence human eating. These factors include time of day, presence of other people, the availability of palatable food, current dieting, emotional state, and concerns about nutrition. Our research indicates that, by the preschool period, whereas responsiveness to energy content remains important, eating has ceased to be exclusively depletion driven, and that other factors begin to influence food intake. As a result, control of eating may be governed by influences that are quite peripheral to the "internal" or physiologically based cues of hunger and satiety. In turn, the influence of "external" factors on the control of food intake can reduce our responsiveness to the energy and macronutrient content of foods.

By late childhood, additional factors have emerged to compete with hunger and satiety and responsiveness to energy density for the control of food intake. For example, about half of 9- and 10-year-old girls in the U.S. report that they have already dieted to lose weight.[9] These observations suggest that for many individuals, the role of energy and macronutrient content of foods as regulators of intake have become peripheral, and intake is controlled by cognitive factors. In short, individual differences in styles of controlling food intake begin to emerge during this stage in development. Among adults, styles of intake control are widely diverse, although not well characterized by researchers. Individual differences in intake regulation include successful restricters, who cognitively control their intake on a chronic basis to maintain weight; and disinhibited "out of control" eaters, who report that they have difficulty stopping eating even when they are no longer hungry, and in whom eating is triggered in the absence of hunger by emotional disturbance or the presence of palatable foods. We are currently pursuing longitudinal research that will provide data on the etiology of these individual differences in styles of intake control.

In the series of experiments described in the remainder of this section, we continued to explore the extent to which children's intake was influence by the energy content of preloads. These experiments also provide additional evidence for caloric compensation, across a variety of preload preparations, delay intervals, and also investigate whether children's responsiveness to energy density can result in learning to anticipate how much to eat of familiar foods, and whether energy density has an impact on children's preferences for foods.

Further Evidence for Caloric Compensation and Learning about Satiety

Following the initial research showing evidence for caloric compensation, we conducted experiments to replicate the findings and determine whether young children (3- to 5-year-olds) were responsive to the energy density of preloads and showed evidence of caloric compensation in the second course of a two-course meal.[10] A second purpose was to determine whether children would learn to associate the energy-density differences in the two preloads with different flavor cues in the preloads, thereby allowing them to learn to anticipate differences in the satiety value of these two foods and subsequently to make anticipatory adjustments in intake. Similar to those preloads used in the experiment from our laboratory described above, puddings were sweetened with either aspartame or sucrose plus LGM to create low- and high-energy density preloads that differed in energy content by 110 kcal.

In this case, children had repeated opportunities to consume the preloads, followed by the self-selected meal, providing opportunities for learning to occur. To test for learning, the two preloads were isocaloric during the extinction test trials, so that any differences in ad libitum consumption were not attributable to differences in the preload densities but to learned association of their caloric consequences with the different flavored preloads. Both experiments provide evidence for caloric compensation, with children eating more following the aspartame-sweetened preloads than following those containing CHO (see FIG. 2 for results of experiment 2). Children in experiment 1 showed evidence of caloric compensation prior to learning, as well as after the series of training trials. In experiment 2, the same pattern was obtained. Taken together, the data of these two experiments and the previous experiment[7] provide evidence for young children's ability to adjust subsequent intake in response to differences in energy density of a food eaten, at least when the energy differences are produced by carbohydrate alterations and the use of aspartame, and when the delay interval between the preload and the self-selected meal is 20 to 30 minutes. Also, children showed evidence that they had learned to anticipate the consequences of eating the high- and low-energy preparations. During extinction when the energy differences were no longer present, they continued to adjust intake in a manner consistent with the previous differences in energy content. These findings provide additional evidence that children can be responsive to the energy density of foods when these differences are produced by the substitution of aspartame for sugar, and that children can learn to anticipate the postingestive consequences of eating foods differing in energy density, and make adjustments in intake accordingly.

Effects of the Timing of Preloads on Subsequent Intake

The extent to which ingested energy has an impact on subsequent intake will differ dramatically with the interval between eating occasions due to the dynamic nature of the absorption and metabolism of nutrients. To begin to understand the time course of the effects of ingested CHO on subsequent intake, we conducted experiments in which the delay interval between the preload and subsequent intake varied. As previously, we examined the effects of high- and low-energy preloads on children's subsequent consumption, where the energy differences were again a result

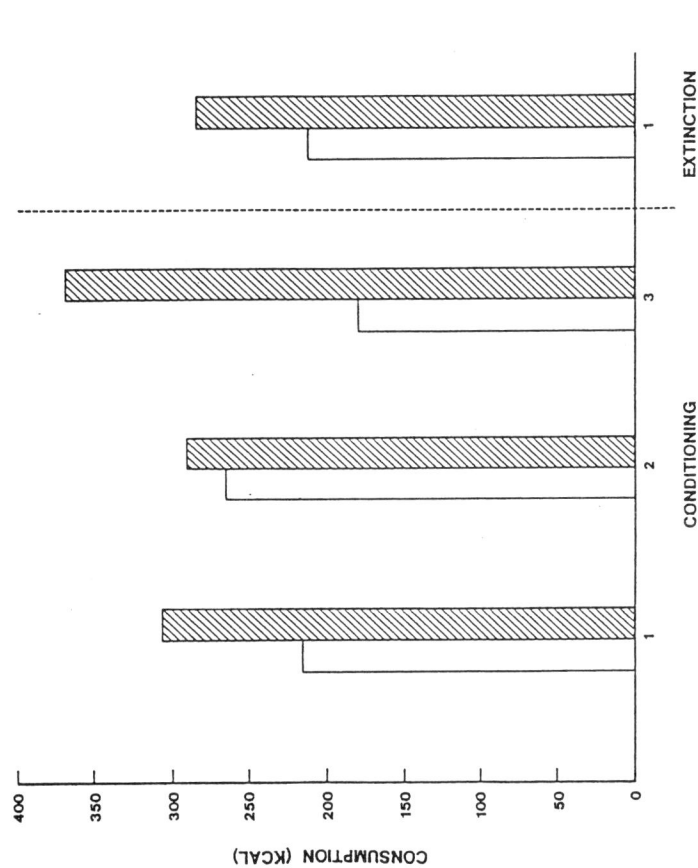

FIGURE 2. Conditioning of flavor cues to consequences, experiment 2: Consumption during training and extinction test snacks following high- and low-caloric density loads. (In extinction test snacks, the flavors previously paired with high- or low-caloric density preloads were both paired with isocaloric, intermediate density preloads). ▨, low-density preload; ☐, high-density preload.

TABLE 3. Experiment 1: Mean Intake following Preloads at 0-, 30-, and 60-minute Delays[a]

Time Delay	Preloads			
	H$_2$O	Asp	Sucrose	LGM + Asp
0	454*	451*	397†	373†
30	521*	458†	459†	394†
60	421*	378*	388*	293†
Overall delays	466*	429†	381‡	353‡

[a] Columns with differing superscripts are significantly different.

of manipulating the CHO content and the use of aspartame.[11] Preloads consisted of fruit-flavored Kool Aid (General Foods) drinks. In this series of experiments, we were especially interested in the time course of the effects of these preloads on subsequent intake; so children were allowed to eat ad libitum at different lengths of time following the preloads: no delay, 30 min, or 60 min. The (200 mL) preloads were either equal volumes of water (0 kcal), or sweetened with aspartame (3 kcal/ 200 mL), sweetened with sucrose (90 kcal/200 mL), or sweetened with aspartame plus LGM (90 kcal/200 mL). Following the preloads, children consumed a self-selected snack, from an array of palatable snack foods. To explore the time course of the effects of preloads on subsequent intake, in experiment 1, children were assigned to one of three delay intervals between the preload consumption and ad libitum consumption: no delay, 30 min, and 60 min. Experiment 2 was a replication, using a completely within-subjects design, so that all children participated at all delay intervals and in all preload conditions. The design of these experiments also differs by including a water control, matched for volume with the other preloads. This control was included because some evidence suggests that fluid ingestion prior to a meal might actually increase food intake. We also included a condition to allow comparison of equicaloric loads using sucrose or LGM as the energy source. We added aspartame to the LGM to equate the sweetness to that of the sucrose- and aspartame-sweetened preloads.

In both experiments, the data reveal only a main effect of preload type and no effect of time delay and no interaction of time delay with preload type. As shown in TABLES 3 and 4, aspartame suppressed intake relative to water, whereas sucrose significantly suppressed intake relative to aspartame. There was no difference between the suppression in ad libitum intake following the sucrose and the LGM plus aspartame load, although the trend in both experiments was for greater suppression following LGM plus aspartame. In experiment 1 (mean age = 55 months), the difference between aspartame and sucrose preloads and between the aspartame and the LGM plus the aspartame preloads was about 90 kcal. Relative to ad libitum consumption following aspartame preload, ad libitum intake was suppressed about 50 kcal after sucrose, and about 80 kcal after aspartame plus LGM. In experiment 2, the sample was younger (mean age = 36 months); the difference between the aspartame and sucrose (aspartame plus LGM) preloads was 60 kcal. Relative to ad libitum consumption following the

TABLE 4. Experiment 1: Mean Intake following Preloads at 0-, 30-, and 60-minute Delays[a]

	Preloads			
Time Delay	H$_2$O	Asp	Sucrose	LGM + Asp
0	371*	350*	290†	253‡
30	391*	353†	300†	288‡
60	367*	346*†	317*	303‡
Overall delays	376*	350†	302‡	281‡

[a] Columns with differing superscripts are significantly different.

aspartame preload, the suppression of ad libitum intake following the sucrose preload was about 50 kcal, and about 70 kcal following the aspartame plus LGM preload. In both cases, there was only a main effect of preload, with children again showing compensation in ad libitum intake in response to energy differences between the aspartame and the more energy-dense preloads. Additionally, there was no effect of time-delay interval between preload and ad libitum intake and no interaction of time delay with preload. We noted significant (although incomplete) compensation for energy in the preloads at all delay intervals up to 60 minutes. These findings indicate that energy from ingested CHO can influence children's subsequent intake, whether the preloads are ingested immediately before the self-selected meal (as would be the case when two-course meals are taken), or when the delay is somewhat longer, as might occur when snacks are taken prior to meals.

Learned Preferences for High-energy Foods

Review of the results of several preloading experiments using aspartame and CHO to alter energy density of preloads, conducted with 3- to 5-year-olds, reveals that (1) children are responsive to energy density and adjust their intake in response to differences in energy density of preloads produced by manipulation of the carbohydrate content of foods consumed; and that (2) children can learn to make such adjustments in an anticipatory way, based on learned associations between foods' sensory cues and energy density. An important question is whether the differing postingestive consequences of high- and low-energy versions of foods can influence children's preferences for those foods. Subsequently, we investigated whether children would learn to prefer energy-dense over energy-dilute versions of the same foods.[12] Research has shown that food preferences and aversions develop as a food's flavor cues are associated with the consequences of ingestion, although the data are more definitive for learned aversions than for learned preferences. In the case of the learned food aversion, foods are avoided and disliked following the association of food flavor cues with the negative GI consequences of nausea and vomiting. Conversely, rats can learn to prefer energy-dense over energy-dilute drinks and foods.[13] There is some evidence that adults can learn to prefer a starch-rich, energy-dense food over a low-energy density version.[14]

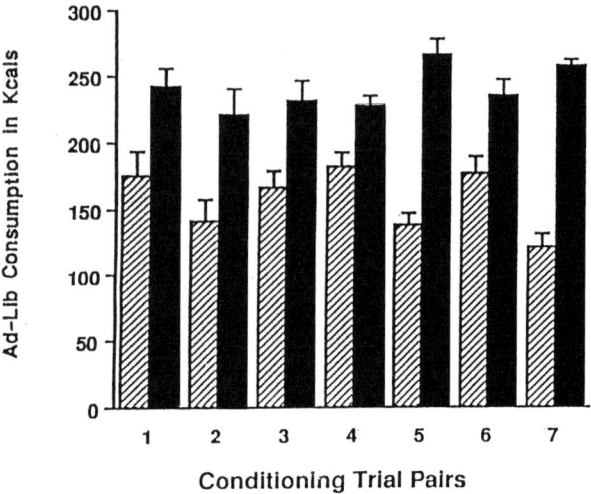

FIGURE 3. Ad lib consumption following high- and low-caloric density drinks. ▨, following high density; ■, following low density.

To investigate children's ability to learn preferences for energy-dense foods, we again provided children with a noncoercive eating context and gave them repeated opportunities to eat high and low energy-dense versions of the same foods or drinks, where differences in energy density were produced through the use of aspartame versus sucrose plus LGM. In the first experiment, high- and low-energy drinks were produced using commercially available "sugar free" and standard versions of the same commercially available drinks (*e.g.*, Tang drink mix), and augmenting the high-energy version with LGM in order to produce drinks that differed substantially in energy density, and using distinctive flavors in the high- and low-energy preparation, with these flavor-energy pairings counterbalanced across participants. In this first experiment, the sugar-free version sweetened with aspartame had 3-5 kcal per 150 mL serving; high-energy versions were sweetened with sucrose and LGM and had 150 kcal/150 mL. Again, our subjects were 3 to 5-year-olds, and over a several week period, they had repeated opportunities to consume, on half the days, a sugar-free, energy-free drink with one distinctive flavor, and a second, high-energy flavor on the other half of the days. Following a 20-30 min delay, the children consumed a snack that they self-selected from among an array of palatable snack foods. Of primary interest in this case were the children's preferences for the drinks and how these preferences changed for the high- and low-energy versions as the children accrued experience with consuming the drinks. Additionally, we were interested in energy intake in the ad libitum portion of the snack, as this provided further evidence on the extent to which the energy content of one eating occasion can influence children's subsequent energy intake. FIGURE 3 shows ad libitum energy intake in the series of meals following high- and low-energy preloads. Also, there was evidence that children learned to prefer the drink flavor consistently high in energy content over the low-energy version. The results are consistent with previous research, indicating that children again adjusted their subsequent intake based on differences in the energy content of a first-course drink (produced by differences between an essentially zero-energy drink, sweetened with aspartame, and a drink using caloric sweeteners—typically a combination of fructose, sucrose, and LGM).

The Impact of Child-feeding Practices on Responsiveness to Energy Density

At least in the absence of attempts by adults to impose external controls on eating, infants[8] and young children can show evidence of responsiveness to energy density in controlling meal size. Because much of children's eating occurs in the presence of adults who may attempt to influence what and how much children eat, we investigated the extent to which children's responsiveness to energy density can be moderated by child-feeding practices.[15] To do this, we used a preloading protocol like those previously described to assess children's responsiveness to energy density in two social contexts differing in the presence or absence of common child-feeding strategies used to control children's eating. The two social contexts included an "internal cues" context in which we trained and monitored teachers to minimize their control over how much and what children ate to give children maximal opportunity to regulate intake. In this condition, we discussed feelings of hunger and satiety in the initiation and termination of eating. In the "external cues" context, we trained adults to focus children on external factors to control their eating, such as how much food was left on the plate and the fact that it was lunchtime, and had teachers reward the children for finishing the portions served to them. In short, the external context incorporated some of the child-feeding practices used by adults in their attempts to control what and how much children eat.

Yogurt preloads differing in energy density were used as preloads, and the energy-density differences were produced by using a nonfat yogurt for the low-energy version and adding LGM to produce the high-energy version. In this case, neither of these yogurts contained aspartame or any noncaloric sweetener. High-energy versions contained 150 kcal/100 g, and the low-energy versions 60 kcal/100 grams. Again, children consumed fixed amounts of these foods and about 20–30 min later ate a self-selected snack.

The results are shown in FIGURE 4. For the "internal context" condition, in which children were allowed to focus on internal cues to control intake, the pattern of findings obtained is very similar to those obtained in the four prior experiments, in which aspartame and CHO were used to vary the energy density of otherwise similar preload drinks or foods. This suggests that differences in ad libitum intake are observed across experiments as a function of differences in CHO or energy content, rather than as that attributable to aspartame content. Additionally, when adults present during the eating occasions focused children on external cues to control eating, all evidence of responsiveness to energy density vanished (see FIG. 4). In summary, these results reveal that (1) the evidence for caloric compensation that we have seen previously is not unique to manipulations involving aspartame to alter energy density; and (2) children's ability to regulate energy intake and to be responsive to energy

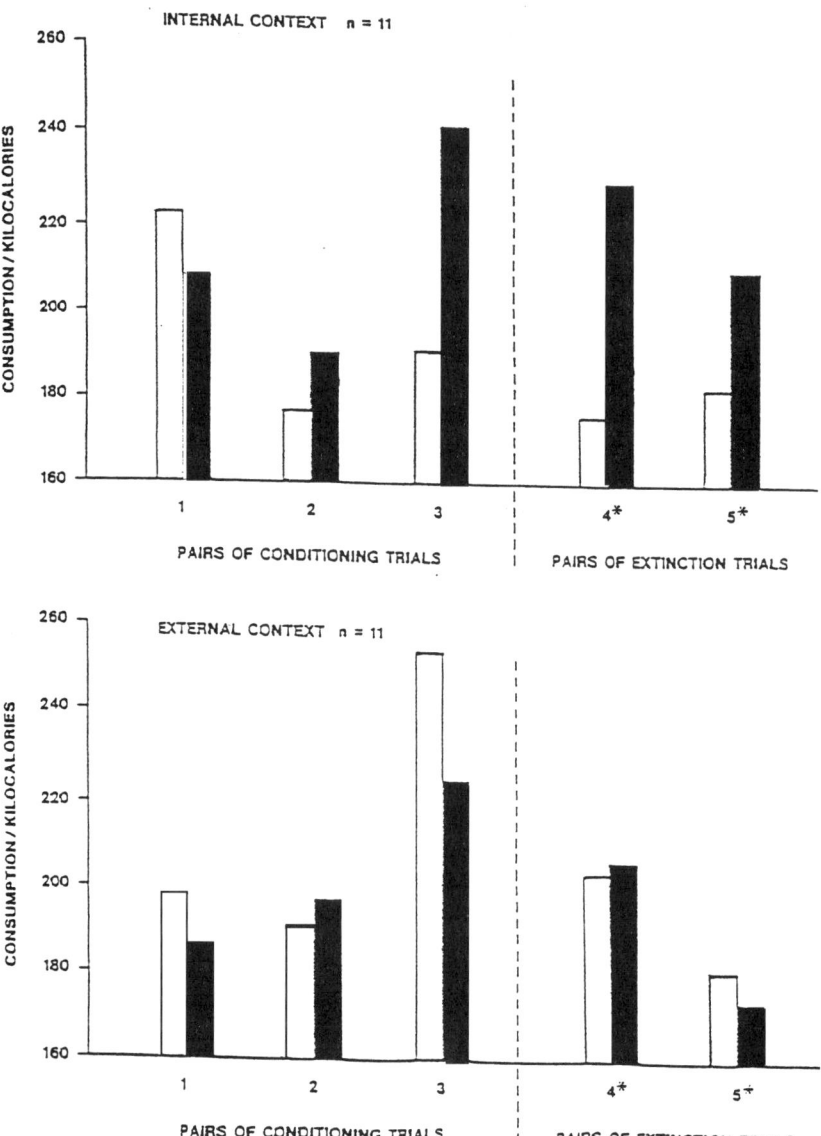

FIGURE 4. Ad lib consumption following high- and low-caloric density preloads during conditioning and extinction, internal and external social contexts. Asterisks indicate that in extinction trials, flavors previously paired with high- or low-density preloads are paired with equal, intermediate preloads. □, high density; ■, low density.

density in controlling their food intake is relatively fragile and can be readily disrupted by child-feeding practices that emphasize attention to aspects of the feeding context other than children's hunger and satiety. The findings also suggest the possibility that individual differences in styles of controlling food intake seen among adults have their beginnings in differences in early child-feeding practices, which can shape a focus on controlling intake in response to either internal or external factors.

The Etiology of Individual Differences in Responsiveness to Energy Density: Diverging Styles of Intake Control

To begin to investigate the question of whether there are individual differences in responsiveness to energy density, and whether any such differences may be linked to familial or individual characteristics, we collected information pertaining to parenting practices, especially those used in child feeding, parental adiposity, dieting history, and also data on the children's adiposity from 77 preschool children and their families.[16] As described previously, we again used a preloading protocol and produced differences in the energy density of the preloads by altering the CHO content, using aspartame to match the low-energy version of the drink for sweetness to the high-energy version, which contained energy from sucrose and LGM. To measure individual differences in caloric compensation among children, we developed an eating index based on the difference in energy intake in the two ad libitum meals, following the high- and low-energy preloads, divided it by the energy difference in the preloads to make this difference proportional to the difference in the preloads, and expressed the resulting value as a percentage, with 100% indicating "perfect," calorie-for-calorie compensation. In this case, the energy difference between the low- and high-energy preloads produced an equivalent adjustment in energy intake in the self-selected meals. The distribution of values of this eating index is shown in FIGURE 5. On average, in the subsequent meal, children typically compensated for about 45% of the energy difference in the preloads, but as shown, there is a high degree of individual variability. Parental control was strongly related to the child's eating index ($r = 0.65$, $p < 0.001$), adding support to the idea that children's responsiveness to energy density can be influenced by parent's child-feeding practices, and that during the early years children may be quite responsive to the energy density of the diet. This responsiveness can be transitory, as other factors may come to control intake. This suggests that the effects of macronutrient substitutes on intake may well differ widely across individuals, depending on whether or not they remain responsive to energy density. If they are responsive, then they may well adjust energy intake to compensate for the missing energy in foods containing fat and sugar substitutes. If they are not responsive to energy content they will not show compensation for energy, but their response will depend on which factors influencing intake are most salient.

The results of preloading experiments indicate that young children can adjust their subsequent intake in response to energy-density differences produced when aspartame is substituted for sucrose or other carbohydrate/caloric sweeteners in an eating occasion that occurs up to one hour prior to eating a self-selected meal. However, whether or not children actually do adjust their intake in response to such alteration of energy and macronutrient content is moderated by the child-feeding

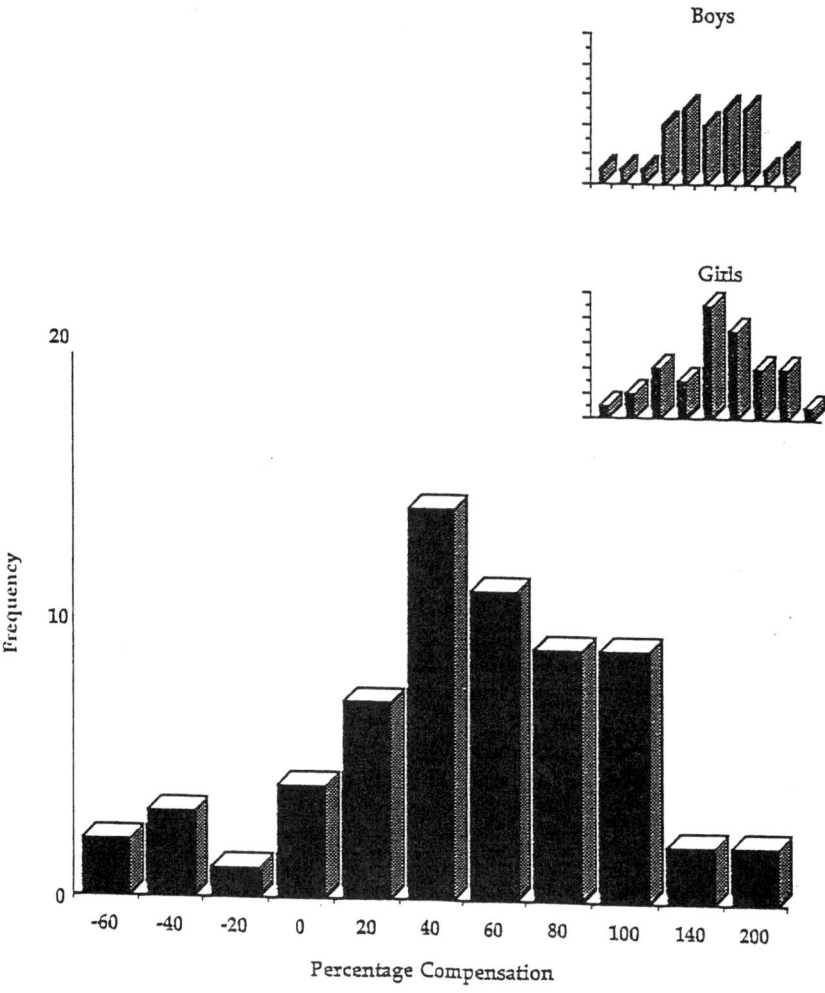

FIGURE 5.

practices imposed on the child, particularly parental attempts to control how much children eat.

The data indicate that children are adjusting their energy intake in self-selected meals following differences in the energy content of a first-course preload, but the question of how they accomplish this at the behavioral level remains. In two experiments[11,17] there were systematic differences in food selection following the different preloads, and these differences in intake were related to the children's preferences for the foods available in the ad libitum meal. The reduction in energy intake following the energy-dense preloads was accomplished primarily by a disproportionate reduction in intake of nonpreferred foods; children tended to maintain their consumption of highly preferred foods in ad libitum intake sessions across all preload conditions. We have not found any evidence that the macronutrient composition of ad libitum meals differed when CHO content was varied to produce alterations in energy content of preloads.

CALORIC COMPENSATION II: USING FAT TO ALTER ENERGY DENSITY

The results of research exploring children's adjustments in energy intake in response to alterations of the CHO content of preloads used to alter preload energy density reveal that when CHO is altered, children can adjust subsequent food intake to compensate for energy differences. However, because the postingestive pathways for absorption and metabolism of fat differ from those of CHO, we cannot draw any conclusions about the potential impact of manipulations of the fat and energy content of foods on children's macronutrient and energy intake. The question of whether children show responsiveness to energy density differences produced by alterations in the fat content of foods is an especially important one because much of the natural variability in the energy content of foods is attributable to differences in fat content, and because diets high in fat have been linked to obesity and increased risk for chronic disease. Unfortunately, the data base relevant to the question of children's responsiveness to alterations in the energy density of foods produced by differences in fat content is even more limited than that based on CHO manipulations.

Caloric Compensation in Infancy: Adjustments in Intake in Response to Alterations of Fat Content of Formula

The initial research on whether or not alterations in fat content produced effects on intake were conducted by Fomon and colleagues with young infants.[8] In a series of experiments conducted during the 1960s, when it was common to put infants on formulas containing skim milk, they varied the fat content of the milks used in formulas fed to infants and noted the changes in the volume of the infants' ad libitum formula intake. These experiments are summarized in TABLE 1. By the time infants were about 6 weeks old, they adjusted the volume of intake so that 24-h energy intake was equivalent for formulas differing in fat and energy content (67 kcal/dL or 133 kcal/dL).

Caloric Compensation and Learned Preferences for High-fat Foods

To explore whether children are responsive to differences in energy density produced by manipulations of the fat content of foods, we conducted two replications of the conditioning protocol;[12] the energy density of the foods was manipulated by altering the fat content. Experiments differ in the ages of the subjects (48 months in experiment 1, 33 months in experiment 2).[18] Differences in energy density were due to differences in fat content; yogurt preparations were matched for CHO and protein

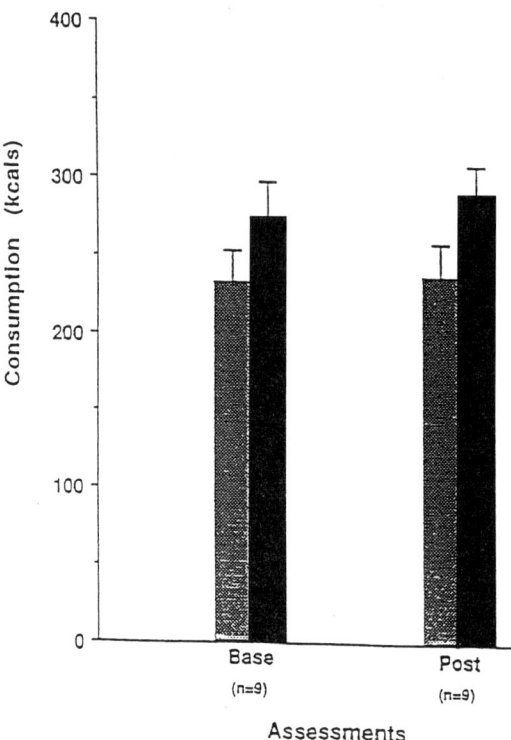

FIGURE 6. Ad lib consumption following high- and low-density yogurts before and after repeated experience (n = 9, p < 0.05). ▨, following high fat; ■, following low fat.

content. No fat substitutes were used; yogurts were prepared with differing levels of added fat. The delay between the preload and the self-selected meal was one hour. In both experiments, there is evidence for caloric compensation (see FIG. 6) and also clear evidence in both experiments of conditioned preferences for the higher-fat version.

The positive findings reported in Johnson, McPhee, and Birch[18] were replicated and extended in research to determine whether children can be responsive to energy-density differences produced by differences in fat content and can learn to prefer high-fat over no-fat yogurt drinks, which were matched for sensory characteristics.[19] We used commercially available fat-free yogurts (Dannon). Twenty-seven 3- and 4-year-olds participated. The energy difference for a 150 mL portion was about 150 kcal, produced by adding fat (canola oil) to the fat-free yogurt. After obtaining initial preferences, a pair of relatively equally preferred flavors of the yogurt drinks was selected for each child. Five fruit flavors were used: banana, cherry, peach, grape, and raspberry. One yogurt flavor was paired with high fat, the other with no fat. Each week for six weeks, following an overnight fast, children consumed a yogurt beverage immediately after arriving at preschool, consuming the high-fat flavor on half the days and the low-fat flavor on the others.

A second group of children participated in a "mere exposure" control condition to assess whether postingestive consequences of the drinks were involved in the formation of these preferences. In this control condition, children tasted but did not actually consume significant amounts of the yogurt drinks. Because the focus of this research was on learned preferences for high-fat foods, we did not obtain data on caloric compensation in subsequent meals. Preferences were obtained once at the beginning and once at the end of a series of conditioning trials in which 150 mL portions were consumed when the children were hungry. Preferences for the yogurt drinks were also obtained on a third occasion after a breakfast, when the children were full, these preference were compared to those assessments when children were hungry. This aspect of the procedure was used to test the hypothesis that learned preferences based on fat/energy content were more clearly expressed when the children were hungry than when they were full.

In the condition where the yogurts were repeatedly consumed, there was clear evidence of learning a preference for the high-fat version over the low-fat version (see FIG. 7). By contrast, no such preference for the high-fat version was learned by the children in the mere exposure control, in which children tasted but did not consume and experience the postingestive consequences of the yogurts. The preferences for the high-fat versions were most clearly expressed when the children were hungry, and these learned preferences persisted for at least two months after the conditioning trials. These results are also consistent with the results of the learning experiments conducted using CHO manipulations.[12] These results are also provocative, because they suggest the possibility that children learn to prefer high-energy versions of foods relative to reduced-energy versions of foods, and also suggest that in the long term, reduced-energy foods produced by the use of macronutrient substitutes may not be well accepted by children. To the extent that these findings reflect children's learning about food as a part of their everyday experience with food and eating, the results could have implications for the long-term acceptance of reduced-energy foods containing macronutrient substitutes.

The Impact of Olestra on Children's 24-hour Energy Intake

Positive energy balance is critical to sustaining children's growth and health, and it is important to determine whether children will adjust their energy intake not only in single meals, but on a long-term basis to compensate for alterations in the macronutrient and energy content of the diet. To address this issue, we investigated whether children could alter their food and energy intake in response to covert changes in the fat and energy content of the diet, produced by the substitution of olestra for dietary fat.[20] Participants were 29, 2 to 5-year-olds. Twenty-four-hour food intake was measured during four, two-day blocks over a four-week period. In this within-subjects crossover design, children consumed foods containing either dietary fat or olestra, a nonenergy fat substitute, during the first three meals of each block (breakfast, morning snack, and lunch). Olestra was substituted for about 10% of the total daily energy intake (14 g). Children consumed six meals each day, and intake was measured for each child by weighing all menu foods before and after all meals. Results indicated that children compensated for the relative energy deficit created by the substitution

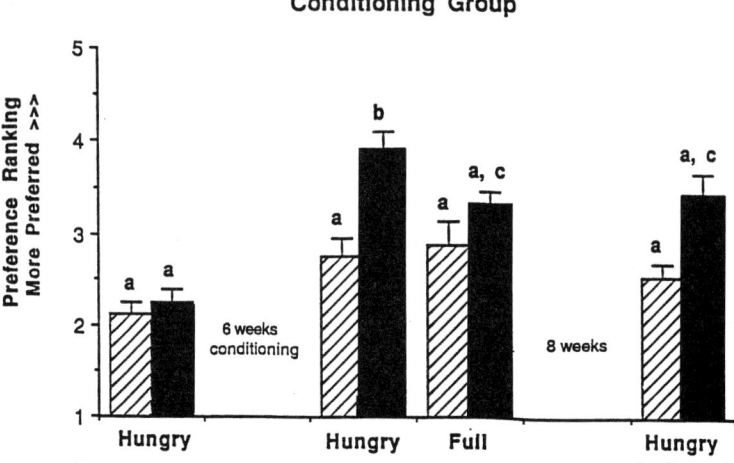
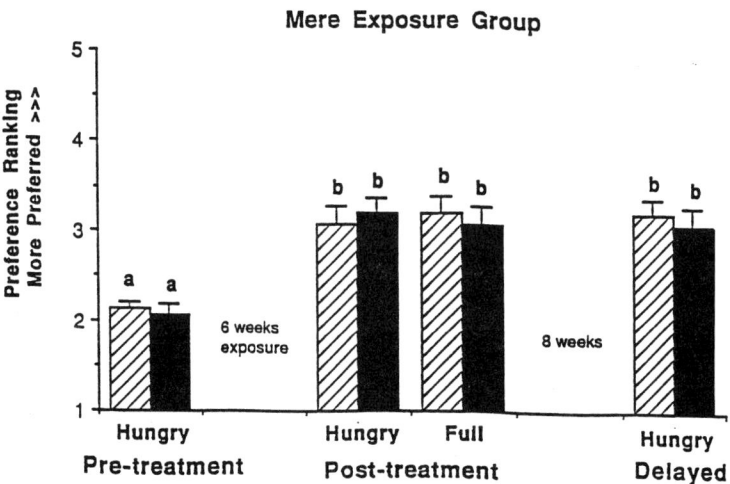

FIGURE 7. Effects of conditioning (n = 12) or mere exposure (n = 15) treatment on 3- and 4-year-olds' preferences for high-fat-(solid column) and fat-free-(striped column) paired flavors. After treatment, children's preferences were assessed both hungry and full.

of olestra for dietary fat. FIGURE 8 shows the cumulative difference in energy intake over the two-day period between olestra and dietary fat conditions. As shown, across the first three meals of the two-day block, when olestra was substituted for dietary fat, the cumulative difference in energy intake between the conditions increased. Following those occasions where olestra was incorporated into the foods, the cumulative difference between the conditions began to decrease. By the end of day two, the cumulative difference in energy intake was reduced to 100 kJ.

In compensating for the energy dilution, children did not show any macronutrient-specific compensation, as shown in TABLE 5. The macronutrient composition of the children's two-day intakes was significantly altered by the substitution of olestra for dietary fat; the percent of energy from dietary fat was significantly reduced on the olestra days (36.4%) compared to the dietary fat days (38.7%), and the percent of energy from carbohydrate intake was increased on olestra (53.3%) versus placebo days (51.5%). Analyses also revealed large individual differences in the extent to which energy intake was adjusted when olestra was substituted for dietary fat.

We noted large individual differences not only in the extent to which children adjusted their intake in the olestra/placebo conditions, but also in how tightly energy intake was regulated over 24-h periods (see FIG. 9). These findings are similar to prior research investigating children's regulation of energy intake over 24-h periods.[21] When we examined the pattern of coefficients of variation for individual meals versus 24-h periods, we saw that the coefficients of variation (CV) for individual meals were quite large relative to those for 24-h energy intake, and that meal-to-meal compensation in energy intake was implicated in producing this pattern of results. In a manner analogous to the compensation we noted in single-meal protocols (in which energy intake at a first-course preload had an impact on intake in the second course), children adjusted their intake across successive meals: meals characterized by relatively high-energy intakes tended to be followed by meals in which energy intake was low. Further, the extent of meal-to-meal compensation varied across children and was related to their CV for total energy intake; children who showed the clearest evidence of meal-to-meal compensation had the smallest CV for total energy intake.

In conclusion, these results indicated that children can adjust their energy intake in response to the replacement of dietary fat by olestra, at least up to 10% of total energy intake. The reductions in the percentage of energy from fat were accomplished without significant reductions in children's energy intake. In this case, caloric compensation occurred in a situation in which the energy density of only some of the foods of the diet were reduced by substituting olestra for dietary fat. The present study provides additional evidence that when allowed to consume what they wish from among a varied array of foods, over 24-h periods, children's 24-h energy intake is relatively consistent. This occurs in part because children are adjusting their intake across successive meals, and that, in fact, this adjustment contributes to the relatively high variability of children's energy intake at individual meals. The evidence for adjustments in energy intake across meals emerged whether or not a fat substitute was present in the diet. Further, children compensated for the reductions in energy but showed no adjustments in their subsequent macronutrient intake; compensation was not fat specific. At least in the absence of adult control and coercion, children

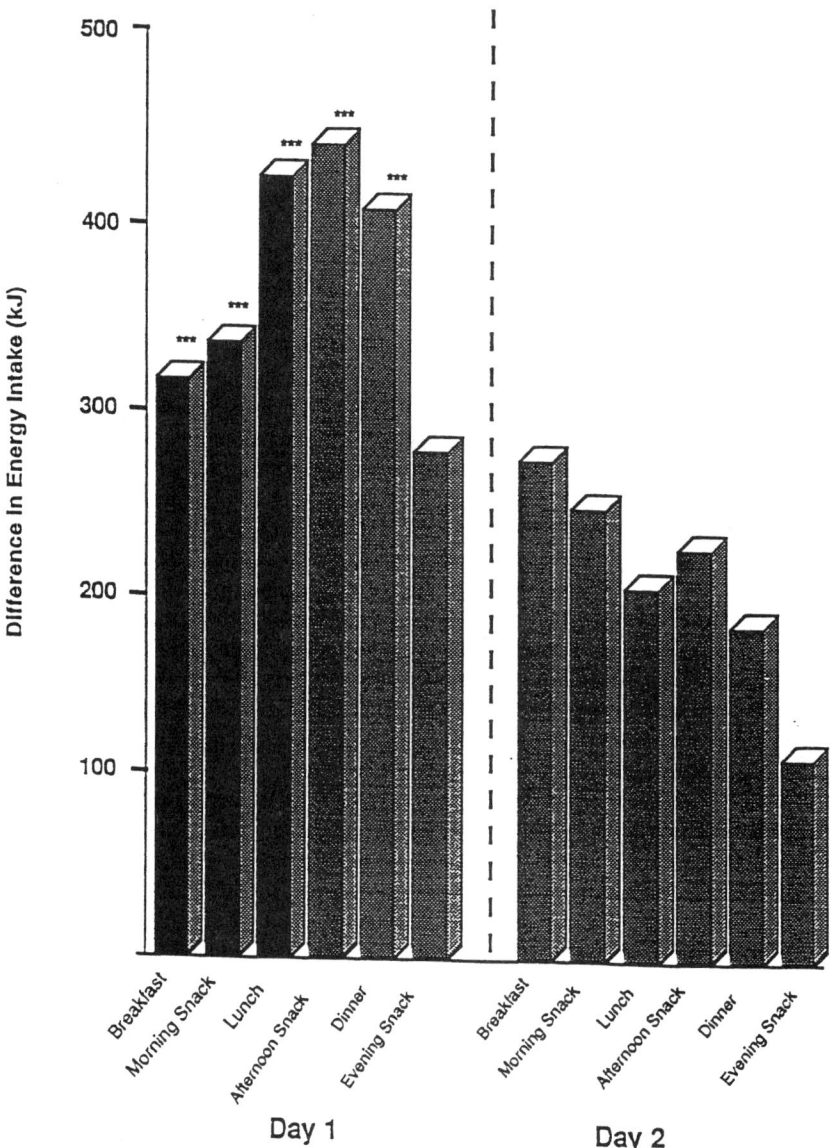

FIGURE 8. Cumulative difference in children's energy intake between placebo and fat-substitute conditions as a percentage of cumulative placebo intake, across eating occasions, over 2-d blocks. The fat substitute replaced dietary fat during the first three meals of day 1. ■, test meals; ***p < .001, **p < .01, *p < .05.

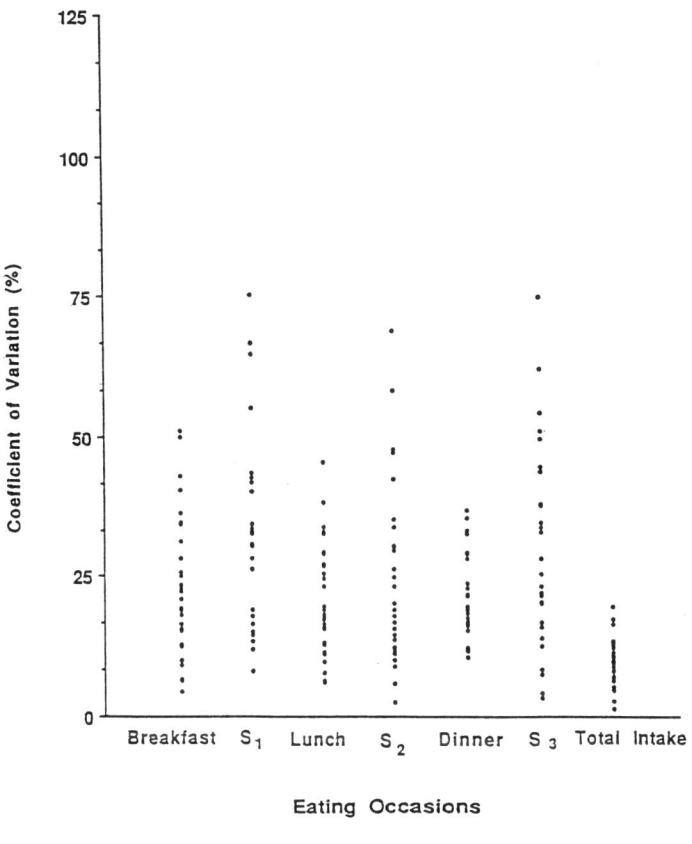

FIGURE 9.

have the capacity to adjust their energy intake at meals to maintain a relatively constant total daily energy intake.

SUMMARY AND CONCLUSIONS

A series of experiments exploring children's responsiveness to manipulations of energy density and macronutrient content of foods have been reviewed to assess the nutritional impact of macronutrient substitutes on children's intake. In these experiments, the focus is on the extent to which the energy content of foods was a salient factor influencing children's food intake, and macronutrient substitutes were used as tools to investigate this issue. Therefore, although several different macronutrient substitutes have been used in this research, we do not have a parametric set of experiments systematically assessing the impact of a variety of macronutrient substitutes. Given this, what can we conclude from the existing data? When the energy

TABLE 5. Forty-eight-hour Macronutrient and Energy Intakes in Fat-substitute and Dietary-fat Conditions

Macronutrient	Fat Substitute	Dietary Fat
Carbohydrate (%)	53.3	51.5[a]
Protein (%)	12.1	11.9
Fat (%)	36.4	38.7[a]
Energy (kJ)	13,573	13,673

[a] Significantly different from fat-substitute condition, $p = 0.0001$.

density and macronutrient content of foods is altered through the use of macronutrient substitutes that reduce the energy content of foods, children tend to adjust for the missing energy, although this adjustment may be partial and incomplete. This suggests the possibility that when macronutrient substitutes are used to reduce the energy content of foods, children's energy intake may be reduced. This adjustment, however, will most likely be less than a "calorie for calorie" reduction. In addition, even among young children, there are individual differences in the extent to which children adjust their intake in response to macronutrient and energy manipulations. The data are more extensive and particularly clear for cases in which CHO manipulations are used to alter energy density, but there is evidence for adjustments in energy intake in response to alterations of the fat content of the diet. The compensation for energy is not macronutrient specific; that is, when the fat content of food is reduced to reduce energy density of foods, children do not selectively consume fat in subsequent meals. This means that manipulations of macronutrient content of foods that reduce foods' energy content may not result in alterations of energy intake, but because these adjustments in energy intake are not macronutrient specific, changes in the overall macronutrient composition of children's diets can be obtained. There does not appear to be anything unique or special about the effects of macronutrient substitutes on children's intake; their effects are similar to those produced by other manipulations of macronutrient and energy content accomplished without macronutrient substitutes (*e.g.*, augmenting foods with fat or carbohydrate to produce macronutrient differences).

The research also indicates that under conditions that minimize adult attempts to control how much and what children eat, children can adjust their food and energy intake in response to the alterations of macronutrient and energy content of foods. Whether or not young children adjust food intake to compensate for energy-density changes depends upon their opportunity to control their own food intake as opposed to having their intake controlled by others. Young children's ability to adjust intake in response to alterations in the energy density of foods can be readily disrupted by the imposition of controlling child-feeding practices that attempt to regulate what and how much children eat. We believe that early experiences, including child-feeding practices imposed by parents, are major factors contributing to the etiology of individual differences and gender differences in the behavioral controls of food intake that can occur in response to the energy content of foods. The extent to which children respond to energy density of the diet has major implications for the effects of fat and sugar substitutes on children's intake. If children who are responsive to energy density consume substantial amounts of foods containing macronutrient substitutes, they should show some adjustments in intake to compensate for reduced energy, so that the impact of macronutrient substitutes on energy intake may be relatively small. However, changes in macronutrient composition of diets might still be accomplished. For children who are unresponsive to energy density, changes in children's energy intake and macronutrient intake have the potential to be greater. However, any general conclusions about the impact of macronutrient substitutes should await the results of population-based research to investigate the impact of macronutrient substitutes on children's intake. Such research must take into account the extent to which children are exposed to, choose, and consume foods containing macronutrient substitutes, as well as individual differences in children's ability to adjust intake in response to the alterations of macronutrient and energy content of foods containing macronutrient substitutes.

REFERENCES

1. AMERICAN ACADEMY OF PEDIATRICS, COMMITTEE ON NUTRITION. 1992. Statement on cholesterol. Pediatrics **90**: 469–473.
2. GAULL, G. E. 1995. Pediatric dietary lipid guidelines: A policy analysis. J. Am. Coll. Nutr. **14**: 411–418.
3. SIGMAN-GRANT, M., S. ZIMMERMAN & P. M. KRIS-ETHERTON. 1993. Dietary approaches for reducing fat intake of preschool-age children. Pediatrics **91**: 955–960.
4. FISHER, J. A. & L. L. BIRCH. 1995. 3–5 year-old children's fat preferences and fat consumption are related to parental adiposity. J. Am. Diet. Assoc. **95**: 759–764.
5. ANDERSON, G. H., S. SARAVIS, R. SCHACHER, S. ZLOTKIN & L. A. LEITER. 1989. Aspartame: Effect on lunch-time food intake, appetite and hedonic response in children. Appetite **13**: 93–103.
6. ROLLS, B. J., S. KIM, A. L. MCNELIS, M. W. FISCHMAN, R. W. FOLTIN & T. H. MORAN. 1991. Time course of effects of preloads high in fat or carbohydrate on food intake and hunger ratings in humans. Am. J. Physiol. **260**: R756–R763.
7. BIRCH, L. L. & M. DEYSHER. 1986. Caloric compensation and sensory specific satiety: Evidence for self regulation of food intake by young children. Appetite **7**: 323–331.
8. FOMAN, S. J. 1993. Nutrition of Normal Infants. Mosby-Year Book, Inc. St. Louis, MO.
9. GUSTAFSON-LARSON, A. M. & R. D. TERRY. 1992. Weight-related behaviors and concerns of fourth-grade children. J. Am. Diet. Assoc. **92**: 818–822.
10. BIRCH, L. L. & M. DEYSHER. 1985. Conditioned and unconditioned caloric compensation: Evidence for self regulation of food intake by young children. Learn. Motiv. **16**: 341–355.
11. BIRCH, L. L., L. MCPHEE & S. SULLIVAN. 1989. Children's food intake following drinks sweetened with sucrose or aspartame: Time course effects. Physiol. & Behav. **45**: 387–396.
12. BIRCH, L. L., L. MCPHEE, L. STEINBERG & S. SULLIVAN. 1990. Conditioned flavor preferences in young children. Physiol. & Behav. **47**: 501–505.
13. SCLAFANI, A. 1995. How food preferences are learned: Laboratory animal models. Proc. Nutr. Soc. **54**: 419–427.
14. BOOTH, D. A. 1985. Food-conditioned eating preferences and aversions with interoceptive elements: Conditioned appetites and satieties. Ann. N.Y. Acad. Sci. **443**: 22–41.
15. BIRCH, L. L., L. MCPHEE, B. C. SHOBA, L. STEINBERG & R. KREHBIEL. 1987. "Clean up your plate": Effects of child feeding practices on the conditioning of meal size. Learn. Motiv. **18**: 301–317.

16. JOHNSON, S. L. & L. L. BIRCH. 1994. Parents' and children's adiposity and eating style. Pediatrics **94:** 653-661.
17. BIRCH, L. L., L. S. MCPHEE, J. L. BRYANT & S. L. JOHNSON. 1993. Children's lunch intake: Effects of midmorning snacks varying in energy density and fat content. Appetite **20:** 83-94.
18. JOHNSON, S. L., L. MCPHEE & L. L. BIRCH. 1991. Conditioned preferences: Young children prefer flavors associated with high dietary fat. Physiol. & Behav. **50:** 1245-1251.
19. KERN, D. L., L. MCPHEE, J. FISHER, S. JOHNSON & L. L. BIRCH. 1993. The postingestive consequences of fat condition preferences for flavors associated with high dietary fat. Physiol. & Behav. **54:** 71-76.
20. BIRCH, L. L., S. L. JOHNSON, M. B. JONES & J. C. PETERS. 1993. Effects of a non-energy fat substitute on children's energy and macronutrient intake. Am. J. Clin. Nutr. **58:** 326-333.
21. BIRCH, L. L., S. L. JOHNSON, G. ANDRESEN, J. C. PETERS & M. C. SCHULTE. 1991. The variability of young children's energy intake. N. Engl. J. Med. **324:** 232-235.
22. FOMON, S. J., L. J. FILER, JR., L. N. THOMAS, R. R. ROGERS & A. M. PROKSCH. 1969. Relationship between formula concentration and rate of growth in normal infants. J. Nutr. **98:** 241-254.
23. FOMON, S. J., L. J. FILER, JR., L. N. THOMAS, T. A. ANDERSON & S. E. NELSON. 1975. Influence of formula concentration on caloric intake and growth of normal infants. Acta Pediatr. Scand. **64:** 172-181.

Beyond Calories: Other Benefits of Macronutrient Substitutes

Effects on Chronic Disease

JUDY S. HANNAH [a]

*Medlantic Research Institute
108 Irving Street N.W.
Washington, DC 20010*

It is well accepted that caloric restriction and weight loss will improve metabolic parameters associated with several chronic diseases. Caloric restriction followed by weight loss will generally reduce LDL and increase HDL cholesterol in hypercholesterolemic subjects, thereby reducing the risk of heart disease. Similarly, hyperglycemia in noninsulin-dependent diabetes (NIDDM) can be improved by weight loss and will result in reductions in medication for many diabetic patients. Yet, many studies, especially in the area of cardiovascular disease, show lipid-lowering effects with low-fat diets independent of any effects on weight. Improvements in lipoprotein concentrations occur when saturated fat calories are replaced with carbohydrate, independent of weight change. Cardiovascular disease, diabetes, and cancer were selected for this review because these three diseases are major contributors to morbidity and mortality in this country, and, in each case, dietary fat has been implicated. The effects of macronutrient substitution on these chronic diseases will be examined using low-fat diets as a model, and evidence for the role of fat substitution or elimination in both the prevention and treatment of these diseases will be presented.

LIPIDS AND ATHEROSCLEROSIS

The data are very strong that macronutrient substitution for fat results in lipid lowering. An elevation in LDL cholesterol is considered to be one of the major risk factors for the development of atherosclerosis.[1] Therefore, cholesterol lowering is the goal, with dietary treatment as the first choice of therapy. The National Cholesterol Education Program (NCEP), first published in 1988 and updated in 1993, developed a primary prevention policy designed to identify people at risk for coronary heart disease and help them to reduce their risk.[2,3] Recommendations of the NCEP have resulted in a standard of care aimed to treat individuals with elevated cholesterol equal to or above 240 mg/dL or an LDL cholesterol of 160 mg/dL or greater. The dietary recommendations urge a reduction in total fat intake to 30%, with an emphasis on lowering the intake of saturated fat to 10% and dietary cholesterol to less than 300 mg/day. If LDL cholesterol is not sufficiently lowered by the step 1 diet, then a more rigorous diet of < 7% saturated fat and 200 mg/day cholesterol is recommended.

---

[a] Tel: (202) 877-5885; fax: (202) 877-3209; e-mail: jsh3@mhg.edu.

It is quite possible that future recommendations could focus on lower total or saturated fat intake. Specifically reducing saturated fat intake is the most important dietary change to achieve LDL cholesterol lowering.

Two early primary prevention trials conducted in this country, the Multiple Risk Factor Intervention Trial (MRFIT) and the Lipid Research Clinics Coronary Primary Prevention Trial (LRC-CPPT), showed that cholesterol lowering through diet intervention reduced the risk of heart disease.[4,5] The dietary recommendations in MRFIT were broad and included a reduction in saturated fat first to 10% and then later to 8% of calories, a reduction in cholesterol to 300 then later to 250 mg/day, and an increase in polyunsaturated fat to 10% of calories.[4] The LRC-CPPT was a pharmacologic intervention study, but the control arm used a diet designed to lower cholesterol 3-5% by decreasing saturated fat and cholesterol intake. This produced decreases in LDL cholesterol of 22 mg/dL during the screening phase of the study, and of 14 mg/dL in men who were later randomized to the trial.[5] The OSLO Diet Antismoking Study was one of the more successful dietary studies, with a 13% cholesterol lowering in the intervention group.[6] The results of a recently completed multicenter feeding study on cholesterol-lowering diets, the DELTA Study, should provide important new information on the effectiveness of diet in a well-controlled situation.[7] Based on the results of these studies and subsequent metaanalyses of a number of studies, the risk of heart disease is expected to be reduced 2% by a 1% reduction in LDL cholesterol.[8,9]

A number of studies have shown not only improvements in lipids and rates of coronary heart disease (CHD) events but also a reduction in the progression of atherosclerosis, and, in some cases, regression of coronary artery disease.[10-12] Reduced stenosis, which is assessed in a variety of ways, generally has correlated with LDL cholesterol lowering, that is, the greater the lowering, the greater the regression. The most positive dietary regression trial was the Diet Lifestyle Study.[10] CHD patients had decreased stenosis when following a low-fat, vegetarian diet with moderate exercise, whereas patients without the dietary intervention had increased stenosis with progression of disease ($p < 0.001$). Because this was a combined diet and exercise program with a relatively strict diet and highly motivated patients, there was a 10 kg weight loss in the treated group. Similarly, Watts et al.[11] showed an increase in coronary luminal diameter and in mean segment widths following a low-fat diet, and Schuler et al.[12] reported that regular exercise and a low-fat diet slowed the progression of coronary disease or reversed it in 77% of the patients versus 52% of the control group after one year. Thus, low-fat diets appear to be effective in preventing heart disease and in reversing atherosclerosis.

Lipid lowering in patients with CHD has been shown recently to reduce mortality from heart disease. These are studies in which pharmacologic agents were used; presumably low-fat diets would also be expected to reduce mortality if the lipid-lowering effect were as large and sustained.[13-15] Two dietary lifestyle interventions have shown reductions in mortality. A 10.5-year follow-up of the MRFIT participants showed a 24% reduction in mortality due to acute myocardial infarction in the treatment group,[16] and the Oslo Study showed a reduction in mortality following treatment after 11 years.[17]

STUDIES ON SUCROSE POLYESTER

There is also the early work using sucrose polyester (SPE), a fat substitute, showing improvements in lipoprotein concentrations in hypercholesterolemic patients. Olestra or Olean, as SPE is being marketed, was originally investigated for use as a lipid-lowering aid for hypercholesterolemic patients. Both 16 and 32 g/day doses of SPE, substituted for an olive oil spread,[18] were found to lower LDL cholesterol by 4-5% in subjects with moderately elevated cholesterol. At the higher dose, mild gastrointestinal side effects were associated with consumption of the product. In another study,[19] one in which the lipid-lowering effects of SPE were examined in obese hypercholesterolemic subjects, LDL cholesterol was reduced by 16% and triglycerides by 20%, both of which were significantly different from the group treated with a low-fat diet alone. In these and most of the SPE studies, lipid lowering was independent of weight loss. Sucrose polyester lowers blood levels of cholesterol in part by reducing its absorption; each gram of SPE increases the excretion of cholesterol 1.3%.[20] Inasmuch as reducing saturated fat intake generally lowers LDL cholesterol on the order of 10%, the use of SPE products may enhance cholesterol lowering through reduced absorption. However, the lipid lowering associated with this specific product, which received FDA approval for use in a limited number of snack foods, may not be duplicated with other fat substitutes.

DIABETES

Two separate issues concerning NIDDM can be influenced by macronutrient substitution: the onset of diabetes and the degree of glycemic control. The prevalence rate for NIDDM is now estimated to be 3.1% in the U.S. population, a threefold increase over the last 35 years.[21] The increasing prevalence of diabetes and the comorbid conditions associated with it, such as CHD, is a major public health concern.

As in the case of heart disease, the primary objective is to prevent diabetes. There is a strong interrelationship between fat intake, obesity, and occurrence of diabetes, and weight loss is desirable for both the prevention of diabetes and its treatment. The effect of a multifaceted approach of weight loss, dietary modification, and exercise will be examined in a recently initiated large multicenter intervention, the Diabetes Prevention Program. Weight loss is the primary objective for the lifestyle change in this program, so it may not be possible to separate the effects of weight loss from a reduction in fat intake.

The consumption of low-fat or fat-free items may, however, improve insulin resistance independent of weight loss. A number of studies have shown that a high intake of dietary fat is correlated with increased fasting insulin, yet most of these studies are cross-sectional in which obesity is also highly correlated.[22-25] Some of the strongest evidence for an independent contribution from dietary fat is from a study in which fat intake, obtained in 24-hour recalls from subjects with impaired glucose tolerance, was shown to be associated with a greater likelihood of developing diabetes. The odds ratio was 6.0 in subjects with the highest fat intake.[26] In addition to these data, the incidence of diabetes in genetically predisposed Native American groups indicates that diet plays a role in the development of diabetes.[27] Native Americans living in Mexico do not have anywhere near the rates of disease as those living in Arizona. However, dietary fat intake and weight cannot be separated in this study.

The type of fat consumed may also affect insulin resistance. Vessby et al.[29] and Storlein et al.[28] found that higher-tissue polyunsaturated fat content is related to increased insulin sensitivity. Therefore, the onset of diabetes may be associated with dietary fat intake.

Previously, low-fat diets have been recommended by the American Diabetes Association for the treatment of diabetic patients.[30] Current guidelines call for a more liberal dietary fat intake in diabetics with elevated triglycerides; however, the consumption of saturated fat is discouraged because it is linked to an increased risk for cardiovascular disease. Thus its avoidance is especially important for diabetic patients. Mortality attributed to CHD is 1.5- to 3-fold higher in diabetics compared to the general population. Although the exact mechanisms for the increased risk for coronary disease in diabetic patients are unknown, one risk factor is the dyslipemia of diabetes, characterized by elevated triglycerides and decreased HDL.[31] The effect of a low-fat, high-fiber diet versus a high-saturated fat diet was examined in 24 diabetic subjects to determine the effects on glucose tolerance, glucose-mediated disposal, and cholesterol concentrations. The diets were fed for 14 days, each in a cross-over design, and were isocaloric.[32] On the high-fat diet, glucose tolerance decreased ($p < 0.01$), and cholesterol concentrations increased ($p < 0.02$). Other metabolic parameters associated with diabetes also deteriorated, indicating that diabetic control and lipid profiles in diabetic patients are improved on a low-fat, high-fiber diet. Therefore, low-fat diets lower cholesterol and may improve glycemic control in diabetic patients.

There is a single study of obese and diabetic patients to whom SPE was given in a 1000-calorie very low-fat diet (period II).[33] Treatment lowered LDL cholesterol 20% in the subjects with normal lipids. Sucrose polyester lowered triglycerides in patients with hypertriglyceridemia, but this lowering was similar to that for the calorie-restricted diet (period III), although more weight loss occurred in period III than II so that exact comparisons are difficult.

In summary, low-fat diets may help prevent or delay the onset of diabetes, independent of weight loss, as well as aid in the treatment of NIDDM. This is especially likely if the diets are also high in fiber.

CANCER

Two of the cancers most commonly reported to be associated with dietary fat intake are colon and breast. Breast cancer is the most prevalent cancer in women, and colorectal cancer is generally listed as the second or third most common type of cancer. Therefore, because incidence of both of these cancers is quite high, the relation with diet is a major public health concern.

Theories of a diet-cancer connection evolved from epidemiological studies showing that increased rates of breast cancer were associated with increased fat consumption.[34] This association has been used to project that a 50% reduction in fat intake could lead to a 2.5-fold reduction in the incidence of breast cancer and a 3-fold reduction in colon cancer.[35] Yet recent reports of the relation between dietary fat and breast cancer risk in postmenopausal women are mixed. A brief review of the literature suggests that the early reports, which were primarily case-control studies,[36,37] found stronger correlations or risk ratios than the more recent prospective studies. The recent studies report risk ratios slightly above 1.0, while the confidence interval commonly includes 1.0.[38,39] Thus, there is currently no conclusive prospective evidence to show that dietary fat intake increases the risk of breast cancer.

The incidence of colon cancer is more strongly linked with dietary factors than is breast. In several prospective trials, a relation between an increased occurrence of colon cancer was associated with a high-fat, low-fiber diet.[40-42] Similar results have been reported in studies in which foods groups, not nutrients, were analyzed. A lower risk of colon cancer was associated with high intakes of fruits and vegetables and low meat consumption in these reports.[43] Thus, a low-fat diet could reduce the risk of developing colon cancer, and studies are currently in progress to examine this issue.

The largest study ever to be conducted in women, the Women's Health Initiative, includes a dietary modification trial designed to determine whether the long-term consumption of a 20% fat diet will reduce the incidence of breast and/or colon cancer as well as heart disease. This primary prevention trial was preceded by two feasibility studies showing that it was possible to instruct women to follow a low-fat diet and make long-term modifications. Both the Nutrition Adjuvant Study and Women's Health Trials showed that it was possible for women to reduce their fat intake by 40-50% and maintain the reduction for up to two years.[44,45] Yet, despite the amount of fat eliminated in these studies, only an average of 3.5 kg weight loss occurred. Preliminary results from the Women's Health Initative show a weight loss of 2.4 kg by the end of the first year of diet intervention, when most of the weight loss would be expected to occur. Thus, an important result of this study will be the separation of the effects of caloric restriction from fat intake on cancer incidence.

Whether a reduction in fat intake will improve the prognosis of subjects with cancer or help prevent the recurrence of cancer is also currently under investigation.[44] The Women's Intervention Nutrition Study is using a 15% fat diet in combination with tamoxifen to determine whether a low-fat diet will decrease breast cancer recurrence and increase survival.[46] Two thousand women will participate for five years. Similarly, the Polyp Prevention Trial is studying 2000 men and women with a history of cancerous polyps, to determine whether a 20% fat diet containing 18 g of dietary fiber diet will reduce the recurrence of disease.[44] Whether significant weight loss occurred in either of these studies is not yet known, but is unlikely; thus the results should clarify the effects of dietary fat reduction in cancer patients. Although there is currently little evidence to support the conclusion that a low-fat diet will prevent the development of, or the recurrence of, cancer, there is no data to suggest that it might be harmful.

In summary, when a low-fat diet is consumed, there is generally an increase in dietary fiber intake, vitamins and minerals, all of which are positive. Therefore, even without significant weight loss, consuming a low-fat diet can generally have positive effects on health without any negative ones.

REFERENCES

1. LOWERING BLOOD CHOLESTEROL TO PREVENT HEART DISEASE: NIH CONSENSUS DEVELOPMENT CONFERENCE STATEMENT. 1985. Arteriosclerosis **5:** 404-412.

2. NCEP EXPERT PANEL. 1988. Report of the National Cholesterol Education Program expert panel on detection, evaluation, and treatment of high blood cholesterol in adults. Arch. Intern. Med. **148:** 36-39.
3. SUMMARY OF THE SECOND REPORT OF THE NATIONAL CHOLESTEROL EDUCATION PROGRAM (NCEP) EXPERT PANEL ON DETECTION, EVALUATION, AND TREATMENT OF HIGH BLOOD CHOLESTEROL IN ADULTS (ADULT TREATMENT PANEL II). 1993. J. Am. Med. Assoc. **269:** 3015-3023.
4. DOLECEK, T. A., N. C. MILAS, L. V. VAN HORN, M. E. FARRAND, D. D. GORDER, A. G. DUCHENE, J. R. DYER, P. A. STONE & B. L. RANDALL. 1986. A long-term nutrition intervention experience: Lipid responses and dietary adherence patterns in the Multiple Risk Factor Intervention Trial. J. Am. Diet. Assoc. **86:** 752-758.
5. GLUECK, C. J., D. J. GORDON, J. J. NELSON, C. E. DAVIS & H. A. TYRPLER. 1986. Dietary and other correlates of changes in total and low density lipoprotein cholesterol in hypercholesterolemic men: The Lipid Research Clinics Coronary Primary Prevention Trial. Am. J. Clin. Nutr. **44:** 489-500.
6. HJERMANN, I., I. HOLME, K. V. BYRE & P. LEREN. 1981. Effects of diet and smoking intervention on the incidence of coronary heart disease. Report from the Oslo study group of a randomized trial in healthy men. Lancet **11:** 1303-1310.
7. GINSBERG, H. 1995. New directions in dietary studies and heart disease: The National Heart, Lung and Blood Institute sponsored multicenter study of diet effects on lipoproteins and thrombogenic activity. Adv. Exp. Med. Biol. **369:** 241-247.
8. HOLME, I. 1990. An analysis of randomized trials evaluating the effect of cholesterol reduction on total mortality and coronary heart disease incidence. Circulation **82:** 1916-1924.
9. MULDOON, M. F., S. B. MANUCK & K. A. MATTHEWS. 1990. Lowering cholesterol concentrations and mortality: A quantitative review of primary prevention trials. Br. Med. J. **301:** 309-314.
10. ORNISH, D., S. E. BROWN, L. W. SCHERWITZ, J. H. BILLINGS, W. T. ARMSTRONG, T. A. PORTS, S. M. MCLANAHAN, R. L. KIRKEEIDE, R. J. BRAND & K. L. GOULD. 1990. Can lifestyle changes reverse coronary heart disease. The Lifestyle Heart Trial. Lancet **336:** 129-133.
11. WATTS, G. F., B. LEWIS, J. N. H. BRUNT, E. S. LEWIS, D. J. COLTART, L. D. R. SMITH, J. I. MANN & A. V. SWAN. 1992. Effects on coronary artery disease of lipid-lowering diet, or diet plus cholestyramine, in the St Thomas' Atherosclerosis Regression Study (STARS). Lancet **339:** 563-569.
12. SCHELER, G., R. HAMBRECHT, G. SCHLIERF, J. NIEBAUER, K. HAUER, J. NEUMANN, E. HOBERG, A. DRINKMANN, F. BACHER, M. GRUNZE & W. KUBER. 1992. Regular physical exercise and low-fat diet: Effects on progression of coronary artery disease. Circulation **86:** 1-11.
13. SCANDINAVIAN SIMVASTATIN SURVIVAL STUDY GROUP. 1994. Randomized trial of cholesterol lowering in 4444 patients with coronary heart disease: The Scandinavian Simvastatin Survival Study. Lancet **344:** 1383-1389.
14. SHEPARD, J., S. M. COBBE, I. FORD, C. G. ISLES, A. R. LORIMER, P. W. MACFARLANE, J. H. MCKILLOP & C. J. PACKARD. 1995. Prevention of coronary heart disease with pravastatin in men with hypercholesterolemia. N. Engl. J. Med. **333:** 1301-1307.
15. SACKS, F. M., M. A. PFEFFER, L. A. MOYE, J. L. ROULEAU, J. D. RUTHERFORD, T. G. COLE, L. BROWN, J. W. WARNICA, J. M. O. ARNOLD, C-C. WUN, B. R. DAVIS & E. BRAUNWALD FOR THE CARE TRIAL INVESTIGATORS. 1996. The effect of pravastatin on coronary events after myocardial infarction in patients with average cholesterol levels. N. Engl. J. Med. **335:** 1001-1009.
16. MORTALITY RATES AFTER 10.5 YEARS FOR PARTICIPANTS IN THE MULTIPLE RISK FACTOR INTERVENTION TRIAL. 1990. Findings related to a priori hypotheses of the trial. The Multiple Risk Factor Intervention Trial Research Group. J. Am. Med. Assoc. **263:** 1795-1801.

17. LEREN, P. 1970. The Oslo Diet-Heart Study: Eleven Year Report. Circulation **42:** 935–942.
18. MELLIES, M. J., R. J. JANDACEK, J. D. TAULBEE, M. B. TEWKSBURY, G. LAMKIN, L. BAEHLER, P. KING, D. BOGGS, S. GOLDMAN, A. GOUGE, R. TSANG & C. J. GLUECK. 1983. A double-blind, placebo-controlled study of sucrose polyester in hypercholesterolemic outpatients. Am. J. Clin. Nutr. **37:** 339–346.
19. MELLIES, M. J., C. VITALE, R. J. JANDACEK, G. LAMKIN & C. J. GLUECK. 1985. The substitution of sucrose polyester for dietary fat in obese, hypercholesterolemic outpatients. Am. J. Clin. Nutr. **41:** 1–12.
20. GLUECK, C. J., R. J. JANDACEK, M. T. R. SUBBIAH, L. GALLON, R. YUNKER, C. ALLEN, E. HOGG & P. M. LASKARZEWSKI. 1980. Effect of sucrose polyester on fecal bile acid excretion and composition in normal men. Am. J. Clin. Nutr. **33:** 2177–2181.
21. KENNEY, S., R. E. AUBERT & L. S. GEISS. 1995. Prevalence and incidence of non-insulin-dependent diabetes. *In* Diabetes in America, 2. NIH Publication No. 95-1468.
22. LOVEJOY, J. & M. DIGIROLAMO. 1992. Habitual dietary intake and insulin sensitivity in lean and obese adults. Am. J. Clin. Nutr. **55:** 1174–1179.
23. MAYER, E. J., B. NEWMAN, C. P. QUESENBERRY & J. V. SELBY. 1993. Usual dietary fat intake and insulin concentrations in healthy women twins. Diabetes Care **16:** 1459–1469.
24. FESKENS, E. J. M., J. G. LOEBER & D. KROMHOUT. 1994. Diet and physical activity as determinants of hyperinsulinemia: The Zutphen elderly study. Am. J. Epidemiol. **140:** 350–360.
25. WARD, K. D., D. SPARROW, P. S. VOKONAS, W. C. WILLETT, L. LANDSBERG & S. T. WEISS. 1994. The relationships of abdominal obesity, hyperinsulinemia and saturated fat intake to serum lipid levels: The Normative Aging Study. Int. J. Obesity Related Metab. Disord. **18:** 137–144.
26. MARSHALL, J. A., S. HOAG, S. SHETTERLY & R. F. HAMMAN. 1994. Dietary fat predicts conversion from impaired glucose tolerance to NIDDM. Diabetes Care **17:** 50–56.
27. RAVUSSIN, E., M. E. VALENCIA, J. ESPARZA, P. H. BENNETT & L. O. SCHULZ. 1994. Effects of a traditional lifestyle on obesity in Pima Indians. Diabetes Care **17:** 1067–1074.
28. BORKMAN, M., L. H. STORLIEN, D. A. PAN, A. B. JENKINS, D. J. CHISHOLM & L. V. CAMPBELL. 1993. The relation between insulin sensitivity and the fatty-acid composition of skeletal-muscle phospholipids. N. Engl. J. Med. **328:** 238–244.
29. VESSBY, B., S. TENGBLAD & H. LITHELL. 1994. Insulin sensitivity is related to the fatty acid composition of serum lipids and skeletal muscle phospholipids in 70-year-old men. Diabetologia **37:** 1044–1050.
30. NUTRITION RECOMMENDATIONS AND PRINCIPLES FOR PEOPLE WITH DIABETES MELLITUS. 1994. Diabetes Care **17:** 519–522.
31. HOWARD, B. V. 1987. Lipoprotein metabolism in diabetes mellitus. J. Lipid Res. **28:** 613–628.
32. SWINBURN, B. A., V. L. BOYCE, R. N. BERGMAN, B. V. HOWARD & C. BOGARDUS. 1991. Deterioration in carbohydrate metabolism and lipoprotein changes induced by modern, high fat diet in Pima Indians and Caucasians. J. Clin. Endocrinol. Metab. **73:** 156–165.
33. GRUNDY, S. M., J. V. ANASTASIA, Y. A. KESANIEMI & J. ABRAMS. 1986. Influence of sucrose polyester on plasma lipoproteins, and cholesterol metabolism in obese patients with and without diabetes mellitus. Am. J. Clin. Nutr. **44:** 620–629.
34. HOWE, G. R. 1994. Dietary fat and breast cancer risks. An epidemiological perspective. Cancer **74:** 1078–1084.
35. PRENTICE, R. L., M. PEPE & S. G. SELF. 1989. A quantitative assessment of the epidemiological literature and a discussion of methodological issues. Cancer Res. **49:** 3147–3156.
36. HOWE, G. R., C. M. FRIEDENREICH, M. JAIN & A. B. MILLER. 1991. A cohort study of fat intake and risk of breast cancer. J. Natl. Cancer Inst. **83:** 336–340.
37. HOWE, G. R., T. HIROHATA, T. G. HISLOP, J. M. ISCOVICH, J-M. YUAN, K. KATSOUYANNI, F. LUBIN, E. MARUBINI, B. MODAN, T. ROHAN, P. TONIOLO & Y. SHUNZHANG. 1990. (Review) Dietary factors and risk of breast cancer: Combined analysis of 12 case-control studies. J. Natl. Cancer Inst. **82:** 561–569.

38. Willett, W. C., D. J. Hunter, M. J. Stampfer, G. Colditz, J. E. Manson, D. Spiegelman, B. Rosner, C. H. Hennekens & F. E. Speizer. 1992. Dietary fat and fiber in relation to risk of breast cancer. J. Am. Med. Assoc. **268:** 2037-2044.
39. Boyd, N. F., L. J. Martin, M. Noffel, G. A. Lockwood & D. L. Trichler. 1993. A meta-analysis of studies of dietary fat and breast cancer risk. Br. J. Cancer **68:** 627-636.
40. Giovannucci, E., M. J. Stampfer, G. Colditz, E. B. Rimm & W. C. Willett. 1992. Relationships of diet to risk of colorectal adenoma in men. J. Natl. Cancer Inst. **84:** 91-98.
41. Neugut, A. I., G. C. Garbowski, W. C. Lee, T. Murray, J. W. Nieves, K. A. Forde, M. R. Treat, J. D. Waye & C. Fenoglio-Preiser. 1993. Dietary risk factors for the incidence and recurrence of colorectal adenomatous polyps. Ann. Intern. Med. **118:** 91-95.
42. Thun, M. J., E. E. Calle, M. M. Namboodiri, W. D. Flanders, R. J. Coates, T. Byers, P. Boffetta, L. Garfinkel & C. W. Heath, Jr. 1993. Risk factors for fatal colon cancer in a large prospective study. J. Natl. Cancer Inst. **84:** 1491-1500.
43. Willett, W. C., M. J. Stampfer, G. Colditz, B. Rosner & F. E. Speizer. 1990. Relation of meat, fat, and fiber intake to the risk of colon cancer in a prospective study among women. N. Engl. J. Med. **323:** 1664-1672.
44. Chlebowski, R. & M. Grosvenor. 1994. The scope of nutrition intervention trials with cancer-related endpoints. Cancer **74:** 2734-2738.
45. Henderson, M. M., L. H. Kushi, D. J. Thompson, S. L. Gorbach, C. K. Clifford, W. Insull, M. Moskowitz & R. S. Thompson. 1990. Feasibility of a randomized trial of a low-fat diet for the prevention of breast cancer: Dietary compliance in the Women's Health Trial Vanguard Study. Prev. Med. **19:** 115-133.
46. Chlebowski, R., G. L. Blackburn, I. M. Buzzard, D. P. Rose, S. Martino, J. D. Khandekar, R. M. York, R. W. Jeffery, R. M. Elashoff & E. L. Wynder. 1993. Adherence to a dietary fat intake reduction program in postmenopausal women receiving therapy for early breast cancer. J. Clin. Oncol. **11:** 2072-2080.

Observations on the Conference Proceedings and Future Research Directions

Luncheon Remarks

CUTBERTO GARZA [a]

Division of Nutritional Sciences
Cornell University
127 Savage Hall
Ithaca, New York 14853-0001

Much of what I am going to say will focus on what I think we don't know. A lot of good data have been presented. I want to thank both the organizers and the speakers for providing much food for thought. I also want to thank the food industry, because many of the technological advances it has made have given individuals like myself an opportunity to think about questions that otherwise may never have come to mind regarding nutrient metabolism and the well-being of our population. For those advances and for showing how quickly it can respond, thank you. It is in this spirit, then, that I will raise some issues and questions.

The first speaker yesterday, Harvey Anderson, listed three major reasons for holding this conference. The first was to consider the rationale for dietary change. The second was to think about the problems in achieving dietary change; I assume he meant both behavioral and metabolic. When we think of barriers to change, most of us focus primarily on behavioral aspects of those barriers. We probably should think also about the types of metabolic issues that were raised throughout the conference. The third reason was to explore the nutritional aspects of macronutrient substitutions. Again, I am assuming that this included both normal adaptive responses, as well as toxicology, although we did not spend a lot of time on toxicological issues.

What Dr. Anderson did not, perhaps, say, because for this audience it is very obvious, but it is not obvious to me, is that there is a special character of macronutrient substitutes that goes beyond characteristics usually associated with food additives. When I think of a food additive, I think of something that one adds to a food to improve the food itself or in the way that it functions. With macronutrient substitutes, the target isn't the food, it is the consumer. Although some speakers were thinking of macronutrient substitutes as food additives, in actuality we are dealing with something quite different. Because the consumer is the target, from my perspective, there is an implied warranty, whether it is explicit or implicit. The implied warranty is that it will be good for their health. Thus we should focus on the predictors of benefit and of risk.

---

[a] Tel: (607) 254-5144; fax: (607) 255-1033; e-mail: cg30@cornell.edu.

Certainly from the regulatory perspective we seem to focus principally on predictors of risk, as opposed to predictors of benefit. We should look beyond factors that focus solely on safety. Throughout the conference I wondered whether we shouldn't search for analogous measures of benefit. That is, we would like to know the estimated exposure, much like we do for a food additive, but in the sense of the dietary changes predicted by the exposure and its potential for benefit as well as risk.

There is a need to understand the mechanisms by which putative benefits may occur. We need to understand the metabolism and pharmacokinetics of the substitutes, if it is partially absorbed, and of nutrients that are affected by them, the individual sensitivities, and the adequacy of the database.

Implicit in all of this is our ability to modify the environment and the food supply much more rapidly than Darwinian selection operates. I bring this up now because the ability of similar genotypes to be expressed as diverse phenotypes in different environments was mentioned several times. I'm not certain that traditional diets will be as profitable to our health under the present environment as they were under the environmental conditions under which traditional diets developed. Although we were warned by some speakers about "techno-fixes," we should not shy away from the technology; rather, we ought to recognize that there is a great need to understand, and to proceed cautiously as our understanding improves.

Therefore, as we examine the rationale for dietary change, obviously there are some strong reasons for improving energy balance. However, I confess that I was confused by some of the presentations. Whether one looked at animal or human data, there seemed to be little doubt that one is more likely to overeat when the energy density of the diet is high. Then, somehow the association between energy density and fat was related to the putative role of dietary fat in causing overeating. What wasn't clear to me was whether presenters were suggesting that high-energy diets tax the regulatory system beyond its ability to maintain a lower set-point for energy intake or whether overeating represents a hedonistic response of the type that Adam Drewnowski raised. Indeed, are they two totally unrelated possibilities?

If we push a set-point below a preexisting threshold by reducing the energy density of the diet, is it forever reset? Will individuals maintain an energy deficit for periods longer than benefits their health? Are we ready to add macronutrient substitutes to freely available foods because of the substitutes' anticipated benefits in reducing energy intakes as a public health strategy to help the 25% of individuals who are consuming, at least by weight standards, too much energy?

Understanding how long a new energy intake set-point is maintained is important. David Levitsky's comments were particularly important in this regard. Our limited understanding of this issue points out how little information we have. Unfortunately this is only one example of a broader problem. The overriding concept this raises is how little we know about what I and others call the biology of interventions.

We have very little difficulty understanding why nutrition is important from a basic biological perspective. We understand fat metabolism. We understand many aspects of energy metabolism from a molecular perspective. We understand the epidemiology of the problem from the perspective that we know who is overweight and where they are.

When we take that information and try to intervene, we run into a series of questions that often are unanswered, because we don't spend the needed resources on the biology of alternative interventions. Barbara Rolls presented some of the best set of questions that could fall under the heading of biology of interventions.

For example, because energy balance is one of the main issues, an omitted topic that came to mind was the role of the GI tract. I found this very surprising given its central role. Its omission left me perplexed.

Beyond the aim of reducing energy intake, macronutrient substitutes are promoted because they are expected to decrease fat intake. It wasn't clear to me if they are expected to reduce total fat or saturated fats. The reason this is important is because if we are to focus on a reduction in cardiovascular disease as a benefit, we miss the important message that reductions in saturated fats are possible. Thus strategies that are developed, if cardiovascular disease is of concern, should target specific fat substitutions, not only the reduction of total fat. In addition to intermediate indicators for cardiovascular disease, other outcomes that relate to specific fats may then become important markers of efficacy.

As I went through the two principal aims—improving energy balance and reducing fat, whether one looked at sugar or at fat substitutes—we seemed to be working under the implicit assumption that a public health strategy was the direction in which to go. This means we will not control their use or necessarily target it, but make substitutes accessible or available to the whole population.

Many of the questions that should be asked pertain to whether substitutes are to be targeted primarily for individuals at particular specified risks. In any case, it is important to consider both the absence of risk and the likelihood of benefit. Indeed, the reason for reducing energy balance, or the reason for changing or altering either total fat intake or the intake of specific fats, is related to specific pathologies.

It is incumbent upon us, to assure that this happens. Thus, postmarket surveillance, in terms of both problems that may emerge because of the use of these products, and the documentation of any benefits, seems appropriate.

Having said that, there is a basic assumption that is made by this strategy. We assume that removing something from a food and changing food patterns yield similar outcomes. The most convincing epidemiologic evidence we have relating diet to health is that there are certain food patterns that result in good outcomes. I have not seen any strong data that suggest that removing a specific component from a food results in the same outcomes. This was brought up by Dr. Katz when he pointed out that the benefits of fat reduction diets and related strategies are likely due to food patterns and thus to the total intake of macro- and micronutrients and other food constituents.

Does this mean that we ought to abandon this specific approach? No. Dr. Peters pointed out that this was one part of a larger package of alternatives. We must, however, be careful, in how this approach is promoted. For example, one aspect that has been left out is the very important physiological role of physical activity. There was some limited attention given to this topic in implementing this approach. I would like to come back to it.

Within the food industry, there are possibly three responses. One is the creation of a new molecule, such as olestra, for achieving better energy balance and/or for reducing dietary fat. The second is applying a new process to an old molecule: Simplesse is a good example of applying a new process to a molecule with which we have much experience. Third, one can expand the use of old processes and apply them to existing molecules; sorbitols and other sugar alcohols are examples of this.

Given that these are among the usual value-added responses industry can make, then we, as a nutrition community, should take the responsibility of examining broader responses and other strategies to achieve the same ends. As public citizens I would hope that the food industry would join us in the nutrition community's investigation of other strategies.

The second major issue we were asked to consider were the problems in achieving dietary change. I found it difficult to separate this from the third charge, that is, a consideration of the nutritional aspects of macronutrient substitutes. It is very difficult to completely separate biology and behavior. Separating biological responses from what people choose to do is particularly difficult in nutrition. Adam Drewnowski's presentation came closest to showing us how difficult this is.

Dr. Drewnowski's presentation suggests that the drive to higher fat intakes is inexorable and that this drive is transcultural, presumably because of the biological link to hedonistic responses we associate with fat. In fact, the preponderance of the evidence, as I mentioned earlier, would suggest that increasing energy density causes us to consume more, and the high correlation between energy density and fat content makes distinctions between these two food characteristics difficult.

One is struck by the heterogeneity of responses among any group of studies in terms of energy balance and the foods that are chosen to achieve it. What is surprising is that no one seemed to have done any follow-up, that is, to characterize subjects by their responsiveness and follow the two ends of any documented spectrum to see what accounts for the differences in responses. We have accepted the heterogeneity and missed wonderful biologic and behavioral opportunities to understand why it is that people respond so differently to apparently similar stimuli. We have accepted the heterogeneity and not pursued understanding the basic biology or the basic behaviors.

I also was struck by the small sample sizes on which we are willing to make public health policies or introduce foods for widespread use. I was struck, for example, by the many investigators who did studies on lean individuals, but chose not to document the voluntary and involuntary strategies used by individuals to stay lean. Part of the explanation of the observed heterogeneity may be explained by the fact that just because all subjects in any study were lean, does not mean that they are genetically or behaviorally comparable. We seem to be assuming a homogeneity in the face of heterogeneity by not pursuing more systematic approaches.

The limited understanding of short- and long-term strategies for maintaining every balance was also very clear. The best example I can offer you is the minimal amount of information we heard of the impact of the aerobic training state on fat oxidation. There are some very good (20- to 30-year-old) data, primarily from Swedish investigators, that show that the better your aerobic training state is, then the lower your RQ (respiratory quotient) is at any given workload. Yet whether investigators were studying Pima Indians or lean individuals in other circumstances, this very basic physical activity parameter was either not examined, or if it was, those data were not presented. We have to be much more careful to look at shorter-term, as well as longer-term strategies, with physical activity and aerobic training states being among strategies of high interest.

Another issue receiving surprisingly little comment was that available technology for detecting energy differences that are physiologically important probably does not exist. If one produced a 50- or 100-calorie intake difference by using macronutrient substitutes in a free-living situation, most dietary methodologies could not provide the needed degree of precision. We need to look much more carefully at the development of new methodologies as products of this type are brought onto the market, in order to better understand the outcomes from functional perspectives.

Another problem is our limited experience and the limited paradigms we have to deal with highly integrated systems. This problem became evident in a variety of ways. We seem to be stuck on reductionist approaches that work wonderfully in the basic sciences. Usually we are expert in isolating a single factor for study in a cell culture or in an animal model and then less expertly presume that one can extrapolate findings to the public arena. We commonly assume that there is such a high degree of external validity that such information is fully transferable and sufficient for action. If that were true, we should have eliminated cretinism and vitamin A blindness in the world. I assure you that we understand the basic biology of both conditions well. Translating that information, though, into the everyday world has proven very difficult.

Although discussants at this meeting stated that under real-life applications this information transfer may not occur, no one presented a systematic breakdown of what was meant by their assertions. Furthermore, there were some suggestions of how this problem could be approached, by observational studies, but no one suggested more sophisticated approaches for determining how integrated systems work. Possibly the best slide that illustrated this problem, although not quite addressed in this way, was from Dr. John Peters; it showed unspecified interactions between genotype and behavior, ending in some sort of functional phenotype.

We therefore tended to focus primarily on "a lumps and bumps type" of physiology, that overemphasizes weight. Several of you made that comment, and I couldn't agree more that more subtle issues require investigation.

Another unaddressed issue is the database and the system that we now have for collecting national dietary information. Many of the questions that I and others raised require an examination of the tails of intake distributions. That is, What are the top and the bottom 5% of our population doing?

We don't have a monitoring system that can provide this type of information, especially if we want to know what subpopulations within our general population are doing. Many issues are not the same for the elderly and the young.

Yet if we are to understand how food patterns are changing and understand how they are affecting the spectrum of changes in health, then having a much better focus on the upper and lower percentiles will be increasingly important. At the present time getting to this level of precision is difficult.

Thus, the current approach of proceeding with caution and limiting the use of new macronutrient substitutes is probably good. I don't think that there is any reason, at least that I heard regarding nutritional implications, to totally restrict the use of these substances. Under the present regulatory scheme used by the FDA, we choose intentionally to err on the side of caution. We should expand postmarket surveillance, in ways that go beyond detecting realized risks, by looking much more carefully at the benefits that we anticipate from this intervention, and by focusing on intermediate indicators to the degree possible.

A third point is that the food industry, with the academic and health care communities, must look at these products as part of a menu of strategies that can be used to achieve health aims related to energy balance and fat intake. We cannot portray macronutrient substitutes as the only solution to either achieving improved energy balance or reducing fat intakes. That was said by a number of presenters, and I applaud this view.

It also is important to reserve the right to be smarter tomorrow than we are today, which means that we need to make sure that research on the various issues raised at this conference is sponsored. We should keep in mind that appromixately 30% of all preventable mortalities in the United States are related to diet and physical activity. Thus there is an enormous opportunity to deal with excess mortality in this country if we get smarter about applying what we know.

The use of macronutrient substitutes is a potentially important strategy. I say *potentially*, because we don't understand the basic biology as well as we should, nor do we understand the biology of intervention as well as we should. The cautious, limited introduction of these products into the current food system permits us the opportunities to look at relevant issues in a responsible way.

Poster Papers

Replacement of Dietary Fat with Fat-free Margarine Alters Vitamin E Storage in Rats

G. V. MITCHELL,[a] E. GRUNDEL,[b] AND
M. Y. JENKINS [c]

*Office of Food Labeling
Center for Food Safety and Applied Nutrition
U.S. Food and Drug Administration
Laurel, Maryland 20708*

The popularity of reduced-fat and fat-free foods has increased among consumers. Some of the high-fat foods (*e.g.*, fats and oils) for which fat-modified alternatives are available are rich sources of vitamin E in the diet. The potential impact of the consumption of fat-modified or fat-free products on the intake and utilization of vitamin E has yet to be clarified. The purpose of this study was to determine the nutritional effects of replacing a high-fat margarine product containing vitamin E with a fat-free margarine in the diets of rats. Fats used in traditional margarines provide 13% of the total α-tocopherol equivalents in the American diet.[1]

Young male (74 ± 0.3 g) and female (70 ± 0.7 g) Sprague Dawley rats (Harlan Sprague Dawley, Indianapolis, IN) were used. Food and water were available ad libitum throughout the study. Rats (10/group) were fed for six weeks a modified American Institute of Nutrition 76 diet containing blends of soybean oil-vitamin E stripped (SO) and vegetable oil spread (VOS) (4.8%: 1.75% and 3%: 4.38%) or diets with the VOS portion replaced by comparable amounts (by weight) of fat-free margarine. The α-tocopherol content in the VOS diets provided a marginally adequate vitamin E intake (33 mg of α-tocopherol per kg). The dietary fat (TABLE 1) and α-tocopherol levels (22-33 mg/kg) of the diets varied as a result of the replacement. The fat-free margarine product was composed of a blend of water, mono- and diglycerides, gelatin, and carbohydrate. At six weeks, food was withheld overnight, and rats were then anesthetized. Plasma α-tocopherol was extracted with hexane.[2] Tissue samples (0.5-1.0 g) were extracted with 2 mL of ethanol and 10 mL of methylene chloride. All α-tocopherol samples were analyzed by HPLC using a fluorescence detector (excitation and emission wavelengths, 290 and 330 nm).

Male rats fed diets containing fat-free margarine consumed significantly more food than the corresponding VOS groups (TABLE 1). The male rats adjusted their food intakes to compensate for the reduced content of dietary energy. The mean food intakes of female rats fed fat-free margarine diets were not significantly different

---

[a] Tel: (301) 594-5829; fax: (301) 594-0517; e-mail: gum@cfsan.fda.gov.
[b] Tel: (301) 594-5819; fax: (301) 594-0517; e-mail: exg@cfsan.fda.gov.
[c] Tel: (301) 594-5830; fax: (301) 594-0517; e-mail: myj@cfsan.fda.gov.

TABLE 1. Food, Energy, and α-Tocopherol Intakes in Male and Female Rats[a]

		Dietary Levels			
Indices	Gender	1.75% VOS[b] (6% fat)[e]	1.75% FFM[c] (4.8% fat)	4.38% VOS (6% fat)	4.38% FFM (3% fat)
Food intake, g	M	666 ± 14	707 ± 14[d]	683 ± 13	756 ± 11[d]
	F	517 ± 12	530 ± 9	536 ± 18	564 ± 9
Energy intake, g	M	2668 ± 54	2746 ± 56	2703 ± 50	2784 ± 42
	F	2069 ± 48	2060 ± 35	2120 ± 71	2085 ± 34
α-Tocopherol intake, mg	M	23.2 ± 0.5	21.8 ± 0.5[d]	23.9 ± 0.5	18.1 ± 0.4[d]
	F	18.1 ± 0.5	16.3 ± 0.3[d]	19.0 ± 0.7	13.6 ± 0.2[d]

[a] Means ± standard errors of values from 9-10 rats/group.
[b] VOS, vegetable oil spread.
[c] FFM, fat-free margarine.
[d] Significantly different from the corresponding VOS group ($p < 0.05$), Student's t-test.
[e] Numbers in parentheses indicate dietary fat levels.

from the corresponding VOS group. However, the slight increases in food intake were enough to maintain energy intake levels comparable to those of the VOS-fed groups of females. The substitution of fat-free margarine did not generally affect growth and tissue weights. One exception was the lower relative weight of the epididymal fat in male rats fed the highest level of fat-free margarine (data not shown). The reduced α-tocopherol intakes of rats consuming the fat-free margarine diets were consistent with the replacement of a margarine containing vitamin E. Liver α-tocopherol concentrations of male rats fed fat-free margarine were significantly reduced (~ 20%) when compared to the corresponding VOS group (TABLE 2). Plasma

TABLE 2. Effect of Dietary Treatments on α-Tocopherol Concentrations in Plasma, Liver, and Heart in Male and Female Rats[a]

		Dietary Levels			
α-Tocopherol concentration	Gender	1.75% VOS[b] (6% fat)[c]	1.75% FFM (4.8% fat)	4.38% VOS (6% fat)	4.38% FFM (3% fat)
Plasma, μg/dL	M	788 ± 23	790 ± 34	977 ± 36	799 ± 57[b]
	F	1060 ± 58	1072 ± 58	1158 ± 66	989 ± 87
Liver, μg/g	M	17 ± 1.0	14 ± 0.6[b]	17 ± 0.8	14 ± 0.7[b]
	F	30 ± 0.8	29 ± 1.0	28 ± 1.5	25 ± 1.4
Heart, μg/g	M	33 ± 1.4	33 ± 1.3	33 ± 1.0	29.5 ± 1.1[b]
	F	38 ± 0.9	39 ± 0.9	36 ± 1.2	34.9 ± 0.8

[a] Means ± standard errors of values from 9-10 rats/group.
[b] Significantly different from the corresponding VOS group ($p < 0.05$), Student's t-test.
[c] Numbers in parentheses indicate dietary fat level.

and heart α-tocopherol concentrations of male rats were also significantly reduced in rats fed the highest level of fat-free margarine when compared to the corresponding VOS group. The plasma, liver, and heart α-tocopherol concentrations of female rats were not significantly affected by the dietary treatments.

Replacement of 20-50% of the dietary fat with fat-free margarine increased the proportions of dietary energy obtained from protein and carbohydrate. All rats compensated for the dilution of dietary energy so that growth, liver, and heart weights were not affected.

Circulating and tissue levels of α-tocopherol were affected more in males than in females when fat-free margarine was fed. The highly significant gender differences in changes in α-tocopherol were probably due to the influence of the sex hormones. Rikans et al.[3] reported gender differences in age-related changes in hepatic α-tocopherol and antioxidant defense enzymes possibly by way of the sex hormones.

Water is the first-listed or main ingredient in the fat-free margarine. The changes in α-tocopherol concentrations in plasma, liver, and heart in male rats are probably related to reduced levels of fat and/or vitamin E resulting from the replacement. The lower levels of tissue α-tocopherol may also reflect reduced absorption and/or changes in transport. It is known that the level and type of dietary fat affect vitamin E absorption and utilization. The functional consequences of the changes in plasma, liver, and heart vitamin E reported here are not known and require further study.

REFERENCES

1. SHEPPARD, A. J., J. A. T. PENNINGTON & J. E. WEIHRAUCH. 1992. Analysis and distribution of vitamin E in vegetable oils and foods. *In* Vitamin E in Health and Disease. L. Packer & J. Fuch, Eds.: 9-31. Marcel Dekker. New York, NY.
2. BIERI, J. G., T. J. TOLLIVER & G. L. CATIGNANI. 1979. Simultaneous determination of α-tocopherol and retinol in plasma and red blood cells by high pressure liquid chromatography. Am J. Clin. Nutr. **32:** 2143-2149.
3. RIKANS, L. E. *et al.* 1991. Sex-dependent differences in the effects of aging on antioxidant defense mechanism of rat liver. Biochim. Biophys. Acta **1074:** 195-200.

Assessment of the Caloric Value of a Fat Substitute Using a New Tracer Method

B. MITTENDORFER,[a] Y. ZHENG, D. CHINKES, AND R. R. WOLFE

Shriners Burns Institute
Metabolism Unit
815 Market Street
Galveston, Texas 77550

METHODS

Seven normal healthy volunteers received the test substance containing 72.9 ± 32 µCi $^{14}C_1$-oleic acid in the fat substitute and 5.23 ± 0.76 g of free $^{13}C_1$-oleic acid served as a control.

The experiment lasted seven days. One day prior to the administration of label, the background enrichment and specific activity of breath and excreta were determined. After the administration of the labeled substances, breath was collected until no more label appeared (approximately 4 days). Excreta were collected for six days. The caloric value was obtained by multiplying the grams of fat in the polyester ingested by the ratio of ^{14}C to ^{13}C in breath as follows:

[N × (MW$_{oleate}$ − 18) × 9 kcal/g] × R = energy from fat in 1 g fat substitute,

where N is the number of fatty acids per gram fat substitute, MW the molecular weight, and R the recovery factor (ratio of ^{14}C excretion to ^{13}C excretion), as determined by breath CO_2 analysis. Eighteen represents the loss of water due to formation of ester bonds.

RESULTS

Percent of label recovery as CO_2 was $7.6 \pm 2.3\%$ $^{14}CO_2$ and $26.1 \pm 6.6\%$ $^{13}CO_2$ of the amount administered when labeled oleic acid was given ($p < 0.05$). This difference in percent recovery indicates diminished fatty acid availability from the fat substitute to $30.4 \pm 3.6\%$ of the amount ingested (FIG. 1). Almost no ^{13}C was recovered in feces, which is consistent with our assumption of complete absorption of the free oleic acid. By contrast, significant amounts of ^{14}C were excreted through feces. Total radiolabel recovery was high, although not complete ($71.7 \pm 22.9\%$) (FIG. 2).

---

[a] Tel: (409) 770 6619; fax: (409) 770 6825; e-mail: bmittend@sbiutmb.edu.

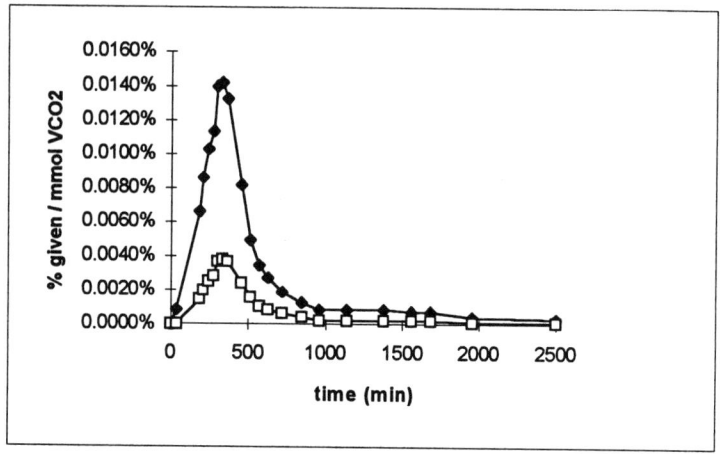

FIGURE 1. Characteristic pattern of recovery of label in breath after ingestion of $^{13}C_1$-oleic acid and the fat substitute labeled with $^{14}C_1$-oleic acid. Data are expressed as the fraction of label administered that is expired per mmol CO_2. ──◆──, ^{13}C; ──□──, ^{14}C.

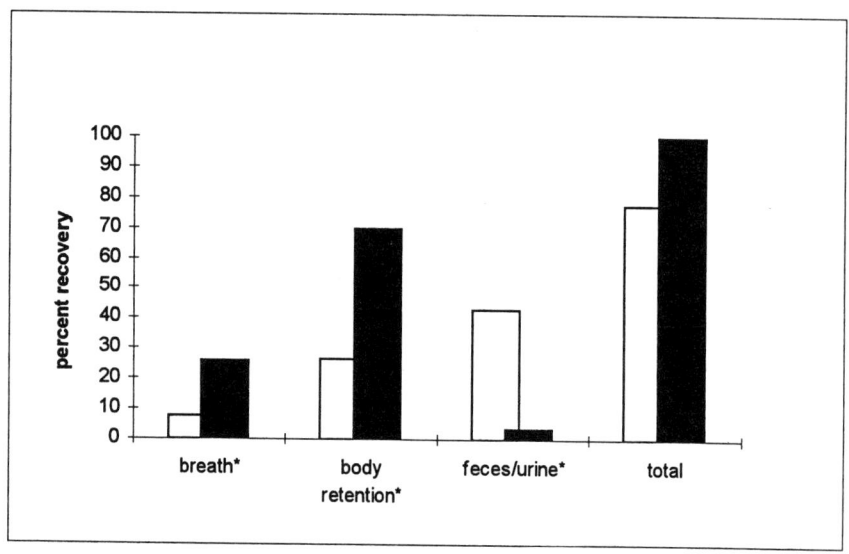

FIGURE 2. The amount of ^{13}C-labeled carbon retained in the body was calculated as the portion of label that did not appear in breath, urine, or feces. Retention of ^{14}C-labeled carbon was assumed to be the same fraction of breath of $^{14}CO_2$ as was the amount of ^{13}C retained. □, ^{14}C; ■, ^{13}C. Asterisk indicates significantly different from ^{13}C ($p < 0.05$).

SUMMARY

We estimated the metabolizable caloric value of the fat substitute to be significantly reduced (30% of a regular fat), by comparing the rate of CO_2 excretion from the labeled fat substitute to the rate of CO_2 excretion resulting from the metabolism of the ingested control substrate with known caloric value in order to estimate the caloric value of the fat substitute. Using the customary approach for determining the metabolizable energy of a partially digested substrate, which includes measuring the amount of substrate that is excreted, and from that deduce the amount absorbed, we would have overestimated the caloric value of the fat substitute.

We feel that the $^{14}C/^{13}C$ ratio method we have used is the preferable means by which to determine the caloric value of a partially absorbed substrate, both because of convenience and, most importantly, accuracy. In conclusion, we demonstrated with this tracer technique that this fat substitute provides one-third of the calories of a regular fat. Therefore, it can be helpful in the reduction of dietary-energy intake.

Oil-soluble Vitamin Content of New Reduced-fat and Fat-free Margarines

Potential Implications for Vitamin E Intake

JEANNE I. RADER [a]

Office of Food Labeling
Center for Food Safety and Applied Nutrition
U.S. Food and Drug Administration
Washington, D.C. 20204

INTRODUCTION

Vegetable oils and their products are among the most significant dietary sources of vitamin E, an antioxidant vitamin postulated to play a protective role in reduction in risk of such chronic diseases as cancer and cardiovascular disease. Margarines provide about 13% of the total α-tocopherol equivalents available in U.S. diets; other sources include mayonnaise, fortified breakfast cereals, shortenings, and cooking oils.[1] Consumers' interest in dietary guidelines advising them to reduce their fat intake has contributed to the development of reduced-fat and fat-free margarine-like products. The purpose of this study was to determine the total fat, vitamin E, and total vitamin A content of these new products. Data of this type are needed before assessments of the nutritional impacts of long-term consumption of such products can be made.

METHODS

All products were purchased locally. Margarines were blended in a dual-speed blender and stored refrigerated in tightly sealed containers. Oils were mixed well before sampling. Fat was determined gravimetrically by Association of Official Analytical Chemists (AOAC) method 922.06.[2]

Saponification and Extraction

Test portions were weighed into round-bottom flasks. To the test portions were added 200 mL of ethanol, 0.5 g of ascorbic acid, and 50 mL of 50% potassium hydroxide solution. The mixture was refluxed for 60 min with an air condenser and cooled to room temperature. The vitamins were extracted with petroleum ether.[3]

---

[a] Tel: (202) 205-5375; fax: (202) 205-4594; e-mail: jir@fdacf.ssw.dhhs.gov.

HPLC Conditions: Tocopherols, Retinol, and β-Carotene

The conditions were as follows: (1) Tocopherols: μBondapak C18 reverse-phase column, mobile phase methanol: water 94 : 6 (v/v); detector, 280 nm; (2) Retinol: μBondapak C18 reverse-phase column, mobile phase methanol: water 90 : 10 (v/v); detector, 325 or 313 nm; (3) β-carotene: LiChrosorb SI-60 column, mobile-phase hexane:propanol 98.3 : 1.7 (v/v); detector, 450 nm. HPLC conditions are described in references 3 and 4. Standards of authentic α-tocopherol, retinol, and β-carotene were carried through all procedures with each set of analyses. Recoveries (percent) for α-tocopherol, retinol, and β-carotene were 94.3 ± 7.4 (n = 24), 95.5 ± 6.1 (n = 23), and 91.2 ± 8.6 (n = 21), respectively.

RESULTS

Composition of the Products

In all margarine products containing 50% or more fat, individual liquid oils, or blends of several liquid oils and partially hydrogenated vegetable oils, were the first-listed ingredient(s) (TABLE 1). Water was the predominant ingredient, and a vegetable oil or a blend of vegetable oils was the second-listed ingredient for products of 20-40% fat content. The most commonly used oils were corn, soybean, and canola or blends of these three oils. No oil component was included in ingredient lists for the two fat-free margarines. Water, skim milk, or modified food starch, or vegetable mono- and diglycerides were listed as the primary ingredients in these products.

Vitamin E

The HPLC system separated the primary isomers of tocopherol (*e.g.*, α, γ, δ). The predominant isomer in the products was γ-tocopherol. The concentrations of α-tocopherol and fat in the products are shown in TABLE 1. The products are listed in order of decreasing fat content and, within groups of products of similar fat content, in order of decreasing α-tocopherol content. Values for fat ranged from <3 to 81 percent. Three of the 19 products contained 11-14% of the daily value (DV) of 30 IU of vitamin E (*i.e.*, 23-30 IU/100 g; 3.22-4.20 IU/14 g serving). Three products contained 5-9% of the DV per serving (*i.e.*, 10-20 IU/100 g; 1.4-2.8 IU/14 g serving). The majority of the products contained <4% of the DV per serving. Products labeled as containing corn, sunflower, and cottonseed oils had the highest levels of α-tocopherol. Those products labeled as containing soybean oil contributed significantly less α-tocopherol. Our findings of α-tocopherol levels in vegetable oils in the order sunflower>canola>corn>soybean are in general agreement with results reported by others.

Vitamin A and β-carotene

Margarines are among the foods with a standard of identity specified in federal regulations. According to the standard, margarines must include not less than 15,000

TABLE 1. α-Tocopherol in Margarines and Margarine-like Products[a]

Product	Ingredient Oils in Order Listed on Label	Fat Percent	Vitamin E (α-tocopherol) IU/100 g	Percent DV/srv
1 Soft margarine	Corn	77.0	30.5 ± 7.3	14.2
2 Unsalted margarine	Corn	78.1	23.9 ± 1.1	11.2
3 Unsalted margarine	Corn/soybn	81.1	10.5 ± 1.2	4.9
4 Margarine	Canol/corn/soybn	80.2	7.6 ± 0.04	3.5
5 Vegetable margarine	Soybn	79.1	5.2 ± 1.6	2.4
6 Blended margarine	Canol/soybn/corn	77.4	4.3 ± 0.5	2.0
7 Vegetable oil spread	Sunflwr/soybn/cotnseed	68.5	23.1 ± 2.0	10.8
8 Vegetable oil spread	Soybn	68.7	6.9 ± 0.5	3.2
9 Corn oil spread	Corn	53.8	12.5 ± 2.3	5.8
10 Vegetable oil spread	Soybn	52.0	5.5 ± 0.1	2.6
11 Vegetable oil spread	Soybn	50.8	3.5 ± 0.8	1.6
12 Light margarine	Sunflwr/soybn/cotnseed	40.7	15.1 ± 1.4	7.0
13 Spread	Soybn	39.1	4.3 ± 0.4	2.0
14 Vegetable oil spread	Canol/soybn/sunflwr/cotnseed	24.8	4.0 ± 1.3	1.9
15 Lower-fat margarine	Canol/corn	35.3	3.1 ± 0.8	1.4
16 Lower-fat margarine	Canol/soy	19.1	4.5 ± 2.3	2.1
17 Fat-free spread	Corn	0	1.0 ± 0.3	0.5
18 Fat-free margarine	None	0	0.6 ± 0.2	0.3
19 Fat-free margarine	None	0	0.5 ± 0.1	0.2
Sunflower oil	Sunflower	100	37.6 ± 1.0	17.5
Blended vegetable oil	Canol/sunflwr/soyb	100	32.7 ± 0.9	15.3
Canola oil	Canola	100	28.4 ± 1.6	13.3
Corn oil	Corn	100	22.4 ± 2.0	10.5
Soybean oil	Soybean	100	9.2 ± 1.0	4.3

[a] Values are means ± SD of 2–11 determinations. Ingredient oils are listed in their order of appearance on product labels. Abbreviations: Canol, canola; soybn, soybean; sunflwr, sunflower; cotnseed, cottonseed; DV, daily value; srv, serving size (14 g). The DV for vitamin E is 30 IU. Vitamin E content was declared on the labels of 2 of 19 products as follows: product 7, label declaration, 15% DV/srv; product 12, label declaration, 10% DV/srv.

TABLE 2. Vitamin A in Margarines and Margarine-like Products[a]

Vitamin A: Analyzed and Label Values

Product	Retinol IU/100 g	Retinol equiv. from β-carotene IU/100 g	Total vitamin A IU/100 g	Label values Vit.A IU/100 g	Label values Percent DV/srv
1 Soft margarine	2,860 ± 670	1,050 ± 210	3,910 ± 880	3,571	10
2 Unsalted margarine	2,990 ± 110	1,020 ± 50	4,010 ± 160	3,571	10
3 Unsalted margarine	1,680 ± 60	640 ± 140	2,320 ± 200	3,571	10
4 Margarine	3,180 ± 110	1,010 ± 40	4,190 ± 150	2,143	6
5 Vegetable margarine	3,200 ± 160	1,260 ± 50	4,460 ± 210	3,571	10
6 Blended margarine	2,020 ± 210	330 ± 0	2,350 ± 210	2,857	8
7 Vegetable oil spread	2,210 ± 170	1,320 ± 230	3,530 ± 140	3,571	10
8 Vegetable oil spread	2,040 ± 109	1,060 ± 170	3,100 ± 280	3,571	10
9 Corn oil spread	3,140 ± 210	650 ± 60	3,790 ± 270	3,333	9.3
10 Vegetable oil spread	3,150 ± 300	670 ± 30	3,810 ± 270	3,571	10
11 Vegetable oil spread	2,790 ± 270	980 ± 70	3,770 ± 350	3,571	10
12 Light margarine	1,610 ± 190	1,140 ± 50	2,740 ± 230	3,571	10
13 Margarine	2,590 ± 180	410 ± 30	3,010 ± 210	3,571	10
14 Vegetable oil spread	2,580 ± 390	400 ± 30	2,980 ± 410	3,571	10
15 Lower-fat margarine	3,040 ± 440	660 ± 30	3,700 ± 460	3,571	10
16 Lower fat margarine	2,410 ± 320	600 ± 0	3,010 ± 330	3,571	10
17 Fat-free spread	2,030 ± 590	620 ± 110	2,640 ± 690	3,333	9.3
18 Fat-free margarine	1,740 ± 230	370 ± 50	2,110 ± 190	3,571	10
19 Fat-free margarine	2,640 ± 10	530 ± 20	3,170 ± 010	3,571	10

[a] Values for retinol and retinol equivalents from β-carotene are means ± SD of 2–11 determinations. Abbreviations: vit. A, vitamin A; DV, daily value; srv, serving size (14 g). The DV for vitamin A is 5,000 IU. Total vitamin A was calculated by summing values for retinol and retinol equivalents from β-carotene. Label values for vitamin A were calculated from label declarations of vitamin A and β-carotene content per serving size of 14 g and were converted to IU/100 g.

IU of vitamin A per pound (*i.e.*, about 3,304 IU/100 g; about 463 IU/14 g serving; about 93% of the DV/14 g serving). Under regulations implementing the Nutrition Labeling and Education Act of 1990, food labels must declare the amount of vitamin A present as a percent of the DV of 5,000 IU. The percent of total vitamin A in the product provided by β-carotene may be declared voluntarily. All margarine products contained vitamin A (added as the palmitate) in concentrations ranging from 6-10% of the DV per serving (TABLE 2). Concentrations of total vitamin A measured in the products were 59-195% of amounts declared on the products' labels. All products listed β-carotene as a colorant. In general, amounts of β-carotene ranged from 20-40% of the total vitamin A content.

CONCLUSIONS

α-Tocopherol content of margarines is highly variable. α-Tocopherol varied among traditional margarines (those of 80% fat content) because of differences in α-tocopherol content of the oils (*e.g.*, corn, canola, soybean) used in their manufacture. Among the higher-fat margarines, products labeled as containing corn and sunflower oils had the highest levels of α-tocopherol. Among oils of similar composition, α-tocopherol content declined with decreasing fat content. Products labeled as containing soybean oil had among the lowest levels of α-tocopherol. Values for total vitamin A (retinol + retinol equivalents from β-carotene) were 59-195% of label values.

Consumers' replacement of margarines with products markedly lower in fat and vitamin E may lead to reduced vitamin E intakes. Food consumption surveys will need to be carefully designed to ascertain impacts on micronutrient intakes of long-term consumption of new reduced-fat and fat-free margarine-like products.

REFERENCES

1. SHEPPARD, A. J., J. A. T. PENNINGTON & J. E. WEIHRAUCH. 1992. Analysis and distribution of vitamin E in vegetable oils and foods. *In* Vitamin E in Health and Disease. L. Packer & J. Fuchs, Eds.: 9-31. Marcel Dekker. New York, NY.
2. ASSOCIATION OF OFFICIAL ANALYTICAL CHEMISTS (AOAC). 1990. Official Methods of Analysis, 15th ed., Association of Official Analytical Chemists, Arlington, VA, sec. 922.06 Fat in Flour, Acid Hydrolysis Method, pp. 780.
3. BUENO, M. P. 1997. Collaborative Study: Determination of retinol and carotene by high-performance liquid chromatography. Food Chem. **59:** 165-170.
4. RADER, J. I., C. M. WEAVER, L. PATRASCU, L. H. ALI & G. ANGYAL. 1997. α-Tocopherol, total vitamin A and total fat in margarines and margarine-like products. Food Chem. **58:** 373-379.

The Evolution of Carbohydrate Intake in the Slovak Republic during the Economic Transformation

ROBERT ŠIMONČIČ [a]

Research Institute of Nutrition
Limbová 14
833 37 Bratislava, Slovak Republic

When studying nutritional trends in the Slovak Republic (SR), we can observe a significant break during the years 1989-1990. Until 1989 we recorded a steady increase in energy intake and basic energetic nutrients as well. From 1980 to 1989 energy intake in the average Slovak citizen increased about 14.5%, while carbohydrate intake went up by about 13.7%. The increased carbohydrate intake was about 54.7 g/person/day. This shows that our diet was too high in its energy content and biologically unbalanced. After introducing economic changes in our country in 1989-1990, there occurred significant changes in consumption of nutrients and foods. Although protein and fat intake slightly decreased and carbohydrate slightly increased, the total energy intake did not change.

TABLE 1 shows trends in consumption of carbohydrate sources in the last six years. At present the greatest portion of carbohydrate intake is represented by cereals. Cereals constitute 56.4% of carbohydrate intake, of which wheat meal and wheat-meal products make up the greatest part. Rye products and rice represent a small part. Sugar and other sweets are the second highest contributors to carbohydrate intake. Other sources of carbohydrates constitute only a small part of carbohydrate intake. Consumption of potatoes (does not reach the RDA) represents 7.2% of energy intake from carbohydrates. Consumption of fruits and fruit products (substantially lower than the RDA) represents 6.4% of energy intake from carbohydrates. During the last six years consumption of milk and diary products (milk, but not butter) has rapidly decreased. There is very low consumption of legumes in Slovakia (only 0.7% of energy intake from carbohydrates). All other sources of carbohydrates are negligible.

The percentage of total intake from protein, fat, and carbohydrates by the latest RDA in the SR is 13.0%, 27.5%, and 59.5%, respectively. In 1995, according to data from the Statistical Bureau of the Slovak Republic (SBSR), it was 11.7%, 33.2%, and 55.1%, respectively. The total energy intake is about 25% higher than recommended. Epidemiological studies carried out at the Research Institute of Nutrition (RIN) showed less satisfactory data. The percentage of total intake of protein,

---

[a] Tel. and fax: 0042 7 373 968.

TABLE 1. Trends in Consumption of Carbohydrate Sources (kg per person per year) and Percent Carbohydrate Contribution in the Slovak Population (SBSR)

	1990	1991	1992	1993	1994	1995	Percent of Carbohydrate Contribution (1995)
Sucrose	42	42	37	34	32	33	20.5
Cereals, flour	116	115	108	104	104	101	56.4
Potatoes	86	91	78	89	72	74	7.2
Fruit and fruit products	54	60	62	64	65	68	6.4
Vegetables and vegetable products	101	110	105	108	107	106	4.0
Milk and milk products	226	212	194	171	166	164	4.0
Legumes	1.7	1.8	1.9	1.8	1.9	2.1	0.7
Other							0.8

TABLE 2. Carbohydrate and Dietary Fiber Intake in the Slovak Population (g per person per day) (RIN)

	Carbohydrate Intake			Dietary Fiber Intake		
Group	Intake g/day	RDA in the SR g/day	Percent of RDA SR	Intake g/day	RDA in the SR g/day	Percent of RDA SR
Men	360	420	88	17	28	61
Women	295	310	95	19	24	79
Boys, 11–14 years	340	368	92	13	20	65
Boys, 15–18 years	440	400	110	18	22	82
Girls, 11–14 years	310	330	94	12	18	67
Girls, 15–18 years	300	316	95	13	18	72

fat, and carbohydrates is 13.0%, 38.0%, and 49.0% for adults, and for children aged 11–18 years, it is similar.

TABLE 2 shows the mean daily intake of total carbohydrates and indigestible carbohydrates (dietary fiber) in the Slovak population and its comparison with the RDA. Carbohydrate intake in adults is slightly lower in comparison with the current Slovak RDA. In children and adolescents, it is mostly lower—about 5–8% of RDA. Dietary fiber intake in our population is about one-third lower than recommended values. When carbohydrate sources were divided into monosaccharides, disaccharides, and polysaccharides, we observed that 20% of carbohydrates were provided by sucrose, 25–30% by other mono- and disaccharides, and 50–55% by carbohydrates such as starch and nonstarch polysaccharides.

Considering the question dealing with improvements of our dietary habits with regard to the quantity and composition of carbohydrate intake, we conclude that a slight improvement of the total carbohydrate diet is required. It is necessary to improve the composition of carbohydrate consumption by increasing dietary fiber intake, increasing potato and fruit consumption, improving the composition of cereal sources (whole grain and low-fat products), and by increasing carbohydrate intake from legumes.

REFERENCES

1. BÉDEROVÁ, A. 1992. Zmeny v stravovaní detí a mládeze v obvode Bratislava II v rokoch 1988–1991. Lek. Obz. **41:** 5, 251–253.
2. BÉDEROVÁ, A., K. BABINSKÁ, T. MAGÁLOVÁ & A. BRTKOVÁ 1995. Vybrané charakteristiky zdravotného stavu mladej generácie z regiónov Rimavská Sobota a Snina. CS. Pediatrie **50:** 10, 597–604.
3. BÉDEROVÁ, A. & K. BABINSKÁ. 1995. Changes in intake of energy and selected nutrients in 1988–1992 in children and adolescents in Slovakia. Current research into eating practices and the contributions of social sciences. AGEV Publications series, vol. 10, suppl. Ernahrungs-Umschau, 55.
4. Statistical Bureau of Slovak Republic. 1996. Consumption of food stuffs in SR in 1995.
5. Statistical Bureau of Slovak Republic. 1996. Nutritional values of food stuffs consumption in SR in 1993 and 1994.
6. BÉDEROVÁ, A., A. BRTKOVÁ, T. MAGÁLOVÁ, M. KUDLÁCKOVÁ & S. TOMOVÁ. 1996. Serum lipid levels and antioxidant parameters in children and adolescents from 6 regions of SR. *In* First International Congress of the Group for Prevention of Atherosclerosis in Childhood 13.–16.10. Budapest.
7. BÉDEROVÁ, A. 1996. Aktuálny spôsob výzivy a spotreba základných zivín vitamínov a minerálnych látok u detí a dospievajúcich v r. 1995. Hygiena. In press.

Weight Gain of Rats Consuming Full-fat versus Reduced-fat Foods[a]

ZOE S. WARWICK,[b] KATHLEEN J. BOWEN, AND MICKA ROY

Department of Psychology
University of Maryland Baltimore County
1000 Hilltop Circle
Baltimore, Maryland 21250

Previous studies comparing the effect of supplemental full-fat and reduced-fat foods on weight gain have yielded inconsistent findings: Sclafani et al.[1] found that rats fed a single high-fat option (cake) gained more weight than rats fed no-fat cake, whereas Harris[2] found no difference in the weight gain of rats fed high-fat versus low-fat cafeteria foods. The purpose of the present study was to further compare the weight gain of rats fed supplemental high-fat foods to that of rats fed the reduced-fat versions of these foods.

METHOD

Two weight-matched groups of male Long-Evans rats (n = 7 or 8 per group, average weight 264 grams) were given an option food daily in addition to Purina chow for 29 days. Group FF received full-fat option foods. Group RF received reduced-fat option foods (TABLE 1). Only one food was provided per day. At the end of 24 hours, the remaining option food was removed, and a different option was given. A control group received only chow. Body weights were measured weekly.

RESULTS

Body weight gains are depicted in FIGURE 1. Repeated measures ANOVA on body weight gain revealed a significant group × days interaction, $F(6,48) = 7.87$. Student-Newman-Keuls post hoc tests, when appropriate, were then conducted to identify significant differences between groups.

CONCLUSIONS

Rats fed either a full-fat option (group FF) or a reduced-fat option (group RF) in addition to chow gained significantly more weight than chow-fed controls. This

---

[a]This work was supported by the Designated Research Initiative Fund, University of Maryland.
[b]Tel. (410) 455-2360; fax: (410) 455-1055; e-mail: warwick@umbc7.umbc.edu.

TABLE 1.

Full-fat Snack Foods		Percent of total kcal		
	kcal/gram	Fat	CHO[a]	Protein
Sandwich cookies (Oreos)	4.9	39	56	5
Mayonnaise (Hellmann's Real)	7.1	100	0	0
Potato chips (Pringles Original)	6.0	59	36	5
Reduced-fat Snack Foods		Percent of total kcal		
	kcal/gram	Fat	CHO	Protein
Sandwich cookies (reduced-fat Oreos)	4.4	23	71	6
Mayonnaise (Hellmann's Light)	3.3	90	10	0
Potato chips (Pringles Original, 1/3 less fat)	5.3	43	52	5

[a] CHO, carbohydrate.

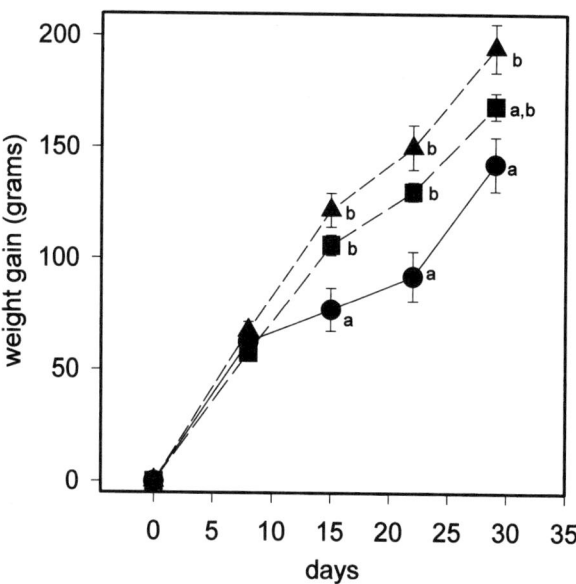

FIGURE 1. Weight gain produced by consumption of full-fat and reduced-fat foods. Weight gain of the three groups studied. Values are mean ± standard error. At each time point, means not sharing the same letter were significantly different. ———●———, chow only; ———■———, reduced-fat foods; ———▲———, full-fat foods.

is consistent with previous studies showing that weight gain can be enhanced by offering supplemental food(s) in addition to chow (*e.g.,* refs. 1 and 3). However, Harris[2] found no difference between the weight gains of rats fed high-fat options, low-fat option, or no options. This discrepancy may be due to the use of a higher-fat (30% of kcal) "control" diet by Harris versus the Purina chow (12% of kcal from fat) used by Sclafani and the present study, or other methodological differences such as the type of options used. Interestingly, rats in Harris' study did show differences in kcal intake, with the high-fat option intake greater than the low-fat option intake, which was greater than the control intake.

Although the difference was not statistically significant, the reduced-fat option rats in the present study gained less weight than the full-fat option rats; by the end of the study, group RF rats had gained 13% less weight than group FF rats. This pattern is consistent with the Sclafani *et al.*[1] study, in which high-fat option rats gained significantly more than no-fat option rats. Possibly the use of a continuously available sweet option (cake) in the Sclafani *et al.* study elicited greater option intake and thus a greater difference, between rats fed full-fat and reduced-fat cake, than in the present method, in which a sweet option (cookies) was available only every third day.

REFERENCES

1. SCLAFANI, A., K. WEISS, C. CARDIERI & K. ACKROFF. 1993. Feeding responses of rats to no-fat and high-fat cakes. Obesity Res. **1:** 173–178.
2. HARRIS, R. B. S. 1993. The impact of high- or low-fat cafeteria foods on nutrient intake and growth of rats consuming a diet containing 30% energy as fat. Int. J. Obesity **17:** 307–315.
3. SCLAFANI, A. & D. SPRINGER. 1976. Dietary obesity in adult rats: Similarities to hypothalamic and human obesity syndromes. Physiol. & Behav. **17:** 461–471.

Index of Contributors

Anderson, G. H., 1-10

Behall, K. M., 142-154
Birch, L. L., 194-220
Bowen, K. J., 251-253

Chinkes, D., 239-241

Drewnowski, A., 132-141

Egan, S. K., 108-114

Finley, J. W., 11-21
Fishell, V., 70-95
Fisher, J. O., 194-220

Garza, C., 229-234
Grivetti, L. E., 121-131
Grundel, E., 236-238

Hannah, J. S., 221-228
Harris, R. B. S., 155-168
Heimbach, J. T., 108-114

James, W. P. T., 44-69
Jenkins, M. Y., 236-238

Kris-Etherton, P. M., 70-95

Leveille, G. A., 11-21

Mela, D. J., 96-107
Mitchell, G. V., 236-238

Mittendorfer, B., 239-241
Morgan, R., 70-95
Moriarty, K., 70-95

Nabors, L. O., 115-120

Pellicore, L. S., 22-28
Peters, J. C., 169-179
Pi-Sunyer, F. X., 29-36
Prentice, A. M., 44-69

Rader, J. I., 242-246
Ravussin, E., 37-43
Rolls, B. J., 180-193
Roy, M., 251-253
Rulis, A. M., 22-28

Sigman-Grant, M., 70-95
Šimončič, R., 247-250
Steffen, D. G., ix
Stubbs, R. J., 44-69

Tataranni, P. A., 37-43
Taylor, D. S., 70-95
Technical Committee on Macronutrient Substitution, xi
Thorsheim, H. R., 22-28

Van der Riet, B. E., 108-114

Warwick, Z. S., 251-253
Wolfe, R. R., 239-241

Zheng, Y., 239-241

OHIO UNIVERSITY LIBRARY

Please return this book as soon as you have finished with it. In order to avoid a fine it must be returned by the latest date stamped below. All books are subject to recall after two weeks or immediately if needed for reserve.

RETURN BY
NOV 1 8 1997

QUARTER LOAN

QUARTER LOAN 07

DEC 0 9 1997

NOV 0 3 1997

RETURNED
JUN 1 4 1999
MAY 1 8 1999

CF